The Bipolar Disorder Survival Guide
Second Edition

Praise for

THE BIPOLAR DISORDER SURVIVAL GUIDE

"A practical, straightforward book that will be a great help to those who have bipolar illness, as well as their families. I could not recommend this book more highly."
—Kay Redfield Jamison, PhD, author of *An Unquiet Mind*

"This book has been a faithful friend in the difficult time since my diagnosis. I particularly appreciate the insights into communicating effectively with doctors, family, and friends after an episode. The charts, lists, and practical tools are amazing for those of us who like to be proactive and organized. But the best part of the book is the quotations from others with the disorder who share their experiences and feelings. I've said some of these exact things myself; seeing them here helps me feel just a little bit less isolated and more hopeful."
—N. B., Boulder, Colorado

"The author's expertise, compassion, and experience are evident throughout.... Well worth reading and remembering."
—*NAMI Advocate*

"*The Bipolar Disorder Survival Guide* is a thorough, research-based book for consumers who would like to learn about their illness and how to manage it."
—*Reintegration Today*

The Bipolar Disorder
SURVIVAL GUIDE

What You and Your Family Need to Know

Second Edition

David J. Miklowitz, PhD

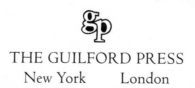

THE GUILFORD PRESS
New York   London

© 2011 The Guilford Press
A Division of Guilford Publications, Inc.
72 Spring Street, New York, NY 10012
www.guilford.com

The information in this volume is not intended as a substitute for consultation with healthcare professionals. Each individual's health concerns should be evaluated by a qualified professional.

Printed in the United States of America

This book is printed on acid-free paper.

Last digit is print number: 9   8   7   6   5   4   3   2   1

Library of Congress Cataloging-in-Publication Data

Miklowitz, David Jay, 1957–
     The bipolar disorder survival guide : what you and your family need to know / David J. Miklowitz. — 2nd ed.
        p.   cm.
     Includes bibliographical references and index.
     ISBN 978-1-60623-983-4 (hardcover : alk. paper) — ISBN 978-1-60623-542-3 (pbk. : alk. paper)
     1. Manic–depressive illness—Popular works.   I. Title.
     RC516.M554 2011
     616.89′5—dc22

                                                                    2010028728

Contents

Part III

PRACTICAL STRATEGIES FOR STAYING WELL

Preface

I first became interested in bipolar disorder in 1982 when, as a predoctoral psychology intern at the University of California, Los Angeles (UCLA), Medical Center, I supervised a bipolar support group with a fellow intern. The assignment was a challenge, but I was immediately struck by how the members of the group—men and women ranging in age from 19 to 50—had discovered, quite independently, how to deal with their illness. They had learned to ask for medical and social support when the early signs of recurrences first appeared, to rely on their significant others for emotional support, and to separate themselves from the disorder and fight its stigma. All of them understood that leading fulfilling lives required more than just taking medications.

The experience inspired me to choose a PhD dissertation on this disorder, specifically about family relationships among late adolescents and young adults who were recently out of the hospital. In the 25-plus years since, I have cared for, or supervised the care of, several hundred people with bipolar disorder—both young and old—and their families in the context of my research studies and clinical practice. People have come to my office in a variety of clinical states, each person with his or her own unique expression of the disorder and unique beliefs about how it should be treated; the factors in his or her genetic, biological, or family background that caused it; and what it meant for the future. Many have had a love–hate relationship with the illness: they have cherished the intensity of the emotional experiences that mania provides but have detested the low periods, the disorder's unpredictability, and the emotional, practical, and financial damage done to their lives.

My long-term collaboration (1979–1997) with the late Michael Goldstein, PhD, of UCLA resulted in the development of family-focused therapy (FFT), an intervention that assists people with the disorder and their family members in coping during the periods after an illness episode. My experimental studies at the University of Colorado, and those with my UCLA colleagues, have shown that people who receive FFT and medications have lower rates of relapse and less severe symptoms than people who receive individual supportive care and medications. Their improvements can be observed for up to 2 years after they begin family treatment. Our most recent work has shown that teens with bipolar disorder benefit from FFT and medications as well, in terms of better recoveries from episodes of illness. These studies, funded by the National Institute of Mental Health and the National Alliance for Research on Schizophrenia and Depression, have included more than 400 people. The participants have varied in age, ethnicity, race, and socioeconomic status. They range from people experiencing their first manic or depressive episode to those who have been ill for most of their lives, from people for whom the disorder poses only occasional life problems to those who are chronically in and out of hospitals, and people in a wide variety of living situations and family contexts.

I wrote this book to respond to a need voiced by virtually everyone with whom I have worked, along with their family members. People with the disorder wish for more understanding from relatives, friends, and coworkers. Their family members, in turn, want to know how best to help their bipolar relative without becoming angry, controlling, or overprotective. Both ask the core question this book attempts to answer: How can people with the disorder achieve better mood stability and lead more fulfilling lives, while taking medications and dealing with the realities the illness imposes?

The second edition of this book reflects my experiences and those of others in working with people with bipolar disorders over the past decade, as well as what the field has learned from the latest research. Much has changed since the first edition, in part because of large-scale studies of pharmacological and psychotherapeutic strategies for people with bipolar depression or mania. For example, the first edition barely mentioned lamotrigine or quetiapine and instead emphasized drugs like carbamazepine, some of which have fallen out of favor. More and more psychiatrists are favoring atypical antipsychotic medications instead of (or in conjunction with) mood stabilizers. There are new findings on the use of antidepressants. And, perhaps most important, there is now considerable evidence regarding the role of psychotherapy as an adjunct to medications for people with bipolar disorder.

This revised edition offers a new chapter on issues for women with bipolar disorder (Chapter 12). We know much more than we used to about the needs of women with the illness: how to manage mood-stabilizing medications when pregnant, during the postpartum, or during the perimenopausal period; how to cope with irregular menstrual cycles, weight gain, or hormone abnormalities; and about side effects that affect women more than men. As with other areas of medicine and other illnesses, women need and deserve to be recognized as different from men so that they can have the best chance of managing their symptoms and leading the lives they want to live.

It is my strong belief that people who do best with the disorder are those who have learned to recognize triggers for their mood cycles and how to minimize the impact of these triggers. They are people who stay close to their recommended medication regimens and have good relationships with their physicians. They have regular therapists or go to support groups. They have learned as much as they can about the illness, go to conferences where the latest findings about the disorder are presented, talk with others who have the illness, and read books and articles concerning the latest treatments. They have learned to accept the disorder but do not unnecessarily limit their personal goals because of it.

At that bipolar support group years ago, I was impressed by the members' ability and willingness to take care of each other as well as themselves. One group member regularly made trips to the local hospital inpatient unit to tell patients with the disorder about the advantages of obtaining medical and psychosocial treatment at the UCLA Mood Disorders Clinic. When a member of the group started to cycle into an episode, others were quickly able to recognize the early warning signs and offer assistance. Members were often blunt with each other but would say things that needed to be said.

I'd like to think of this book as performing the same function as that support group. It is my sincere hope that after reading it, you will feel less alone in your struggles, realize that there are effective treatments available, and have at your fingertips strategies to prevent mood swings from ruling your life. I hope this book will tell you the things that need to be said and that you'll use them to your benefit, even if you don't always want to hear them. Most of all, I hope you and your family members will become convinced that you can lead a full life and achieve many of your personal goals despite having the disorder.

A Word of Thanks

Many people deserve my heartfelt appreciation for supporting me in writing this book and for providing friendship and mentoring over the past several decades. I feel especially grateful to my collaborators, Ellen Frank and David Kupfer of the University of Pittsburgh School of Medicine, for their clinical wisdom and their encouragement of my research. The illness management tools outlined in this book—education, relapse prevention, effective communication and problem solving, relying on social supports, and social rhythm stabilization—in many ways reflect a synthesis of FFT principles and their interpersonal therapy approach to helping people cope more effectively with bipolar disorder.

Many teachers and close colleagues have been inspirational throughout my career and have strongly influenced how I think about clinical problems, including Michael Goldstein, Ian Falloon, Keith Nuechterlein, Raymond Knight, Connie Hammen, W. Edward Craighead, Gary Sachs, Michael Thase, Steve Carter, Lyman Wynne, Robert Liberman, Michael Gitlin, David Wellisch, and Kay Jamison. My graduate students and postdoctoral fellows at the University of Colorado were often the first to suggest clinical strategies for working with individuals or families, and their research has often influenced the direction of my own. They have included Elizabeth George, Teri Simoneau, Dawn Taylor, Jeff Richards, Tina Goldstein, Eunice Kim, Vicky Cosgrove, Kim Mullen, Jed Bopp, Chris Hawkey, Aimee Sullivan, Natalie Sachs-Ericsson, Jennifer Wendel, Kristin Powell, and Aparna Kalbag. Colleagues with whom I collaborated at UCLA in the late 1980s hold a special place in my heart, including Margaret Rea, Angus Strachan, Martha Tompson, Jim Mintz, and Amy Weisman.

I have greatly enjoyed my friendship and research collaboration with psychiatrists David Axelson and Boris Birmaher (University of Pittsburgh), Kiki Chang and Manpreet Singh (Stanford), Robert Kowatch and Melissa DelBello (Cincinnati Children's Hospital and University of Cincinnati), and Chris Schneck, Cheryl Chessick, Michael Allen, and Marshall Thomas (University of Colorado School of Medicine). I feel very grateful to my friends and collaborators in the Department of Psychiatry at the University of Oxford, United Kingdom: Guy Goodwin, John Geddes, and Mark Williams. Each has taught me something unique about bipolar disorder and psychotherapy. I would like to extend special appreciation to several friends and colleagues who commented on early drafts of this book and, in many cases, suggested additional material: Lori Altshuler, Melissa DelBello, Cheryl Chessick, Richard Suddath, Joseph Goldberg, Sheri Johnson, and Sona Dimidjian.

Many thanks go to members of my family—my spouse, Mary Yaeger; my daughter, Ariana; and my brother, Paul Miklowitz, and his family—all of whom have brought me great joy and reminded me that life is not just about work. My mother, Gloria Miklowitz, a children's author who has published over 70 books, has been a source of inspiration during the often difficult process of writing this book. The memory of my father, Julius Miklowitz, a professor who taught me the value of research, hard work, and a life of learning, has guided me throughout my academic life.

Finally, I would like to express my sincere gratitude to two of the most talented, patient, and knowledgeable editors in the universe—Kitty Moore and Chris Benton of The Guilford Press. Their imprint appears throughout the book. Without their encouragement, tenacity, support, and great senses of humor, this project would never have come to fruition.

I have enjoyed writing this book and wish you success in your personal journey through the ups and downs of bipolar disorder.

Part I

The Experience and Diagnosis of Bipolar Disorder

1

How This Book Can Help You Survive—and Thrive

Why Do You Need This Book?

- To understand the symptoms, diagnosis, and causes of your bipolar disorder
- To learn about effective medical and psychological treatments
- To learn self-management techniques to help you deal with mood cycles
- To improve your functioning in family and work settings

Martha, 34, ended up in the hospital after storming out of the house, in which she lived with her husband and two school-age children, and spending a disastrous night in a town over two hours away. Her problems, however, had started about two weeks earlier, when she became unusually irritable with her husband, Eric, "slamming about the house," as he described it, and becoming easily provoked by the minor infractions of their children. She then began to sleep less and less and was increasingly preoccupied with many ideas for a new dot-com business she planned to start. Despite this intense focus, Martha seemed very easily distracted. She also began speaking very rapidly.

Her problems came to a head when she left the house in a fury shortly after dinner one night and impulsively took a bus to a gambling casino about 100 miles away. By her account, she met a man at a bar the same night and went to bed with him. The next morning she called her husband, crying, and explained what had happened. Needless to say, he was quite angry and drove to the casino to pick her up. He arrived at the agreed-upon place and time, only to find that Martha was not there, so he returned home—where he found his wife, disheveled, sleep deprived, and angry. After sobbing for several hours, she finally agreed to go with him to be evaluated at a local hospital. She was admitted to the inpatient unit and given a diagnosis of bipolar I disorder, manic phase.

Bipolar disorder is a mood disorder that affects at least one in every 50 people—and as many as one in 25 by some estimates—and puts them at high risk for the kinds of problems in their family, social, and work lives that Martha suffered. People with bipolar disorder are also at high risk for physical problems, alcohol and substance use disorders, and even suicide. Fortunately, there is much hope. With medications, psychotherapy, and self-management techniques, it's possible to control the rapid shifts in mood from manic highs to severe depressive lows (called *mood disorder episodes*), prevent future episodes from occurring, decrease the impact of environmental triggers, and cope effectively so that you can enjoy a full life.

Whether you have already been diagnosed with bipolar disorder, think you might have this illness, or are concerned about someone who has it, this book will help you understand the disorder and learn to manage it effectively. In the following chapters you'll find up-to-date information on the nature of the disorder, its causes, medical and psychological treatments, and the lifestyle changes you can make to help manage the disorder. The information should be relevant to you whether you have been treated on an inpatient basis, like Martha, or on an outpatient basis, which is becoming more and more common.

Understanding the Facts about Bipolar Disorder: Its Symptoms, Causes, Treatment, and Self-Management

The inpatient physician who saw Martha diagnosed her as bipolar very quickly and recommended a regimen of lithium, a mood-stabilizing medication, and risperidone (Risperdal), an atypical antipsychotic medication. After only a few days it was clear that she was responding well. But when her doctor made plans to discharge her, Martha confronted him with a litany of questions and worries she had about everything that was happening to her. Why was she being given "this death sentence" (her diagnosis) and "drugged and disposed of so quickly"? Why was she being labeled manic, when most of what she had done, she felt, could be attributed to her personality or interpersonal style? "I've always been assertive," she complained to her doctor, her husband, and almost everyone else she saw. "Since when is everything I do a mental illness?" Her doctor responded with sympathy but offered insufficient information to satisfy Martha. Under considerable pressure to get people in and out of the hospital quickly, he left her with a list of medications to take but little understanding of what had happened to her or what to expect once she got home.

If you were in Martha's position, in all likelihood you would find the hospital experience as confusing and frustrating as she did. In my experience, people with bipolar disorder and their family members usually are hungry for information about the disorder, particularly during or after a manic or depressive episode, whether or not the episode involves hospitalization. Of course, people with the disorder have an easier time assimilating information about it once they are over the worst of their symptoms. But even during the hospitalization, Martha and her husband would have benefited a great deal from some basic facts: how her doctors knew she had the illness, how the symptoms are experienced by the person with the disorder versus everyone else, and the course of the illness over time. They would have benefited from knowing what to expect after she was discharged from the hospital, including her risks of cycling into new episodes. Without this information, it was difficult for Martha to put her experiences in context. As a result, she began to doubt the accuracy of the diagnosis and, by extension, the wisdom of complying with her prescribed treatments.

A major assumption of this book is that understanding the facts about your disorder will help you accept it and live with it. Important questions that often go unanswered because mental health providers simply don't have time include:

- ■ "What are the symptoms of bipolar disorder?"
- ■ "Who am I apart from my disorder?"
- ■ "Where did the illness come from?"
- ■ "How do I know when I'm becoming ill?"
- ■ "What triggers my mood cycles?"
- ■ "What can I do to minimize my chances of becoming ill again?"
- ■ "How do I explain the illness to other people?"
- ■ "What can I expect from my future?"

By the end of this book, I hope you'll have gotten useful answers to these questions, together with a more complete understanding of bipolar disorder, a new grasp of who you are and how bipolar disorder fits into your life, and a wealth of illness management techniques. I also hope to leave you

> **Effective prevention:** Being able to put your illness in an informational context helps you prevent or at least minimize the damage associated with future recurrences of the disorder and set appropriate goals for your immediate and long-term future.

knowing where to turn when the future brings new challenges and you need additional information and advice.

Adjusting to the Aftermath of an Episode

Martha left the hospital with prescriptions for lithium and risperidone and an appointment to see a new doctor 2 weeks later. Upon discharge she had agreed to follow the recommendations of the inpatient staff to continue taking her medications, but she knew little about what the medications were doing or exactly what was being medicated. She felt shaky, agitated, and irritable, and became mentally confused. These uncomfortable sensations were largely the result of continuing symptoms of her disorder, but in the absence of any information to the contrary, Martha assumed her confusion was due entirely to the lithium.

She then noticed her mood start to drop, gradually at first. She felt numb, disinterested in things, tired, and unable to sleep even though she desperately wanted to. She began to spend more time during the day "sleep bingeing" to try to catch up from the night before. She awoke in the afternoon feeling worse and had difficulty with her usual responsibilities, such as making dinner or helping the children do their homework. She dreaded interacting with her neighbors. The idea of committing suicide crossed her mind for the first time. She felt guilty about the impact of her disorder on her children and wondered whether they would be better off without her.

Martha developed an upper respiratory infection, which kept her up late at night coughing. Compounding this stress, the neighbors were having work done on their house, and she was awakened from her fitful sleep by noise early in the morning. Her sleep became more and more inconsistent, and her daily and nightly routines—when she went to bed and when she woke up—began to change from day to day.

About a week after being discharged from the hospital, Martha's mood escalated upward again. Her thoughts began to race, and she started to think again about the dot-com business. Then, in what she later described as a "flash," she decided that all of her problems—not just the mental confusion but also her cycling mood, her sleep disturbance, and her lethargy—were caused by the lithium. Without checking with a physician or telling anyone, she lowered her lithium dosage. When she saw no apparent negative results, she discontinued it altogether. She stopped her risperidone next. Martha became severely irritable again, began to sleep less and less, and finally ended up back in the hospital only 3 weeks after her discharge.

Martha's story is all too common. Because the nature of the disorder was not explained fully to her, she thought of the episode as a sort of "nervous breakdown" requiring only temporary medication. She did not understand that the illness could be recurrent. In Chapters 2, 3, and 4, you will become familiar with the expected course of bipolar disorder over time and the various forms that mood recurrences can take. This knowledge can help you stick to a treatment and self-management plan that may help stave off recurrences.

Martha also would have benefited from knowledge of the factors that we believe cause the cycling of bipolar disorder: a complex interplay of genetic background, individual biochemistry, and life stress, as discussed in Chapter 5. Many people who have bipolar disorder burden themselves with guilt and self-blame because they believe their mood disorder is caused solely by psychological factors or even sheer weakness of character. Martha could have avoided such self-blame if she had known that her dramatic mood shifts were associated with biological imbalances of brain neurotransmitters and the function of nerve cell receptors. Her experiences would have made more sense to her in the context of her family tree: her mother had depression and her paternal grandfather was hospitalized once for "mental anguish" and "exhaustion."

Knowing about the biological causes of your disorder will also clarify why consistency with your medications is essential to maintaining good mood stability. Martha knew that she needed to take medications, but not why. Chapters 6 and 7 deal with medication treatments for bipolar disorder. There are many drugs available nowadays, in various combinations and dosages. Doctors have to be constantly updated on which treatments to recommend to which patients, since the accepted treatment guidelines for this disorder change so rapidly. You will feel more effective in managing your disorder if you can openly communicate with your physician about which medications are most effective for you, their side effects, and the mixed emotions you may feel about taking them.

Self-Management Strategies

Beyond taking medications and meeting with a psychiatrist, there are good and bad ways to manage your disorder. Self-management involves learning to recognize your own individual triggers for episodes and adjusting your life accordingly. This book will teach you a number of self-management tools that will probably increase the amount of time that your moods remain stable. For example, Martha would have benefited from sleep–wake monitoring or staying on a regular daily and nightly routine, including going to bed and waking at the same time, strategies described in Chapter 8. Likewise, keeping a mood chart (discussed in Chapter 8) would have provided a structure for tracking the day-to-day changes in her emotions and revealed how these changes corresponded with fluctuations in sleep, consistency with her medication regimen, and stressful events. Recall that Martha's worsening mood was precipitated by a respiratory infection and the appearance of neighborhood noise, which were stressful and disrupted her sleep–wake patterns. In addition to recognizing these events as triggers, Martha and her husband could have developed a list of early warning signs that would alert them to the possibility of a new episode of mania. In Martha's case, these signs included irritability and a sudden interest in developing a business. Chapter 9 provides a comprehensive overview of possible early warning signs of mania.

When Martha first started becoming depressed, certain behavioral strategies might have kept her from sinking further, including behavior activation exercises and cognitive restructuring techniques, introduced in Chapter 10. She would have had the support of knowing that suicidal thoughts and feelings—a common component of the bipolar syndrome—can be combated through prevention strategies involving the support of close friends and relatives, counseling, and medications, as described in Chapter 11. She would have understood some of the differences between women and men during the depressed phase (for example, the role of the menstrual cycle and the influence of the postpartum period or menopause), and how to manage some of the health complications that affect women who take mood-stabilizing medications, as discussed in Chapter 12.

Coping Effectively in the Family and Work Settings

Martha spent 5 more days in the hospital but this time was discharged with a clearer follow-up plan. She met the physician who would see her as an outpatient to monitor her medications and blood serum levels. The inpatient social work team also helped arrange an outpatient appointment with a psychologist who specialized in the treatment of mood disorders. This time, she felt better about the hospitalization experience but was quite wary of what would happen once she was back at home.

After her discharge, Martha spoke with close friends about what had happened. They were sympathetic but said things like "I guess everybody's a little bit manic–depressive" and "Maybe you were just working too hard." When she disclosed to one friend that she was taking lithium, the friend said, "Don't get addicted." Although she knew her friends were trying to be supportive, these messages confused her. Was she really ill or just going through a tough time? Were her problems really an illness or just an extreme of her personality? Hadn't the physicians told her that medications were meant to be taken over the long term?

Martha's husband, Eric, seemed unsure of how to relate to her. He genuinely cared about her and wanted to help but frequently became intrusive about issues such as whether she had taken her medications. He pointed out minor shifts in her emotional reactions to things, which formerly would have escaped his notice but which he now relabeled as "your rapid cycling." Martha, in turn, felt she was being told she was "no longer allowed to have normal emotional reactions." She told him, "You can't just hand me a tray of lithium every time I laugh too loud or cry during a movie."

At other times Eric became angry and criticized her for the deterioration in her care of the children. Indeed, she didn't have enough energy to take them to their various activities or get them to school on time. She didn't feel up to the social demands of being a parent. "You aren't trying hard enough," Eric said.

"You've got to buck up and beat this thing." At other times he would tell her she shouldn't take on too much responsibility because of her illness. Martha became confused about what her husband expected of her. What neither understood was that most people need a low-key, low-demand period of convalescence after a hospitalization so that they can fully recover from their episode of bipolar disorder.

Her children eyed Martha with suspicion, expecting her to burst into irritable tirades, as she had done prior to her first hospitalization. She began to feel that her family was ganging up on her. The family stress during the aftermath of her episode contributed to her depression and desire to withdraw.

Given the economic pressure her family was under, Martha decided to immediately return to her part-time computer programming job, but felt unable to handle the long commute. When she arrived at work, she stared at the computer screen. "The programs I used to know well now seem like gobbledygook," she complained. She finally told her boss about her psychiatric hospitalizations. He seemed sympathetic at first but soon began pressuring her to return to her prior level of functioning. She felt uncomfortable around her coworkers, who seemed edgy and avoidant as they "handled me with kid gloves." The shifts in work schedules, which had been a regular part of her job before, started to feel like they were contributing to her mood swings.

Martha had significant problems reestablishing herself in her home, work, and community following her hospitalization. People who develop other chronic medical illnesses, such as diabetes, cardiac disorders, multiple sclerosis, or hypertension, also have trouble relating to their partner, children, other family members, friends, and coworkers. When you reenter your everyday world following a mood episode, even well-intentioned family members don't know how to interpret the changes in your behavior (for example, your irritability or lack of motivation). They often mistakenly think that you are acting this way on purpose and could control these behaviors if you only tried harder. As a result, they become critical, evaluative, and judgmental. They may also mistakenly think you can't take care of yourself and try to do things for you that you are more than capable of doing yourself. For example, they may try to actively manage your time, direct your career moves, telephone your doctors with information about you, constantly question you about your medications, or become vigilant about even the most minor changes in your emotional state.

In the workplace you may find your employer initially sympathetic but impatient. Your coworkers may be guarded, suspicious, or even scared. In addition, you may feel that you can't concentrate as well on the job as you did before you became ill. These difficulties are all a part of the convalescent period that follows an episode. In all likelihood, your concentration problems will diminish once your mood becomes stable. But it can be quite upsetting to feel like you're not functioning at the level at which you know you can.

As you are probably aware, bipolar disorder carries a social stigma not associated with medical illnesses. Even though bipolar disorder is clearly a disorder of the brain, and its genetic and biological underpinnings are well documented, it is still treated as a "mental illness." Many people still erroneously believe it is related to your personal choices or morals. As a result, you may feel alienated from others when they find out about your disorder.

On the hopeful side, there is much you can do to educate your family, coworkers, and friends about the nature of your illness. Certainly, people will respond to your disorder in ways that you will find uncomfortable, but their reactions will vary, at least in part, with how you present it to them.

Chapter 13 is devoted to exploring ways of coping effectively in the family and workplace. You'll learn how to talk to your family, friends, and coworkers about your disorder so that they know how best to help you and don't perpetuate their misconceptions with you (as was the case for Martha). You'll learn specific strategies for communicating effectively with your family so that disagreements about the disorder don't escalate into unproductive and stressful arguments.

> **Effective prevention:** One objective of this book is to familiarize you with the role of family and other social factors in contributing to, or ameliorating, the cycling of your bipolar disorder.

Martha: Epilogue

Martha's first year after her two hospitalizations was quite difficult, but now, several years later, she is doing much better. She found a psychiatrist with whom she feels comfortable. She is taking a regimen of lithium, divalproex sodium (Depakote), and a thyroid supplement. Her mood and behavior still shift up and down, but her symptoms are no longer incapacitating. For example, she reacts strongly to disagreements with her husband and still has periods of feeling down or unmotivated. In part due to her willingness to commit to a program of mood stabilizing medications, she has not needed the intensive inpatient treatment she received initially.

Martha and Eric have improved their relationship. They regularly see a marital therapist, who has helped them distinguish how the disorder affects their relationship, how conflicts in their relationship affect the disorder, and what problems in their family life are unrelated to her illness. Together they have developed a list of the signs of her oncoming episodes and what steps to take when these signs appear (for example, calling her physician for an emergency appointment to prevent hospitalization). Her children have become more accepting of her moodiness, and she has become more enthusiastic about parenting. She has had frustrations in the workplace, and finally came to the conclusion that "I'm just not a nine-to-fiver." She decided to try freelance work, which, although not as financially lucrative, has reduced her stress and given her predictable hours.

Martha now has a better understanding of the disorder and how to manage it. For example, by keeping a mood chart she has learned to distinguish—for herself as well as for other people—between her everyday, normal mood swings and the more dramatic mood swings of her bipolar illness. She has learned to maintain a regular sleep–wake cycle. She recognizes that keeping her disorder well controlled is the key to meeting her own expectations of herself. She is now more comfortable trusting and enlisting the support of her husband and friends when she feels depressed or suicidal.

Martha recognizes that her disorder is recurrent, but also feels that she is more in control of her fate. In summing up her developing ability to cope with the disorder, she said, "I've learned to accept that I've got something biochemical that goes haywire, but it's not the sum total of who I am. If I could change one thing about myself, it'd be other people's moods and how they affect me, even when it's their problem and not mine."

Above all, this book is about hope. If you've just been diagnosed with bipolar disorder, or even if you have had many episodes, you probably have fears about what the future holds. Martha's story—while perhaps representative of only one form of the disorder and one type of life situation—captures some of the ways that people learn to live with bipolar illness. *A diagnosis of bipolar disorder doesn't have to mean giving up your hopes and aspirations.* As you will soon see, you can come to terms with the disorder and develop skills for coping with it and still experience life to its fullest.

How This Book Is Organized

This book is divided into three sections. In the remaining chapters (2–4) of this section, "The Experience and Diagnosis of Bipolar Disorder," you'll learn about the symptoms and recurrent nature of the disorder from your own vantage point as well as that of your relatives and the physician who makes the diagnosis. You'll become familiar with the behaviors considered to be within the bipolar spectrum and learn what to expect from the diagnostic process. Chapter 4 offers you tips on how to cope with the diagnosis and addresses the question many people ask themselves: "Is it an illness or is it me?"

In Part II, "Laying the Foundation for Effective Treatment," Chapter 5 provides an overview of the genetic, biological, and environmental determinants of the disorder. You'll come to see how the disorder is not *just* about biology or *just* about environment but an interaction of the two. Chapter 6 discusses medications for treating the biological aspects of the disorder (mood stabilizers, antidepressants, second-generation [atypical] antipsychotics, and newer, nontraditional agents), including their effectiveness, how we think they work, and their side effects, as well as the role of psychotherapy in helping you cope more effectively with mood swings and their triggers. Chapter 7 deals with the issue of accepting and coming to terms with a long-term program of medication. For people with bipolar disorder—and many other recurrent illnesses—taking medications regularly and for the long term poses many emotional and practical challenges. In this chapter you'll learn why taking medications consistently is so important and why some of the common arguments for discontinuing medications (for example, "I don't need to take medications when I feel well") are erroneous.

Part III, "Practical Strategies for Staying Well," starts with "Tips to Help You Manage Moods and Improve Your Daily Life" (Chapter 8), strategies for derailing the upward cycle into mania (Chapter 9), and how to recognize and handle depression (Chapter 10). I devote a special chapter to dealing with suicidal thoughts and feelings (Chapter 11), which, for many people with bipolar disorder, is a constant source of pain. You'll learn ways to get help from others when you're suicidal and some things you can do to manage these feelings on your own.

Chapter 12 is brand new to this second edition, and it contains a wealth of up-to-date information and advice just for women, on how bipolar affects and is affected by the reproductive cycle, how to have a healthy pregnancy in the context of mood symptoms and medications, and how bipolar disorder and its treatments affect women's health in unique ways. The last chapter, "Succeeding at Home and at Work: Communication, Problem-Solving Skills, and Dealing Effectively with Stigma," is designed to help you handle the family, social, and work stress that usually accompanies the disorder and to educate others about the challenges you face.

2

Understanding the Experience
of Bipolar Disorder

Though bipolar disorder is very difficult to diagnose, the textbook descriptions of it make it sound like it shouldn't be so hard. After all, what could be more dramatic than shifting between extraordinarily manic behavior, feeling on top of the world and supercharged with energy, to feeling depressed, withdrawn, and suicidal?

Consider a surprising fact: On average, there is an 8-year lag between a first episode of depression or manic symptoms and the first time the disorder is diagnosed and treated (Lewis, 2000; Post & Leverich, 2006). Why should it take so long for a person with the disorder to come to the attention of the mental health profession? In part, the answer is that the behaviors we summarize with the term *bipolar disorder* can look quite different, depending on your perspective. But even when people agree on how a person's behavior deviates from normal, they can have very different beliefs about what causes the person to be this way. Consider Lauren, who has bipolar disorder:

> Lauren, a 28-year-old mother of three, describes herself as an "exercise junkie." In the past three weeks, a typical day went like this: Once she got the kids off to school, she rushed to the gym, where she worked out on an exercise bicycle for up to two hours. Then, she grabbed a quick yogurt and went hiking for most of the afternoon. She would pick up her kids from school, make dinner for them, and spend the majority of the evening on the stairmaster. But she did not consult her psychiatrist until, by the end of the second week, she had become exhausted and unable to function. At this point she left the children with their grandparents and spent several days sleeping. She admitted to having had several cycles like these.

Now consider how Lauren, her mother, and her doctor describe her behavior. Lauren summarizes her problems as the result of being overcommitted. "It's incredibly difficult to take care of three kids, maintain a household, and try to stay healthy," she argues. "My ex-husband is of very little help, and I don't have many friends who can help out. Sometimes I push myself too hard, but I always bounce back." Her mother feels that she is "irresponsible and self-centered," would "rather be exercising than taking care of her kids," and questions whether her children are getting enough guidance and structure. Lauren's doctor has diagnosed her as having bipolar II disorder.

Who is right? Lauren thinks her behavior is a function of her environment. Her mother describes the same behaviors as driven by her personality attributes. Her psychiatrist thinks she has a biologically based mood disorder. These different perspectives pose a problem for Lauren, because they lead to very different remedies for the situation. Lauren feels that others need to be more supportive. Her mother thinks Lauren needs to become more responsible. Her doctor thinks Lauren needs to take a mood-stabilizing medication.

Almost every patient I have worked with describes his or her behavior differently from the way a doctor or family member would. Consider Brent, who has been having trouble holding jobs. He says he is depressed but feels most of it is due to being unable to deal with his hypercritical boss. As a result, he thinks he needs to switch jobs and find a more permissive work environment. His wife, Alice, thinks he is manic and irritable, not depressed, and that he needs long-term psychotherapy to deal with his problems with male authority figures. She also thinks he drinks too much and needs to attend Alcoholics Anonymous meetings. Brent's doctor thinks he is in a postmanic depressive phase and would benefit from a combination of medication and couple therapy.

Psychiatrists and psychologists usually think of bipolar disorder as a set of symptoms, which must be present in clusters (that is, more than one at a time) and last for a certain length of time, usually in "episodes" that have a beginning phase, a phase in which symptoms are at their worst, and a recovery phase (see the box "What Is a Bipolar Episode?"). The traditional approach to psychiatric diagnosis described in Chapter 3 follows this line of reasoning. In contrast, people with the illness often prefer to think of bipolar disorder as a series of life experiences, with the actual symptoms being of secondary importance to the factors that provoked them. Family members or significant others may have a different perspective altogether, perhaps one that emphasizes the patient's personality or that views the deviant behavior in historical perspective (for example, "She's always been moody"). Although they are often quite different, there is a degree of validity to all three points of view.

In this chapter you'll gain a sense of the different perspectives people take in understanding bipolar mood swings and how these different perspectives can lead to very different feelings about which treatments should be undertaken. These perspectives include the personal standpoint, as described by patients who have the disorder; the observers' viewpoint, which usually means parents, spouses, or close friends; and the doctor's viewpoint. Questions to pose to yourself when reading this chapter are:

- "How do I experience swings in my mood?"
- "Are they similar to the ways others with bipolar disorder experience them?"
- "How do I understand my own behavior?"
- "How is my understanding different from the way others perceive me?"
- "How do I see myself differently from the way my doctor sees me?"
- "What kinds of problems arise from these differences in perceptions?"

Understanding these varying perspectives will be of considerable use to you, whether you are on your first episode or have had many episodes, in that you will gain some clarity on how your own experiences may differ from those of people without bipolar disorder. You may also come to see why others in your family or work or social environment think you need treatment, even if you don't agree with them.

Nuts and Bolts: What Is Bipolar Disorder?

Let's begin by defining the syndrome of bipolar disorder. Its key characteristic is extreme mood swings, from manic highs to severe depressions. It is called a mood disorder because it profoundly affects a person's experiences of emotion and *affect* (the way he or she conveys emotions to others). It is called *bipolar* because the mood swings occur between two poles, high and low, as opposed to unipolar disorder, where mood swings occur along only one pole—the lows.

In the manic "high" state, people experience different combinations of the following: elated or euphoric mood (excessive happiness or expansiveness), irritable mood (excessive anger and touchiness), a decreased need for sleep, grandiosity (an inflated sense of themselves and their abilities), increased talkativeness, racing thoughts or jumping from one idea to another, an increase in activity and energy levels, changes in thinking, attention, and perception, and impulsive, reckless behavior. These episodes alternate with intervals in which a person becomes depressed, sad, blue, or "down in the dumps," loses interest in things he or she ordinarily enjoys, loses weight and appetite, feels fatigued, has difficulty sleeping, feels guilty and bad about him- or herself, has trouble concentrating or making decisions, and often feels like committing suicide.

Episodes of either mania or depression can last anywhere from days to months. Some people (about 40% by some estimates; Calabrese et al., 2004) don't experi-

---

What Is a Bipolar Episode?

■ A set of symptoms that go together, with a beginning *prodromal* phase, a middle *acute* phase, and a final *recovery* phase.

■ The *polarity* of an episode can be depressed, manic, hypomanic, or mixed.

■ Episodes can last anywhere from a few days to several months.

■ Some people switch polarities in the middle of an episode (e.g., from depressed to manic or from manic to mixed).

---

ence depressions and manias in alternating fashion. Instead, they experience them simultaneously, in what we call *mixed episodes,* which I'll talk about in the next chapter.

Episodes of bipolar disorder do not develop overnight, and how severe the manias or depressions get varies greatly from person to person. Many people accelerate into mania in stages. Drs. Gabrielle Carlson and Frederick Goodwin (1973) observed that in the early stages of mania, people feel "wired" or charged up and their thoughts race with numerous ideas. They start needing less and less sleep and feel giddy or mildly irritable (*hypomania*). Later they accelerate into a full-blown mania, marked by euphoria, anger, impulsive behaviors such as spending sprees, and intense, frenetic periods of activity. In the most advanced stages, the person can develop mental confusion, delusions (beliefs that are irrational), hallucinations (hearing voices or seeing things), and severe anxiety. Not everyone experiences these stages, and many people receive treatment before they get to the most advanced stage.

People also spiral into depression gradually, although its stages are less clear-cut. For some, severe depressions arise when they were otherwise feeling well. In others, major depression develops on top of ongoing, milder depressions called *dysthymias* (see Chapter 10).

The periods in between manic and depressive episodes are symptom free in some people. For others, there are symptoms left over from previous episodes, such as sleep disturbance, ongoing irritability, or dysthymic or hypomanic disorders. A 13-year study found that people with bipolar disorder spend an average of one-third of the weeks of their lives in states of depression, about 9% in states of mania, about 6% in mixed or rapid cycling states, and about 53% in *euthymic* or normal mood states (Judd et al., 2002). Most people experience problems in their social and work life because of the illness.

About 1% of the general population has bipolar I disorder, marked by swings from extreme depression to extreme mania. Another 1% has bipolar II disorder, in which people vary from severely depressed to hypomanic, a milder form of mania. New cases of bipolar disorder have been recognized in young children and in the elderly, but the typical age at first onset is around 18 (Merikangas et al., 2007). Bipolar disorder is generally treated with a range of drugs in combination with psychotherapy:

- Mood stabilizers (e.g., lithium carbonate, divalproex sodium [Depakote], or lamotrigine [Lamictal])

- Atypical antipsychotics (e.g., quetiapine [Seroquel], risperidone [Risperdal], or aripiprazole [Abilify])

- Antianxiety agents (e.g., clonazepam [Klonopin] or lorazepam [Ativan, Temesta])

- Antidepressants (e.g., sertraline [Zoloft], paroxetine [Paxil], bupropion [Wellbutrin], or citalopram [Celexa]) (see Chapter 6 for a discussion of the risks associated with antidepressants)

Different Perspectives on Mania and Depression

As noted, the symptoms associated with bipolar mood disorder can be experienced quite differently by the person with the disorder, by an observer, and by a physician. The disorder primarily affects *moods* and *behavior.* Your moods cannot always be observed by others, although you will usually be aware of them. Likewise, you may not always be aware of your behavior or its impact on others, while others (family, friends, or doctors) are acutely aware of it. When people look at and evaluate the same set of behaviors or experiences through different lenses, you can imagine how much room there is for interpretation and misinterpretation.

You may be quite articulate in describing what you are feeling and thinking. When in a manic phase, your thoughts may flow rapidly and life may feel exotic and wonderful. You may speak more than usual and more freely reveal your inner thoughts. An observer, such as a family member, usually focuses on your behavior, which he or she may describe as too outspoken, boisterous, verbally hostile, dangerous to yourself or others, or impulsive in ways that negatively affect others (for example, spending or investing your money suddenly). Your doctor is usually attuned to whether your mood and behavior are significant departures from your normal state, taking into account such things as whether the symptoms have lasted for a period of time, how intense they are, and whether they cause impairment in your functioning.

In the following sections, I will describe mania and depression from these three perspectives. I will focus on the personal experiences that really define episodes of bipolar disorder, which are summarized in the sidebar on page 18.

Roller-Coaster Mood States

"How can I ever make plans or count on anything or anybody? I never know how I'm going to feel. I can be up and happy and full of ideas, but then the littlest things set me off. I'll drink a cup of tea and it doesn't match my expectation of how hot it should be, and I'll just react—I'll cuss, scream—I'm bitterly volatile … I'm afraid of my own moods."

—A 30-year-old woman with bipolar I disorder

Most people with bipolar disorder describe their moods as volatile, unpredictable, "all over the map," or "like a seesaw." Mood states accompanying bipolar disorder can be irritable (during either depression or mania), euphoric, elevated or excessively giddy (during mania), or extremely sad (during depression).

Effective prevention: Moods and behaviors associated with bipolar disorder look different depending on one's perspective. Family and friends may react to changes in your behavior, you may focus on your mood state or sleep, and doctors may be comparing your mood and behavior at any moment to what is normal for you or other patients they have seen. Understanding these different perspectives can prevent misinterpretation and delays in diagnosis and treatment.

You may agree that you have variable mood states, but your explanation for these mood states may be quite different from those of your doctor, family members, or friends. People with bipolar disorder often get angry when their doctors bring out a list of symptoms and ask them how many they have had and for how long. They find themselves reluctantly agreeing that they suffer from irritable moods but also know the triggers for these moods that other people may not see.

Experiences of Manic and Depressive Episodes

■ Roller-coaster mood states (euphoria, irritability, depression)

■ Changes in energy or activity levels

■ Changes in thinking and perception

■ Suicidal thoughts

■ Sleep problems

■ Impulsive or self-destructive behavior

"When I'm mad, nobody better get in my face. I feel like crushing everything and everybody. Every little thing will provoke me. I hate everybody, I hate my life and want to kill myself in some really dramatic way. It's like a sharp-edged, pointed anger, like a burning feeling."

—A 23-year-old woman with bipolar II disorder

Family members, when describing the emotional volatility of their bipolar sibling, child, or parent, tend to emphasize the intimidation they feel in the face of sudden outbursts that they don't feel they've provoked. Consider this interchange between Kirsten, age 21, and her mother, after Kirsten had railed at her mother just minutes earlier.

Kirsten: I wanna come back and live with you. I can handle it.

Mother: But you're not in a good place right now. Look how angry you just got.

Kirsten: But you told me I wasn't ready to take care of myself! Of course I exploded!

Mother: And you're not. I can tell because you're overreacting to me, and that tells me you're probably not better yet.

It's hard to think of your mood swings as evidence of an illness, especially when every emotional reaction you have seems perfectly justifiable, given what's just happened to you. To Kirsten, her angry outburst seemed perfectly justified, because her mother had questioned her competency. Her mother knows what her daughter is like when she's well and sees her irritability as a departure from this norm.

In contrast, the elated, euphoric periods of the manic experience feel exceptionally good to the person with the disorder. Kay Jamison has written extensively about the wondrous feelings that can accompany manic episodes and how the desire to sustain these feelings can lead a person to resist taking medications (Jamison, 1995, 2005). Not all people with bipolar disorder experience their high moods as euphoria, however. For example, Beth, age 42, described her mood during manic episodes as "the sudden awareness that I'm not depressed anymore." Seth, age 27, described his manic states as "tired but wired."

To others, your euphoria or high mood may seem strange or clownish, and they may not share it with you, but they are unlikely to be as disturbed by it as they are by your irritability. To your relatives, especially those who have gone through one or more previous episodes with you, euphoric mood is worrisome to the extent that it heralds the development of a full-blown manic episode.

Now consider how you experience depression. Would you describe it as an intense sadness ... a numbing feeling ... a feeling of being removed from others ... a lack of interest in things you ordinarily enjoy? One man put it bluntly: "My depressions eat me alive. I feel like I'm in a fish tank that separates me from other people. It's all just hopelessness, and I don't see any future for myself."

In contrast, a family member, friend, or lover might see your depression as self-inflicted. People who are close to you might feel sympathetic at first but then get irritated and annoyed. They may think you're not trying hard enough or could "make this all go away if you had the right mental attitude." You will probably experience these reactions as unpleasant and lacking in empathy.

What does the doctor look for? To determine whether the diagnosis is correct (if you are being diagnosed for the first time), or whether you are experiencing a recurrence of the disorder (if you've been diagnosed before), your doctor will evaluate whether your mood states are different, in terms of degree or intensity, from those of "normal" people. Do your moods—euphoric, irritable, or depressed—get out of hand and stay out of hand for days at a time? Do your mood swings cause problems in your social, work, and/or family life? The questions listed in the sidebar on the next page will figure prominently in your doctor's evaluation of whether your mood states are problematic from a clinical perspective.

Changes in Energy and Activity Levels

If someone asked you to describe your symptoms, you might not focus on your mood fluctuations. In fact, many people who are asked about their mood states answer with descriptions of their energy and activity levels instead. They're more conscious of what they do or don't do than of how they feel. They focus on the great increases in energy that they experience during the manic or mixed phases or the decreases in energy they experience during the depressive phases.

One way to understand these fluctuations is to think of bipolar disorder as a dysregulation of drive states as well as of mood. Changes in normal motivational drives, such as those that govern eating, sleeping, sex, interacting with others, and achievement are part and parcel of the bipolar pendulum. The normal drives that guide our behavior become intensified in mania and diminished in depression. These changes in drive states, of course, can have a tremendous impact on one's daily life and productivity.

> "I feel like I have a motor attached. Everything is moving too slowly, and I want to go, go, go. I feel like one of those toys that somebody winds up and sends spinning or doing cartwheels or whatever ... and to stop feels like being in a cage."
>
> —A 38-year-old woman with bipolar I disorder

Consider the increases in energy level that accompany manic episodes. For Lauren, this surge took the form of an intense drive to accomplish a particular activity

---

Questions a Doctor Might Ask to Distinguish Bipolar Mood Swings from Normal Mood Variability

- ■ "Do your mood swings cause problems in your social or family life?"

- ■ "Do your mood swings lead to decreases in your work productivity that last more than a few days?"

- ■ "Do your mood states last for days at a time with little relief, or do they change when something good happens?"

- ■ "Do other people notice and comment when your mood shifts?"

- ■ "Do your mood changes go along with noticeable changes in thinking, perceiving, sleeping, and/or energy or activity levels?"

- ■ "Do your mood swings ever get so out of hand that the police have to be called or a hospitalization becomes necessary?"

If your answer to most of these questions is yes, then it is likely that your mood swings go beyond the normal range.

(exercising and getting in shape). For Cynthia it took the form of a strong desire for social contact and stimulation. When manic, she would call people all over the country whom she hadn't spoken to in years, double- and triple-schedule her social calendar, and become bored quickly with the company of others. Jolene's took on a sexual quality: Accumulating as many sexual partners as possible felt to her like a physical need. Ted felt the drive in relation to food: "I couldn't stuff enough things in my mouth. They [the nursing staff at the hospital] put this entire chicken in front of me and I, like, inhaled it."

Quite often, increases in activity are accompanied by grandiose behavior. This is behavior that most people would consider dangerous, "over the top," unrealistic, and associated with inflated (sometimes delusional) beliefs about one's powers or abilities.

> "I walked into a real fancy restaurant with my mother and started jumping around and running, and there were these chandeliers on the ceiling. I thought I was Superman or something, and I leapt up to grab onto one of them and started swinging on it."
>
> —A 21-year-old man with bipolar I disorder

Grandiose behaviors usually go along with high or euphoric feelings, but not invariably. You may experience an inflated sense of self-confidence and then feel impatient and irritable because others seem slow to go along with your ideas or plans. Grandiose behavior is detrimental not only because of its associated health risks but also because it leads to feelings of shame, which can compound your depression in the aftermath of a manic episode. In the case of the young man just quoted, the police were called in, a scuffle ensued, and a hospitalization followed. Although he later related the incident with a degree of bravado, he admitted to feeling quite embarrassed by his public behavior.

For every example already given, you can imagine what a counterexample would look like during the depressed phase. In depression, you may become unusually slowed down, like you're "moving through molasses." The most mundane of tasks feels like it requires tremendous effort. Your appetite is usually diminished. Typically, the last thing a depressed person wants is sex, and exercise has even less appeal. Socializing seems like an unpleasant chore and requires too much concentration and mental energy.

When drive states are heightened in hypomania and mania, important things can be accomplished and significant plans for personal advancement can be put into place. Unfortunately, the depressive aftermath of these heightened drive states can make the plans seem difficult or even impossible to accomplish. The inability to carry out plans that were hatched while manic can become a source of despair while depressed. A 19-year-old man with bipolar disorder described the switch from mania to depression like this: "I'm like a porpoise. I fly high up in the air and then I yell, 'I'm going down again!' And then I go underneath the water, and all the air, sunshine, and the ocean breeze just vanish."

What Do Others See?

Carol, a 20-year-old, had had several episodes of bipolar disorder. Her older sister described her manic, activated behavior this way:

> "She gets involved in these creative projects that we all want to support, like hand-painting dishes or making soap sculptures and trying to sell them. But then she seems to take it too far. She tries to sell them on the Web, and then she gets all riled up and frantic and starts staying up all night on the computer—and then she crashes and all the projects get dumped."

The rapid changes in energy and activity that accompany highs and lows are often a source of family conflicts. To observers, your activated behavior while manic may look attractive or encouraging at first, especially if you were formerly depressed. But it loses its charm as you become more and more manic and your behavior begins to look frenetic and purposeless. Observers (for example, family members) are usually unaware of the feeling of purposefulness that you may be experiencing. Family members or friends may become angry about your agitated, driven quality and apparent lack of concern for others. In the extreme manic states, family members become worried that you will hurt yourself or someone else. In parallel, they may become frustrated with your inactivity during depressed phases and give you "pep talks" that can contribute to your feelings of guilt or inadequacy.

To a doctor, your increases in activity are the surest clue that hypomania or mania has set in, but he or she will probably look for evidence that your behavior is consistently activated across different situations. The mere fact that you have taken on extra work projects is not usually enough to point to mania. So your doctor may ask you how many telephone calls you've made, how many hours you've worked, how much sleep you've gotten, how much money you've spent, how many social engagements you've arranged, or how much sex activity and drive you've had. He or she may also base judgments about your state on how you behave in the interview room: whether you can sit still, whether you answer questions rapidly or interrupt a lot, or whether you wring your hands, pick at things, or constantly fidget. Likewise, your physician will look for *psychomotor retardation* (being slowed down in your physical movements) and blunted facial expressions during depressions.

A key point to remember here is that, to you, the increases in energy and activity that accompany manic episodes may feel good, productive, and purposeful. To others, including your doctor, they may be seen as pointless, unrealistic, or signs of a developing illness. During depressions, you may feel unable to do even the most basic of things, like showering, dressing, or eating; but others may unfairly accuse you of being lazy. These different perceptions will cause conflict between you and them, but it's important to be open to their perspectives while also explaining your own.

Changes in Thinking and Perception

"My mind feels like I'm in one of those postcards of the city that are taken at night, with the camera moving. Lights feel like they have tails, the whole world is zooming—I love it. My mind is so full of thoughts that I feel like I'm going to burst."

—A 26-year-old woman with bipolar I disorder

Manic and depressive moods almost always involve changes in your thinking. During mania this involves the speeding up of mental functions (racing thoughts) and the verbal expression of one thought after another in rapid-fire fashion (flight of ideas). Many experience the world differently: colors become brighter and sounds become intolerably loud. Mental confusion can accompany the most advanced stages of mania: the world begins to feel like a Ferris wheel that is spinning out of control.

During mania, your memory can seem extra crisp and clear, you feel brilliantly sharp, one idea can be easily related to another, and you can recall events in vivid detail. However, this apparent improvement in memory is often illusory; people experiencing mania think they remember better than they actually do. In fact, attention and concentration can become quite impaired during mania. You cannot keep your mind on any one thing at a time because your mind is trying to process too many things at once. Your attention can become easily distracted by mundane things like random noises, the facial expressions of others, or the feeling of your clothing against your skin.

As mania spirals upward, your thoughts can become increasingly jumbled and even incoherent. Others to whom you speak may be unable to understand you. They will probably try to keep you focused and ask you to slow down. You will probably find these interactions annoying and have the reaction that others seem slow, dumb, and uninteresting.

Some people develop hallucinations (perceptual experiences that are not real) and delusions (unrealistic, mistaken beliefs) during mania. *Grandiose delusions* are especially common, such as thinking you are exceptionally talented in an arena in which you have had no formal training, believing you have exceptionally high intelligence, feeling like you know what others are thinking, believing you have special powers, or thinking you are a major public figure or even God:

> *"[As I was cycling into mania], I got this idea in my head that I should throw a party for everyone I knew. As the days wore on, I believed that all my doctors— everyone who had ever treated me—were going to come. Before long, I thought Bruce Springsteen was coming, and so was Beyoncé, and I heard the voice of God telling me, 'Go to Dennis [ex-boyfriend]; he wants you.'"*
> —A 19-year-old bipolar woman

Delusions and hallucinations are particularly scary to significant others, who view them as the most concrete sign of "craziness." Doctors will be especially attuned to these symptoms and will also be on the lookout for less dramatic signs of distorted thinking. Consider the following exchange between a psychologist and a 20-year-old man who was coming off the crest of his manic high. The man sat with a law book in his lap, arguing that he could pass the bar exam without going to law school and would sue anyone who challenged him:

Doctor: Have you had any unusual thoughts or experiences this past week?

Patient: No, not really.

Doctor: Any feelings like you have special powers or that you're a famous person? Last week you were thinking a lot about God and having—

Patient: (Interrupts.) Well, that was last week! *(Laughs.)* No, I don't think of myself that way, but I'm more like a young god, kind of like a teacher. *(Giggles.)* I think I have a lot to offer others.

The client above was still delusional. His thinking frequently g
with others, especially his parents, who were mostly concerned at
hold a job. They were angered by his unrealistic beliefs in himsel
schemes for fighting the educational system.

In contrast, during depression it's hard to focus on even o
experience the slowing down of mental functions as difficulty concentrating or making simple decisions. Colors seem drab. Disturbances of memory are common: you
may have difficulty recalling telephone numbers you use regularly, remembering
appointments, or following a television program because of trouble holding recent
events in your memory.

Ruminations, in which a person thinks about a certain event again and again,
are a frequent accompaniment to depression. Ruminations during the depressive
phase are often self-recriminating. For example, Margie became preoccupied with
the thought "Was Paul [her boss] insulted when I didn't sit next to him at the meeting?" Similarly, Cameron described: "When I was manic I jokingly asked my friend
if his wife was 'hot,' and I couldn't stop thinking about how stupid that was when I
got depressed." Depressive ruminations frequently include guilt or shame, or feeling
worthless, hopeless, or helpless. They can become all encompassing and affect one's
day-to-day functioning. When Patrice became depressed, she found herself "rehears-
ing like a mantra" statements like "I suck … I hate myself … I'm such a bitch."

Suicidal Thoughts

Ruminations often take the form of suicidal preoccupations—thoughts about
the various ways one could kill oneself. These ruminations are most common during
depressive or mixed episodes but can also be present during mania. Depending on
how desperate a person feels, he or she may act on these thoughts or impulses, often
with dire consequences.

Friends and family members will be particularly upset and scared by your suicidal thoughts, if voiced to them, and will do their best to help you deal with these
thoughts, although they may not know what to say or do. Your therapist or physician
is also likely to ask about them (for example, "Are you having any thoughts of hurting or killing yourself, as many people do when they're down?"). If you have never
had suicidal thoughts before and have them now, you may feel afraid to express them.

> **Effective prevention:** Telling your doctor—or a trusted friend or family member—about any suicidal thoughts you have may help alleviate those thoughts.

You may fear that the physician will hospitalize
you immediately. This is certainly one treatment
option, but not the only one. Others may include
psychotherapy, modifications of your medication
regimen, and/or various forms of community or
family support.

Take the chance of discussing these feelings
with your physician or therapist—you may find

at some of these thoughts dissipate after you've shared them with someone else. You may also learn that mental health professionals are more helpful at such times than you would have expected. I will discuss suicidal feelings and actions in more detail in Chapter 11.

Sleep Disturbances

Virtually all people with bipolar disorder experience disturbances of sleep during their mood swings. When you get manic, you may feel no need to sleep. Sleeping feels like a waste of time, especially when so many things can get accomplished in the middle of the night! During depression, sleep can feel like the only thing that is welcomed. When you are depressed, you may sleep many more hours than usual (for example, 16 hours a day) and become unproductive and unable to function outside of the home (hypersomnia). Alternatively you may have insomnia and find that sleep eludes you. You may lie awake at night tossing and turning, thinking about the same problems over and over again, and then feel exhausted the next day. Sleep can feel frustratingly out of your reach.

Are sleep problems a symptom of bipolar disorder, or do they actually cause problems in mood? It appears that they are both symptom and cause. Most people have changes in mood when they have trouble sleeping, but people with bipolar disorder are particularly vulnerable to changes in the sleep–wake cycle (Harvey, 2008). I'll say more about sleep disruptions and mood states in Chapter 5.

Your doctor will probably ask you about sleep disturbances, with emphasis on whether the problem is falling asleep, waking up in the middle of the night, or waking up too early. He or she may ask you to keep track of your sleep if you have trouble recalling the nature of your disturbances. If you have a spouse, he or she may be affected by your sleep patterns—when one person can't sleep, others often can't as well. Your own irritability, as well as that of your family members, can be a function of lack of sleep or inconsistent sleep habits.

Impulsive, Self-Destructive, or Addictive Behaviors

What do you usually do when you start to feel manic? When you are loaded with energy, you may feel like you have to have an outlet. Ordinary life moves too slowly. Perhaps as a result, when people get manic, they often lose their inhibitions and behave impulsively. Many of these impulsive behaviors can be threatening to one's life or health, such as driving recklessly on the freeway, performing daredevil acts, or having unprotected sex with many different partners. Martha's impulsive behavior (Chapter 1) was a major cause of the marital problems she had after her manic episode.

Some people make unwise decisions, like spending a lot of money indiscriminately. Kevin was 34 and lived with his father. When manic, he convinced his father to liquidate part of his IRA, which Kevin invested wildly in various commodities. Most of the money disappeared. His family, understandably, was livid; his older brothers refused to talk to him anymore. Prior to this incident, Kevin had been making plans to move out on his own. But his father insisted he pay the money back before he agreed to help finance Kevin's attempts to become independent.

Carl, age 40, spent tremendous amounts of money on home improvements. He installed elaborate fireplaces, impractical bathroom fixtures, and eye-catching but gaudy paintings. His partner, Roberta, with whom he cohabitated, became increasingly frustrated about their dwindling finances, and their conflicts intensified. In Roberta's view, Carl was unwilling to recognize his mania as the source of the problem.

Self-destructive behavior can take many forms. Many people turn to alcohol or drugs during manic episodes. Substance use problems and addictive behaviors are not essential symptoms of bipolar disorder, but they can become intertwined with mood disorder symptoms in such a way that each worsens the other. Alcohol is often sought as a means of bringing oneself down from the high state and quelling the anxiety, confusion, and sleep disturbance that typically go with it. Some use cocaine, amphetamine, or marijuana to heighten and intensify the euphoric experiences of mania. During a depression, alcohol or drugs are usually craved as a means of dulling the pain, or what we call self-medicating. More than any other associated condition, drug and alcohol abuse makes the course of your bipolar disorder much worse (Weiss et al., 2007). Mark described the role alcohol played in his depressions as follows:

"When I'm down, drinking for me is like a security blanket. When I'm feeling my worst, the bottle is there in the closet, like an old friend. I don't think about what it's doing to my body, only that I need to numb myself out. Sometimes, just knowing there's a bottle in the cabinet is enough to make me feel better. I just can't stop myself. I keep blowing it."

Another person with bipolar disorder, Thad, was less clear on why he drank when he was manic. While in the hospital, he summarized it like this: "I don't know what it is with me and booze (*smiling*). I know it's not funny, but whenever I get that way [high, manic], I just seem to need to tie one on."

Family members may be more bothered by your drug and alcohol use than your mood swings. They may even define your problems as alcohol or drug related and reject the bipolar diagnosis, thinking it is a way for you to justify continuing to drink. They may be incorrect about this, but your doctor will need to conduct a thorough diagnostic assessment to be sure (see Chapter 3).

Your doctor will probably be skeptical of the bipolar diagnosis unless there is concrete evidence that your mood swings occur when you do not use drugs or alcohol. Jeff, for example, had had several manic episodes before he developed problems with alcohol, and the bipolar diagnosis seemed justified. On the other hand, Kate's alcohol problems developed well before there was any evidence of mood swings, and her mood episodes—although characterized by typical bipolar symptoms such as irritability, sleep disturbance, lethargy, suicidality, and impulsiveness—were eventually attributed to the effects of alcohol intoxication.

Summary: Different Perspectives

As you already know or have just seen, people with bipolar disorder have distinct experiences that comprise their mood disorder. Varying emotional states and changes in energy, judgment, thinking, and sleep characterize the swings between the poles. Family members or significant others are not likely to understand these widely fluctuating experiences (unless they have bipolar disorder themselves) and are likely to focus on how your behavior affects them and other family members. Most psychiatrists will be less interested in the meaning of these experiences to you than in the symptoms you've had that are consistent or inconsistent with the bipolar diagnosis, or that point to specific treatments (see Chapter 6).

These different perspectives may be a source of frustration for you, because you may feel like others don't understand you or aren't interested in your inner life. Likewise, your family members, and perhaps your doctor, will be frustrated if you seem to be oblivious to or unconcerned about the effects of your behavior on others. These disparate perceptions can be a source of conflicts over the treatment plan: You may feel that you've had profound experiences, but others only seem interested in labeling you as a sick person. Many people with bipolar disorder, out of frustration over these issues, reject the notion that they are having symptoms and also reject the diagnosis and its associated treatments (see Chapters 3 and 4). Others are fortunate enough to be able to communicate effectively with their doctor and family members, who correspondingly make attempts to understand these private experiences. The hope, of course, is that you will find a treatment regimen that will stabilize your mood without minimizing the significance that these personal experiences have held for you.

Whether you are having your first episode or have had many, the first step in obtaining optimal treatment for yourself is to get a proper diagnosis. Chapter 3 deals with this very important issue by answering the following questions:

■ How is the disorder actually diagnosed by mental health professionals?

■ What symptoms and behaviors do doctors look for?

■ What can you expect during the diagnostic process?

■ How will your doctor elicit information from you to determine the diagnosis?

In describing the diagnostic criteria, I'll touch on the important issue of *border conditions:*

- How do you know if you have bipolar disorder versus some other psychiatric illness?
- Does the diagnosis give a reasonable explanation for your behavior?
- If not, are there other diagnoses that fit you better?

3

Into the Doctor's Court
Getting an Accurate Diagnosis

The endless questioning finally ended. My psychiatrist looked at me, there was no uncertainty in his voice. "Manic–depressive illness." I admired his bluntness. I wished him locusts on his lands and a pox upon his house. Silent, unbelievable rage. I smiled pleasantly. He smiled back. The war had just begun.
—Kay Redfield Jamison, *An Unquiet Mind* (1995, p. 104)

You're not alone in feeling that mania and depression are very personal and intense experiences. Nor are you alone if you are wary of any stranger's ability to understand what you're going through, no matter how highly qualified as a medical professional. Many people experiencing bipolar symptoms postpone seeing a doctor for as long as possible because they already feel thoroughly misunderstood. Others receive a diagnosis but reject it out of hand. Still others grudgingly accept a diagnosis of bipolar disorder but then express their resistance by refusing to comply with their treatment regimen. If you fit into any of these categories, I hope you'll reconsider the benefits of a professional diagnosis.

No diagnostic label can completely capture your unique situation. In fact, you may feel offended by the diagnostic label because it is incomplete, impersonal, or simply doesn't do justice to your life experiences. But these labels do serve a purpose. First, using standardized labels allows clinicians to communicate with each other. If I refer a client of mine to another mental health professional and say that "she has bipolar I disorder, mixed episode, with mood-incongruent psychotic features," there is a high likelihood that this other doctor will know what to expect. This common language serves you well should you switch doctors, as so many of us do today. Second, an accurate diagnosis is important to selecting the right treatment. If you are misdiagnosed as having depression alone, for example, your doctor might recommend a standard antidepressant medication such as fluoxetine (Prozac), sertraline (Zoloft), or bupropion (Wellbutrin) without a mood stabilizer like lithium (see Chapter 6). If you are actually bipolar, this treatment regimen could make you swing into mania. Likewise, if you were diagnosed as bipolar when the real problem is attention-deficit/hyperactivity disorder (ADHD), you might not benefit from the mood stabilizer you would be given. An accurate diagnostic label helps doctors treat the whole syndrome that is affecting you rather than just the symptoms you are reporting right now.

Diagnoses also help you prepare for the challenges the future might hold. Will you have another episode? Will you be able to go back to work? How will you know when you're getting sick again? Knowing that you have bipolar disorder makes you and your doctor privy to all of the information that researchers and clinicians have gathered from the experiences of thousands of people like you. For example, you can expect to have another episode soon if you don't take medication, and you may need to wait for a while after an episode before going back to work full time.

> **Effective solution:** An accurate diagnosis leads to a clearer prognosis, which may make it easier to manage your life and minimize the disabilities that bipolar disorder can cause.

The Criteria for a Diagnosis of Bipolar Disorder

Psychiatrists and psychologists rely on the fourth edition of the *Diagnostic and Statistical Manual of Mental Disorders* to make diagnoses (DSM-IV-TR; American Psychiatric Association, 2000). Note the term *manual* in the title: A clinician should be able to pick up the manual and decide whether a patient meets the criteria for a specific psychiatric illness. Applying these diagnostic criteria reliably (that is, being able to tell one disorder from another) cannot be done quickly or haphazardly: it requires considerable training, experience, and skill on the part of the mental health professional.

The first edition of the DSM was published in 1952; other editions were published in 1968, 1980, 1987, and 1994 (with a text revision, DSM-IV-TR, in 2000). DSM-V is planned for 2013. Each version has been informed by the research and observations of many investigators and clinicians and by experiences elicited from numerous patients with psychiatric disorders. No diagnostic manual is perfect, and not everyone agrees with the premises of the DSM. In my opinion, DSM-IV-TR is an extremely useful manual, and no one has created another diagnostic system that provides a reasonable alternative.

Your doctor will first identify which symptoms you have (for example, sleep disturbance, irritability), how severe these symptoms are, and how long they have lasted. From your particular pattern of symptoms, he or she will then determine if the diagnosis of bipolar disorder—as outlined in DSM-IV-TR—fits you. If it does, your doctor will then be concerned with which kind of bipolar disorder you have: Is it bipolar type I or II? Do you have rapid cycling?

Bipolar I Disorder

The box on this page describes the major subtypes of bipolar disorder listed in DSM-IV-TR. For bipolar I disorder, you must have had at least one manic or mixed episode, with elated mood and three other associated symptoms of mania (grandiose thinking, decreased need for sleep, pressured speech, increased activity or energy level, racing thoughts, flight of ideas, distractibility, or impulsive behavior) that lasted a week or more and/or required that you receive emergency treatment. If your mood was irritable and not elated, four or more associated symptoms are required.

The DSM–IV Subtypes of Bipolar Disorder

Bipolar I disorder

■ At least one lifetime episode of manic or mixed disorder

■ Although not required for the diagnosis, at least one lifetime episode of major depressive disorder

Bipolar II disorder

■ At least one lifetime episode of hypomanic disorder

■ At least one lifetime episode of major depressive disorder

Bipolar disorder not otherwise specified (NOS)

■ Multiple manic episodes with impairment of functioning that do not meet the DSM-IV-TR duration criteria or that fall one symptom short of the required number of symptoms

Bipolar disorder with rapid cycling

■ Meets criteria for bipolar I or bipolar II disorder

■ Four or more episodes of major depressive disorder, manic disorder, mixed disorder, or hypomanic disorder in any 1 year

---

Note how these symptoms capture the essence of the subjective experiences of mania described in Chapter 2: the roller-coaster mood states, increases in activity and drive, changes in thinking and perception, and impulsive or self-destructive behaviors.

You may find yourself reacting negatively to how reductionistic the symptom labels are: what you see as clear insights and the energy to get important things done may be labeled by DSM-IV-TR as grandiosity, for example. Your reactions are certainly understandable. These symptom labels are shorthand for very complex life experiences and mood states, much like the diagnostic label itself.

DSM-IV-TR requires at least 1 week of manic symptoms for bipolar I disorder, unless hospitalization or other emergency treatment was necessary, in which case there is no time requirement. There must also be evidence that you showed deterioration in your work or family life (for example, major family arguments, loss of your job). In most cases, a person with bipolar I disorder will also have had, at some point in life, a minimum 2-week period with five or more symptoms of major depressive illness (depressed mood, loss of interests, weight loss or a change in appetite, loss of energy or fatigue, motor agitation or retardation, loss of concentration, feelings of worthlessness, insomnia or hypersomnia, suicidal thoughts or actions) during which there was a deterioration in everyday functioning.

People with bipolar I disorder can experience episodes of mania and depression in different sequences. Some people have manias followed by depressions followed by periods in which their mood returns to normal (*euthymic* mood). Other people have depressions followed by manias, which are then followed by euthymic mood. Other people have rapid cycling states, which I'll talk more about later.

If you have had a manic episode but no depressions, your doctor will still diagnose you with bipolar I disorder. This is because he or she assumes that a depression will eventually occur if the disorder is not treated adequately. As I mentioned in Chapter 2, people diagnosed with bipolar I disorder can also have mixed episodes, or what some physicians refer to as *dysphoric mania*. According to the DSM-IV-TR, this means that you have met the criteria for major depressive disorder and mania nearly every day for at least a week. Some people describe mixed mania as the "tired but wired" feeling. You can feel extraordinarily pessimistic and hopeless, fatigued, and unable to concentrate, but still feel "revved," anxious, irritable, driven, and sleep deprived, with your thoughts moving very rapidly.

Bipolar II Disorder

In bipolar II disorder, a person alternates between major depressive episodes and hypomanias. Hypomanias are milder forms of mania that may not last as long as full manias (the minimum requirement for the diagnosis is 4 days), but the number of symptoms required is the same (that is, three if the mood is elated, four if the mood is irritable). People with hypomania experience the first of the three stages of mania described in Chapter 2, but they do not go beyond this: they have sleep problems, irritability, increased activity, and an inflated sense of themselves, but not to the dangerous levels of the fully manic person. Generally, hypomanic episodes do not cause big problems in your work, family, or social life, but you may still experience some interpersonal difficulties when in this state (for example, more arguments with your spouse or kids). Hypomanias do not require hospitalization.

Hypomanic episodes can be quite enjoyable to the person experiencing them. In general, others will be baffled and put off by your energetic, hypersexual, and driven quality when hypomanic (for example, they may tell you to "chill out"). Your family members or friends may also be relieved by what they perceive to be the disappearance of the depressive states that often precede the energized one. Consider Heather, who had bipolar II disorder:

> Heather, age 36, was a professional conference coordinator. She described herself as almost always depressed. When she went through her divorce, contact with her soon-to-be ex-husband "felt like a drug I needed—it was the only thing that kept me alive." She became suicidal at that time. But soon after, she began planning a conference for a group of architects, and started dating one of them. The work and the new relationship "wired me ... I got my energy back. I stopped sleeping and staying in my condo so much of the time ... went walking my dog at 2 A.M. People told me I seemed much better, like I had my old self back, but I knew I was going overboard."

Keep in mind what different diagnostic subtypes may mean for your treatment. If you have bipolar II instead of bipolar I disorder, your illness may be less severe. But you still need to be careful: hypomanias, while fun and exciting, can herald the development of a severe depression, or even of rapid cycling, especially if you are not protected by mood-stabilizing medications. Ongoing depressions appear to be the major difficulty experienced by people with bipolar II disorder, with one study finding that patients spent 37 weeks depressed for every 1 week they spent hypomanic (Judd et al., 2003).

Bipolar Disorder Not Otherwise Specified (NOS)

DSM-IV-TR has a "hedge" category called bipolar NOS. This category usually is reserved for people who have had several manic episodes that do not meet the full duration criteria (7 days for mania unless controlled by emergency treatment) or that fall short of the minimum number of required symptoms. Some definitions require you to have had a major depressive episode as well. So, for example, Shelley, 31, had had three hypomanic episodes with irritability, decreased need for sleep, distractibility, and pressure of speech that each lasted 1–2 days; her single depressive episode came after the birth of her first child.

Estevan, age 46, had lengthy, unremitting periods of depression that his doctor originally labeled as *dysthymic disorder*. His diagnosis was changed to bipolar NOS when he had two brief manic episodes marked by elated mood, grandiosity, and decreased need for sleep, along with a sudden deterioration in his functioning. Both episodes remitted quickly but, sadly, were followed by a return to his depressive state.

Bipolar NOS is most frequently used to describe children or adolescents whose cycling pattern looks much like an adult bipolar I cycle, but whose episodes are frequent and very short (for example, lasting a day or less). Although this symptom pattern may sound like it could characterize almost any child, it is actually fairly rare when combined with the requirement of functional impairment. About 30% of kids who have the NOS diagnosis "convert" to bipolar I or II disorder in 4 years, and about 58% do if they have a first- or second-degree relative with bipolar I disorder. They also experience substantial impairments in their school and social functioning (Birmaher et al., 2009). So, bipolar NOS can be used to help identify children who are at risk for developing the full syndrome.

Rapid Cycling

Rapid cycling can accompany either bipolar I or II disorder. In rapid cycling, people quickly switch back and forth from mania or hypomania or mixed disorder to depression, with four or more distinct episodes in a single year. In other words, you have many episodes in a short period of time. Some people have *ultra-radian cycling,* which means switching from one mood pole to the other within a single 24-hour period.

If you have rapid cycling, you may have to go through quite a bit of trial and error with your medications until you find something that works. Your doctor may want to rule out other factors that may contribute to your mood swings, like thyroid abnormalities. The good news is that rapid cycling appears to be a time-limited phenomenon (Coryell, 2009; Schneck et al., 2008): people do not rapidly cycle their whole lives. I'll talk more about frequent cycling in Chapter 6 on drug treatments.

The Progression of Bipolar Episodes

Many people—including those who have not yet been diagnosed with bipolar disorder and those who have but are in doubt about it—find the diagnostic criteria just discussed confusing. Many clinicians do as well! You may wonder whether having only one or two of these symptoms qualifies you for the diagnosis or what it means if you had one symptom in January, none in February and March, and a different symptom in April.

One of the keys to making the diagnosis of bipolar disorder is to think in terms of clusters of symptoms that cycle together in episodes. There must be evidence that you have had time-limited periods of mood disorder that alternate with periods of functioning fairly normally or that alternate with intervals in which you experience the opposite pole of the illness (for example, manic episodes that are followed by depressive episodes). As I mentioned in Chapter 2, episodes are intervals when your mood, activity level, thinking patterns, and sleep all change at the same time (see the figure on this page). Consider, Tom, a 46-year-old with bipolar disorder:

> Tom described both depressive episodes and mixed episodes. As his depression developed over several weeks, he experienced sadness and loss of interests in his usual activities, but a mild paranoia with anxiety also developed. He began to feel that no one in his family was on his side and that they were talking about him behind his back. As he progressed into a mixed episode, his depression worsened and so did his anxiety and paranoia, but he also developed an irritability and anger that he expressed inappropriately. In one case, he broke some dishes; in another, he kicked in a door. His family members became scared of him. His sleep deteriorated, and his thoughts took on a rapid, ruminating quality ("I think about death and that there's no future—doesn't seem like there's anything I or anybody can do"). These periods usually lasted at least a week but often longer. As he recovered from his mixed episode—usually after his medication dosage had been increased or a new medication added—he would feel less hopeless, his thoughts would slow down, and he became easier for others to communicate with. Nonetheless, he continued to feel anxious, sad, and easily irritated by others. He began to see how his behavior affected his family and that at least some of his paranoid feelings were unfounded.

Notice how, in Tom's case, a single episode progressed in stages. Some symptoms (his hopelessness and paranoia) changed more rapidly than others (his sadness and anger). The length of bipolar episodes varies from person to person.

It may not always be possible to tell when you are finished (the recovery phase)

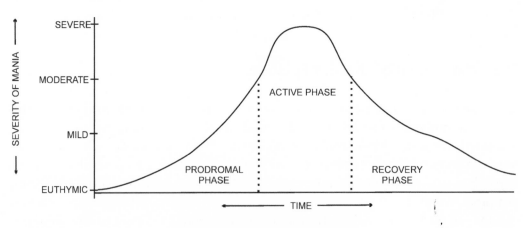

The phases of a manic episode.

with an episode or developing a new one. If you have had a number of episodes already, you probably are more attuned than most people to what it feels like to be ill versus well. But if you're on your first episode, you may be unclear as to when you're back to normal or what it feels like to be getting sick again. As you'll see when we discuss self-management techniques, knowing your prodromal phase symptoms (the signs that an episode of mania or depression has begun) and when to get emergency treatment help protect you against further escalation of the disorder.

Diagnostic Self-Evaluation as a Starting Point or a Backup Check

The self-administered checklist that follows is a starting point in determining whether your diagnosis is correct. If you have never seen a psychiatrist but think you might need to, the checklist will orient you to the kinds of symptoms your doctor will ask about. If you've already received the diagnosis of bipolar disorder and are suspicious of it, the list provides your doctor with a backup check. The checklist is not a diagnostic instrument: just because you endorse the items does not mean that you have the disorder, only that you've had symptoms of mania and depression that you and your doctor will want to discuss. Likewise, if none of the symptoms sounds familiar, you may still have the disorder but you and your doctor will want to discuss other diagnoses as well.

In filling out the checklist, and in discussing the symptoms with your physician, keep in mind that these symptoms must co-occur during the same period of time. If you had sad mood at one time in your life, racing thoughts at another, and insomnia during another period, that is not the same thing as having an episode of major depressive illness or a manic or hypomanic episode.

What the Doctor Will Want to Know: Steps toward Diagnosis and Treatment

Many of my patients have come to me feeling that their initial diagnosis was made too hastily. Either they became victims of the managed care rush to make diagnostic and treatment decisions or they were never asked about elements of their life story that, to them, seemed critical to an understanding of their mood problems.

Whether you have already been diagnosed and wish to review whether your case has been handled correctly, or you are preparing for your first evaluation, understanding the sequence of steps in the diagnostic and treatment process will help. These steps include the diagnostic referral, reviewing your prior medical records, and the diagnostic interview.

As I review the steps in the diagnostic process, keep in mind that your doctor

Bipolar Symptoms: A Self-Administered Checklist

DEPRESSION[1]

Has there ever been a period of time lasting two weeks or more when you were not your usual self and you experienced five or more of the following:

	Yes	No
Felt sad, blue, or down in the dumps?	✓	
Were uninterested in things?	✓	
Lost or gained more than 5% of your body weight?	✓	
Slept too little or too much?		✓
Were slowed down or sped up in your movements?	✓	
Felt fatigued or low in energy?	✓	
Felt worthless or very guilty about things?	✓	
Were unable to concentrate or make decisions?	✓	
Thought about killing yourself or making plans to do so?		✓

MANIA OR HYPOMANIA[2]

Has there been a period of time when you were not your usual self and you: *NO*

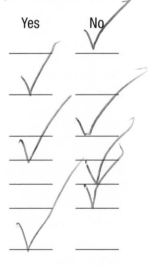

	Yes	No
Felt so good or so hyper that other people thought you were not your normal self or you were so hyper that you got into trouble?		✓
Were so irritable that you shouted at people or started fights or arguments?	✓	
Felt much more self-confident than usual?		✓
Got much less sleep than usual and found you didn't really miss it?	✓	✓
Were much more talkative or spoke much faster than usual?		
Had thoughts racing through your head or couldn't slow down your mind?		
Were so easily distracted by things around you that you had trouble concentrating or staying on track?	✓	

(cont.)

---

[1]Adapted by permission from the criteria for major depressive and manic episodes of the DSM-IV text revision (DSM-IV-TR; American Psychiatric Association, 2000). Copyright by the American Psychiatric Association.

[2]Adapted by permission from Hirschfeld et al. (2000). Copyright by the American Psychiatric Association.

Had much more energy than usual?

Were much more active or did many more things than usual?

Were much more social or outgoing than usual, for example, telephoning friends in the middle of the night?

Were much more interested in sex than usual?

Did things that were unusual for you or that other people might have thought were excessive, foolish, or risky? *NoComment*

Spent excessive money that got you or your family into trouble?

If you checked yes to more than one of the above, have several of these ever happened during the same period of time?

How much of a problem did any of these cause you—like being unable to work; having family, money, or legal troubles; getting into arguments or a fight? Please check one response only.

No problem _____   Minor problem _____

Moderate problem_____   Serious problem _____

---

will base your diagnosis largely on the symptoms you have recently experienced. How you developed these symptoms (also called the *etiology* of your disorder) is really a different question. You may feel that these symptoms are not the product of a biochemical imbalance as much as current stressors (for example, having just broken off a relationship) or childhood issues (for example, traumatic events such as physical or sexual abuse). If your doctor is doing his or her job, these psychological issues will be addressed later in treatment, after the diagnosis has been established and after the two of you have agreed on a medication treatment plan. If your doctor does not do psychotherapy, you may want to ask him or her for a referral so that you receive simultaneous treatment with a therapist.

Step 1: The Diagnostic Referral

The first step in getting a proper diagnosis is to find the right doctor. If you have private insurance, you may be able to see someone who specializes in mood disorders. If it is unclear whether a doctor is a specialist, you should feel free to ask. You can also obtain information about who in your area treats persons with mood disorders from the American Psychiatric Association (888-35-PSYCH; *apa@psych. org*) or from the books in the "America's Top Doctors" series (for example, Connolly, 2009).

If you have a managed care plan or no insurance, you may not have a lot of choice about whom you see. Hopefully, your plan will direct you to a mental health professional who has at least some experience in mood disorders. But this may

39

require some detective work on your part. Nancy, for example, thought she might have bipolar disorder and wanted to see a psychiatrist but was confused by the number of doctors listed in the Yellow Pages who purportedly treated mood problems. She called several but could reach only their receptionists, who gave her information like "Dr. Rosen sees mainly adults" or "She has a general psychiatry practice." She finally discussed the matter with her general practitioner, who referred her to a psychiatrist in town who was covered by her insurance plan and, although not a specialist, was known to have experience in the treatment of mood disorders.

In today's managed care system, your initial diagnostic evaluation may not be done by a psychiatrist. Many insurance plans have an intake worker who determines the need for follow-up psychiatric care. However, this does not mean your care will be inferior. Mental health professionals from other disciplines (e.g., psychology, social work, nursing) are often well trained in diagnostic methods. There is a good chance that this intake worker will refer you to a psychiatrist if there is any suspicion that you have bipolar disorder, and he or she will almost certainly do so if you have had prior mood disorder episodes. But if you don't feel that this initial evaluation was adequate or led to appropriate follow-up care, be assertive with your health care program in asking for follow-up appointments.

Step 2: Reviewing Your Records

The doctor you do see will probably want to review any prior medical records that other doctors have for you. The records usually contain previous diagnoses (which may or may not include bipolar disorder), your previous medications (including how well you responded and if you experienced side effects from them), relevant blood tests, and information about your medical, social, and family history.

Your doctor will ask you to sign a "release of information" form, which allows him or her to gain access to these records. Of course, you can refuse to sign this release, but refusing is not in your best interest. Even if you feel your previous psychiatric care was flawed, it will help your new doctor to know about these flaws, as well as what treatments were tried and why they were discontinued. Your doctor will not necessarily recommend the same treatments as you've had in the past.

If this is your first visit to a mental health professional, you may not have prior medical records. If you have had other psychiatric consultations, you may wonder why your new doctor needs to conduct a new diagnostic evaluation and can't simply review your medical records. There are many reasons why medical charts are inadequate for determining your diagnosis, treatment, or prognosis. First, medical charts are often sketchy. They contain comments like "patient complains of depression" without specifying the severity of this depression, whether other symptoms co-occurred, or whether the depression occurred in discrete episodes. Chart notes are often written by professionals focused on other aspects of your medical or psychiatric history (for example, an endocrinologist evaluating thyroid functioning) rather than your bipolar disorder. So think of the prior medical records as supplemental information that may help your doctor clarify the diagnosis. The majority of his or her judgments will come from the face-to-face diagnostic interview.

Step 3: What to Expect from the Diagnostic Interview

The diagnosis of bipolar disorder is established through a clinical interview, in which you will be asked whether you have experienced certain symptoms over a given period of time. If your doctor conducts a comprehensive interview, he or she will ask not only about your mood disorder symptoms but also whether you have ever had psychotic symptoms (for example, hallucinations), drug or alcohol abuse, anxiety symptoms, eating disorder symptoms, or other problems.

Filling out the self-administered checklist from the last section may help your doctor obtain some of this information more efficiently. Because the checklist is based on DSM-IV-TR, it may parallel some of the questions your doctor will ask. You can give it to him or her at the beginning of the first interview as a way of ensuring that he or she follows up on certain symptoms that may concern you.

During this interview, your doctor will probably want to know not only which symptoms you've experienced but also which symptoms typically go together with other ones (that is, in discrete episodes), the severity of these symptoms, and their duration. Your doctor has a threshold in mind for how severe and how impairing a symptom must be before it is considered part of the bipolar syndrome. For example, when asking about "loss of energy or fatigue," your doctor will want to know such things as whether you've been unable to go to work because of fatigue, or whether you have trouble doing housework. When asking about insomnia, he or she may want to know how many nights of the week you have trouble sleeping and whether your lack of sleep impairs your ability to drive, concentrate at work, play sports, or conduct any of your usual activities. In many ways bipolar symptoms are just exaggerations of normal mental, behavioral, and emotional processes, and some degree of variability in mood, sleep, or activity level is part of the human condition. Your doctor has to establish whether your symptoms meet a criterion of severity or impairment.

Interviews can be quite subjective, and there is always the possibility that the way your doctor asks you the questions, and the way you answer them, will affect the final diagnosis. Consider the following interchange that occurred between a doctor and a person with bipolar disorder. Notice that this doctor probes carefully for certain symptoms, and the patient, correspondingly, gives useful examples of his experiences and behavior.

> *Doctor:* Did you ever have a weeklong period when you felt very happy or very irritable?
>
> *Patient:* No, not really.

Doctor: Or when you felt very grouchy or easily provoked?

Patient: No.

Doctor: How about feeling charged up and full of energy?

Patient: Yes.

Doctor: What was that like?

Patient: Well, in March I was running at full tilt, full of, like, all sorts of ideas. I thought I could develop a weather-monitoring system that could be operated from my basement.

Doctor: How were you sleeping at the time?

Patient: Not at all! I didn't need to, and I got resentful when people told me I should.

Doctor: Resentful? Tell me more.

Patient: Well, nobody appreciated what I was trying to do. Everybody seemed like they were moving slowly. One time, I practically bit this guy's head off for knocking on my door when I was in the middle of a project. And I yelled at my kids a bunch of times because they kept interrupting me.

In this example, the doctor has found evidence of irritable mood and other manic symptoms in this patient's history. Had the doctor not done this probing, evidence of this manic syndrome might not have emerged.

The diagnostic interview will take at least an hour or two. If you have a particularly complicated set of symptoms, your doctor may request several sessions to be reasonably sure of the diagnosis. A long interview can be tedious, especially if you've been through one before, but in most cases you'll find that your and the doctor's time has been well spent. The information you provide will inform a careful diagnosis, which will almost certainly translate into better treatment.

Does the Diagnosis Fit? Could You Have Another Disorder Instead?

If you are having your first problems with depression or mania, and possibly even if you have had numerous episodes of mood disorder, you will probably want to discuss the accuracy of the diagnosis with your doctor. Does the diagnosis give a reasonable explanation for the kinds of problems you've had with your mood states, behavior, and relationships with other people? Could you have another disorder instead? You may wonder whether the mood swings you experience are really a part of your personality (see Chapter 4). You may believe that you have a different psychiatric disorder or no disorder at all. Alternatively, you may believe, rightfully, that you have another psychiatric disorder in addition to bipolar disorder.

Bipolar disorder can be difficult to tell apart from other disorders that share features in common with it. In this section, I discuss the problem of misdiagnosis. I also discuss the disorders that are often confused with bipolar disorder and how they differ from it. Sometimes these disorders are diagnosed alongside of bipolar disorder (*comorbidity*).

What Can You Do If You Think You've Been Misdiagnosed?

There are many reasons why bipolar disorder can be hard to distinguish from other disorders. First, moods can vary for any number of reasons, which can include hormones, personal stress, sleep problems, personality disturbances, diseases of the brain, or ingestion of drugs or alcohol. Second, people with the disorder often have trouble describing their mood states to others and giving accurate histories of their disorder. Third, mental health professionals are not always adequately trained to recognize the more subtle forms of the disorder (for example, mixed states, rapid cycling, mild depressions, hypomania).

Diagnostic confusion can also occur because of the diagnostic criteria themselves. Certain symptoms are characteristic of more than one disorder. Psychotic experiences (for example, grandiose delusions) can occur in other disorders, such as schizophrenia. Problems with distractibility occur in mania and in ADHD. Sleep disturbance and irritability can occur in recurrent depression and anxiety disorders as well as bipolar disorder. Lastly, mood variability is a key feature of borderline personality disorder.

Try to be as patient as you can with the diagnostic process. The common use of DSM-IV-TR and improved training in the recognition of mood disorders make diagnosis more reliable than it used to be. Nonetheless, errors inevitably occur. Your physician may need to observe you during an episode and once you have recovered to be sure of your diagnosis. If you have strong doubts about the diagnosis you have been given, getting a second opinion is a good idea.

If you do seek a second opinion, be prepared to be asked some of the same questions about your symptoms that you were asked the first time. Tell the new psychiatrist why you think you have some disorder other than bipolar and, specifically, why you don't think the diagnostic criteria for bipolar disorder fit. Alternatively, if you think that bipolar is the correct diagnosis but you've been diagnosed with something else, tell the new physician why you believe this. Bring along a close family member, significant other, or

Effective solution: If you're not convinced the diagnosis is correct, ask questions:

■ What is the rationale behind the doctor's opinion?
■ What diagnostic criteria does the doctor think apply to you?
■ Is the doctor considering other diagnoses, and if not, why not?

trusted friend. This person can offer a different perspective on your symptoms and life experiences, which may be quite useful to the mental health professional who makes the diagnosis.

Most of all, it's important to work collaboratively with your doctor. Relate what you can about your history and report events and symptoms as accurately as possible, even if what you are reporting is sometimes embarrassing or painful to talk about. Try to see things from the doctor's perspective.

Comorbid Disorders

The term *comorbidity* refers to the co-occurrence of two or more psychiatric disorders in the same person. Many people have more than one DSM-IV-TR psychiatric disorder. In clinical practice, people are often given multiple diagnoses, sometimes because they have more than one disorder and sometimes because the clinician isn't sure which diagnosis best applies and therefore diagnoses more than one.

What does it look like when a person has two or more comorbid disorders? Consider Elena, a 49-year-old woman who has been diagnosed with bipolar II disorder and ADHD.

New research: A carefully designed large national survey of psychiatric disorders in the general population—the National Comorbidity Survey, Revised—concluded that 45% of people with one psychiatric disorder report two or more disorders (Kessler et al., 2005). People with bipolar disorder most frequently reported comorbid ADHD, anxiety disorders, or alcohol or drug abuse disorders.

Elena had several long-lasting depressive episodes, during which she had had difficulty holding a job. Her hypomanic periods were characterized by irritability, racing thoughts, and sleep disturbance. Her husband, Chris, was understanding of her depression but became enraged at the fact that when he tried to talk to her about her job situation, Elena's eyes would glaze over and she seemed not to be listening. Chris also complained that she made a lot of careless mistakes: when she sent her résumé to prospective employers, there was often a page missing or the printing was slanted. She also frequently forgot appointments with her doctors and prospective employers. Her forgetfulness and inattention seemed to characterize her behavior most of the time, even when she wasn't depressed.

In Elena's case, the codiagnosis of bipolar disorder with ADHD led her physician to recommend a regimen that included a mood stabilizer and dextroamphetamine (Adderall), a drug designed to improve attention and concentration.

The sidebar on page 46 lists disorders that are often comorbid with bipolar disorder or confused with it diagnostically. ADHD, borderline personality disorder, and cyclothymic disorder can all be codiagnosed with bipolar disorder. The others require that the clinician make a decision between these diagnoses and bipolar disorder.

Attention-Deficit/Hyperactivity Disorder (ADHD)

Do you have ...

■ difficulty paying attention to details?
■ trouble with making careless mistakes in work or other activities? *Never*
■ trouble listening to others?
■ problems with organization?
■ distraction? *go to hell!!*
■ forgetfulness?

ADHD is a childhood-onset disorder characterized by difficulty attending to tasks. A child who has ADHD with hyperactivity or impulsivity will fidget, blurt out answers to questions, have difficulty remaining seated, and talk excessively (American Psychiatric Association, 2000). Notice how similar these symptoms are to mania! Distinguishing childhood-onset bipolar disorder from ADHD, or distinguishing adult bipolar disorder from the continuation of ADHD first diagnosed in childhood, is extremely difficult. And it is possible to have both. Some studies have found that as many as 90% of children and 30% of adolescents with bipolar disorder also have ADHD, although not everyone agrees on these figures (Pavuluri et al., 2005).

Even among adults, distinguishing bipolar disorder from ADHD is important, because the primary drugs for treating ADHD are stimulants such as methylphenidate (Ritalin) or amphetamine/dextroamphetamine. These drugs are not usually given to people with bipolar disorder unless accompanied by a mood-stabilizing agent like lithium or valproate. You'll learn more about these medications in Chapter 6. Ritalin, like many stimulating drugs, may increase the chances of experiencing a manic or hypomanic episode.

There is currently a trend among mental health professionals to codiagnose bipolar disorder and ADHD, particularly in children. There are no separate diagnostic criteria for bipolar disorder in children, and, unfortunately, this trend sometimes leads to imprecision. It is possible to have both bipolar and ADHD, and many people do, but there are also ways to tell them apart.

First, the cognitive problems associated with ADHD do not change much from day to day or week to week, unless the person is taking Ritalin or a similar psycho-

Psychiatric Disorders Often Confused with Bipolar Disorder

■ Attention-deficit/hyperactivity disorder (ADHD)

■ Borderline personality disorder

■ Cyclothymic disorder

■ Schizophrenia or schizoaffective disorder

■ Recurrent major depressive disorder

■ Substance-induced mood disorder

stimulant medication. People with ADHD have fairly constant problems with attention, distractibility, and organization, regardless of their mood state. In contrast, people with bipolar disorder may become impulsive and have difficulty attending, but mainly when they are in the midst of a manic, mixed, or depressed episode. For example, Teri, age 37, worked successfully as a graphic artist during her periods of mood stability. Only when she was depressed was she unable to concentrate on her design layouts. Nick, age 52, was a successful computer programmer who was known among his colleagues for his ability to stick with difficult problems and solve them. But when he had mixed episodes, he would become unfocused and distractible, jumping from one task to another without gaining closure on any of them.

ADHD is not accompanied by the extreme highs and lows of mood states that are the hallmark of bipolar disorder. It is not typical for people with ADHD to experience elated highs, goal-directed behavior, hypersexuality, decreased need for sleep, or grandiosity (Geller et al., 1998), or to experience deep depressions alternating with periods of stable mood.

ADHD is usually associated with difficulty in school settings. When you were in school, were you fairly consistently able to keep your mind on class activities? Have you generally functioned well in tasks that require concentration and sustained effort since then? If the answer to both of these is yes, it is unlikely that you have ADHD, although a thorough answer to this question requires cognitive testing. If you think you might have ADHD, raise the possibility with your doctor and ask for a separate evaluation of that condition. In addition to medications for ADHD, there may be "cognitive rehabilitation" programs in your area that you can enroll in to help you develop strategies for improving your attention and concentration. If you'd like more information on ADHD, take a look at the National Institute of Mental Health's website (*www.nimh.nih.gov/health/publications/attention-deficit-hyperactivity-disorder/complete-index.shtml*).

Borderline Personality Disorder

Do you have ...

■ difficulty defining for yourself who you are or who you want to be? *Yes*

■ a history of very intense and unstable relationships with people? *No*

■ a history of making great efforts to keep people from abandoning or leaving you? *Don't care or give a shit*

■ frequent periods of feeling empty or bored? *never*

■ difficulty controlling angry outbursts?

■ a history of impulsive or reckless behavior that involves sex, spending money, substance abuse, or eating? *Past in texas and chicago*

■ a history of self-destructive acts (for example, self-cutting)?

Personality disorders are long-lasting patterns of disturbance in thinking, perceiving, emotional response, interpersonal functioning, and impulse control. The hallmarks of borderline personality disorder are instability in mood, relationships, and one's sense of self or identity. People with borderline disorder feel chronically empty and bored, have terrible trouble being alone, and frequently make suicidal gestures or threats. They tend to have remarkably reactive moods and quickly become intensely sad, anxious, or irritable in response to events involving close relationships. These mood states tend to last for only a few hours or, at most, a few days. Borderline personality disorder generally continues throughout adulthood, unless the individual seeks treatment.

Carla, age 27, called her boyfriend up to 10 times a day. When she did, she often raged at him for "not being there for her" and, if she couldn't reach him, accused him of being with another woman. When alone, she would feel like she was disappearing, and feel intolerable cravings to smoke, eat, drink alcohol, vomit, or cut herself with glass. She tried to hurt herself in minor ways several times, but never severely enough to threaten her life. These problems had continued for several years, despite the fact that she was in psychotherapy and had tried various forms of antidepressant medication.

There are several parallels between borderline personality disorder and bipolar disorder, particularly the rapid cycling forms, but there are also discernible differences. In borderline personality disorder the changing mood states are usually very short-lived and a reaction to being rejected or even just slighted by people with whom the person is closely affiliated. In fact, the disturbances in people with borderline personality are often visible only when one observes their romantic relationships. They tend to idealize and then devalue those with whom they become close, and they go to great lengths to avoid what they experience as being abandoned.

People with borderline personality disorder do become depressed and often meet full criteria for a major depressive episode at some point in their lives. But they do not develop the full manic or mixed affective syndrome unless they also have a bipolar disorder. Between 10 and 40% of people with bipolar disorder also meet the diagnostic criteria for a borderline personality (George et al., 2003; Goldberg & Garno, 2009).

Why is it important to know if you have borderline personality as well as (or instead of) bipolar disorder? Currently, there are no agreed-on drug-treatment guidelines for people with borderline personality or those with both borderline and bipolar disorders. It is generally believed that people with both disorders are more *treatment refractory,* or have more trouble responding or adhering to mood-stabilizing drugs. If you are having trouble finding the right combination of medications, and if some of the preceding features fit you, it is possible you have this complicating condition. If you have been misdiagnosed with borderline personality disorder when your real diagnosis is bipolar II disorder, you might do better with medications like lamotrigine (Lamictal) or quetiapine (Seroquel) than with antidepressants like fluoxetine (Prozac) (John & Sharma, 2007).

If you think you might have borderline personality disorder, it is especially important for you to consider certain structured forms of psychotherapy in addition to medications. Various forms of therapy have research support for borderline personality disorder, most notably *dialectical behavior therapy,* a form of therapy that combines cognitive and behavioral strategies with Zen Buddhist mindfulness practices (Linehan et al., 2006).

Cyclothymic Disorder

Do you have ...

- short periods of feeling active, irritable, and excited? *Never*
- short periods of feeling mildly depressed? *Yes*
- a tendency to alternate back and forth between the two? *Don't Know*

To make matters even more complicated, you can have a fluctuating form of mood disorder marked by short periods of hypomania alternating with short, mild periods of depression. To have cyclothymic disorder, you must have alternated between high and low periods for at least 2 consecutive years and never been without mood disorder symptoms for more than 2 months at a time (American Psychiatric Association, 2000). How is this different from bipolar II disorder? Consider the following vignette:

Katherine was a 30-year-old woman who, since adolescence, had experienced a pattern of alternating between 3-day periods during the week in which she cried a lot and felt sad and less interested in things, followed by weekends in which she would feel irritable, energetic, and talkative. She had never been hospitalized for either her depressive or hypomanic symptoms, nor had she been suicidal or unable to concentrate, or lost significant amounts of weight. Her boyfriend sometimes complained about her moodiness and rage. Although it was more difficult for her to work when she was depressed, she had never lost a job because of it.

Katherine received a diagnosis of cyclothymic rather than bipolar disorder. Had her depressions been worse and/or required hospitalization, her diagnosis would have been changed to bipolar II disorder with cyclothymic disorder. One can be diagnosed with both!

The psychiatrist Hagop Akiskal from the School of Medicine at the University of California, San Diego, views cyclothymia as a disturbance of temperament that predisposes people to bipolar disorder (Akiskal et al., 2006; see also Chapter 4). In fact, cyclothymia has a lot in common with bipolar I and II disorders in terms of its pattern of inheritance and its presumed biology. Cyclothymia is listed in DSM-IV-TR as a mild form of bipolar disorder. About one in every four people with cyclothymia progresses to bipolar I or II disorder (that is, they develop full-blown manic episodes, longer hypomanias, or major depressive episodes) over periods of 2 to 4 years (Birmaher et al., 2009; Kochman et al., 2005).

There are very few studies on the ideal treatments for bipolar II disorder versus cyclothymia. As a result, psychiatrists tend to treat them in a similar way, with mood stabilizers like lithium, lamotrigine, or divalproex. Nonetheless, people with cyclothymia can sometimes function without medication because their disorder is generally less severe and less impairing. For some, the label *cyclothymia* feels less frightening than *bipolar II disorder,* even though they have many similar features.

Schizophrenia

If you are a person with schizophrenia, you will experience some of the following symptoms:

■ Delusions, such as believing that you are being followed, your thoughts are being controlled by an outside force, your thoughts are being stolen or altered in some way, or that someone (or some organization) wants to hurt you

■ Hallucinations, in which you hear a voice or see a vision

■ Lack of motivation, apathy, and disinterest in seeing anyone

■ Loss or "blunting" of emotions

■ Very jumbled or confused communication and thinking

It can be quite difficult to distinguish bipolar disorder from schizophrenia, especially when a person is first seeking treatment or has his or her first hospitalization. People with schizophrenia do not have multiple personalities, as is commonly believed. Instead, they have delusions (mistaken, unrealistic beliefs) or hallucinations (sensory experiences, like voices, without a real stimulus). They can experience severe depressions, but often their biggest problem is being cut off from their emotions (flatness or blunting of affect). People with bipolar disorder can also have delusions and hallucinations; these are typically (but not invariably) of a manic, grandiose type (for example, "I have finely tuned extrasensory perception") or of a depressive sort (for example, "The devil tells me I am to be punished for my bad deeds").

According to DSM-IV-TR criteria, you have bipolar disorder instead of schizophrenia if, during your episodes, you experience severe swings of emotion and energy or activity levels, and your delusions or hallucinations (if they occur at all) do not appear until after the onset of your mood swings. If your delusions and hallucinations develop before your mood swings and/or persist after your depressive or manic symptoms clear up, you would more likely be diagnosed with schizophrenia or *schizoaffective disorder,* a blend of the schizophrenia and mood disorder categories.

These distinctions are important in relation to your prognosis. The long-term outcome for schizophrenia—in terms of number of hospitalizations, ability to work, and other quality-of-life indicators—is worse than for bipolar or schizoaffective disorder (Harrow et al., 2000). There are also implications for treatment. If your diagnosis is schizophrenia or schizoaffective disorder, your physician will probably start you on drugs like ziprasidone (Geodon), olanzapine (Zyprexa), or risperidone (Risperdal) before introducing lithium or other mood stabilizers (see also Chapter 6). These are newer antipsychotic drugs with mood-stabilizing properties. The doctor may also recommend an older line of "typical" antipsychotics like chlorpromazine (Thorazine) or haloperidol (Haldol). If the doctor feels your bipolar diagnosis is accurate but that you have psychotic symptoms or severe agitation, he or she may recommend one of these drugs along with a mood-stabilizing agent. Consider the experiences of Kurt, age 19:

> Kurt believed there was a "gang of nine" that roamed the planet and was looking for him. He described his "self" as a "shell" that was gradually deteriorating and would eventually be taken over by this gang. When he began to be preoccupied with the gang of nine, he would become revved up, irritable, easily provoked to tears, speak a mile a minute, and stop sleeping. He was hospitalized because his thinking became increasingly bizarre and his parents became afraid of him. When his older brother visited him in the hospital, Kurt ran up to him, threw his arms around him, began crying, and screamed, "Thanks for saving me!" After hospital treatment with Haldol, he calmed down considerably and began sleeping again. But he continued to believe a gang was following him and that its members were waiting for him to be discharged from the hospital.

Notice that Kurt's primary disturbance is in his thinking processes rather than his mood. He continued to be preoccupied with his delusional beliefs even after his mood and sleep problems improved. He was given the diagnosis of schizoaffective instead of bipolar disorder. These diagnostic distinctions are among the most difficult to make reliably. Often, people with these unclear patterns of symptoms have to be observed across several episodes, and try many different medications before their diagnosis becomes clear.

Recurrent Major Depressive Disorder

Have you had major, severe periods of depression that have come and gone, but no obvious signs of mania or hypomania? It may seem simple to distinguish people with only recurrent depressions (unipolar depression) from those who have both depressions and manias, but it is actually quite difficult. In the most common situation, a person has had repeated episodes of major depression, and then undergoes a brief period (a few days) of feeling "wired," "up," and "ready to take on the world." Is this bipolar II disorder? Or simply the high most of us would feel after coming out of a long depression?

A true hypomanic episode involves an observable change in functioning from a prior mood state. A hypomanic person sleeps less, feels mildly or moderately elated or irritable, and has racing thoughts or becomes talkative. If this state lasts for days at a time, and others have commented on it, a hypomanic episode (and bipolar disorder) is suspected. In contrast, a person who simply feels good after being depressed, but who has few or none of the other symptoms in the hypomanic cluster, probably has *unipolar depression.*

Some people have *agitated depression,* which can look a lot like a bipolar mixed episode. Bethany, age 37, had major depressive episodes in which she became anxious, restless, and unable to sit still. Her main feeling was one of dread rather than the optimism or confidence usually characteristic of hypomania or mania. Her doctor diagnosed her with major depressive disorder.

A history of bipolar disorder in your family provides additional evidence for the bipolar over the unipolar diagnosis. As mentioned earlier, if your doctor cannot be certain if you have unipolar depression or bipolar disorder, he or she will probably recommend that you take a mood stabilizer before an antidepressant.

Substance-Induced Mood Disorder

Are all of the following true for you?

▪ You have had an episode of depression or mania.

▪ These symptoms developed after you took a street drug, drank a large quantity of alcohol over several days or weeks, or began taking an antidepressant or some other medication that affects moods.

- ▪ Your mood symptoms subsided shortly after you stopped drinking alcohol or taking the drug.

- ▪ You have not had previous manic or depressive episodes, except those brought on by alcohol or drugs.

Manic and depressive symptoms can be mimicked by certain drugs of abuse. Cocaine, amphetamine ("speed"), methamphetamine, heroin, Ecstacy, and LSD have all been known to create manic-like states, often with accompanying psychosis. Amphetamine, in particular, has been known to produce irritable, hyperactivated, delusional states. It is unlikely that alcohol abuse or dependence will directly cause a manic episode, but it can certainly contribute to a spiraling depression.

DSM-IV-TR distinguishes mood disorders that are brought on by external substances from those that are due to a person's inherent physiology. Mood disorders that are the direct function of substances are usually short-lived, disappearing more quickly than non-substance-related mood disorders, and are usually treated through detoxification and chemical dependency programs. Sometimes they abate without treatment. However, substances can contribute to the onset of the first episode of bipolar disorder, which then takes on a course of its own. It is not uncommon for persons with bipolar disorder to say that their first manic episode began shortly after they began experimenting with drugs.

As I discussed in Chapter 2, you can have both a mood and a substance use disorder, with one influencing the course of the other. Mood swings make you more likely to take drugs or alcohol, and drugs or alcohol can worsen your mood swings. About 60% of people with bipolar disorder have had an alcohol or substance use disorder at some point in life—a rate that is much higher than the general population rate of 10–20% (Kessler et al., 2005; Regier et al., 1990; Weiss et al., 2007). So, even if you originally sought treatment for a mood problem, your doctor may still diagnose a substance or alcohol use disorder and recommend that you take part in a 12-step program (for example, Alcoholics Anonymous) or individual therapy (such as motivational enhancement therapy) designed to help you overcome chemical dependency problems.

Your doctor will probably assess the sequence of your mood symptoms and drinking or drug use: Do you usually get depressed and then drink? Does it ever happen that you drink and then get depressed? Do you use cocaine or marijuana and then get manic, or is it the reverse? Usually, he or she will not be able to tell for sure if you have both a bipolar and a substance abuse problem until you have remained sober or drug free for a period of time. Again, your close relatives and significant others may be of help here. For example, your spouse may be able to recall how and when your behavior started to shift in relation to when you took certain substances.

An important case of substance-induced mood disorder is mania, hypomania, or rapid cycling that develops after taking antidepressants. Karine, in the example below, showed symptoms that strongly mimicked a mixed episode, but her symptoms remitted once the antidepressant was withdrawn. DSM-IV-TR requires that the bipolar syndrome not be diagnosed until at least one manic, mixed, or hypomanic episode has occurred without provocation by antidepressants or other substances. If you do become manic or hypomanic because of antidepressants, you may indeed have bipolar disorder, but more evidence will be required.

Karine, age 48, had been severely depressed and anxious for about a month after the death of her father. She had never had a manic or a hypomanic episode. Her physician had put her on an antidepressant, but it did not make her depression better; in fact, her anxiety got worse. Her physician then gave her a different kind of antidepressant.

> "At first, I felt great. I could focus on things like never before. I no longer needed cigarettes to keep my mind on my work. But then my mood started to go up and down like a seesaw. My sleep got worse and worse—I woke up almost every hour. I felt wired, but then my depression came back. I started feeling really irritable and worried, and I couldn't stop my ruminations, which were like a DVD playing on fast-forward. I had to take Ambien (a sleep medication) nearly every night. I couldn't stand it."

Her physician took her off the antidepressant gradually. Her mood continued to fluctuate for a few weeks but then returned to a milder state of depression. She was eventually treated successfully with lamotrigine (a mood stabilizer) and psychotherapy. Her rapid cycling was considered an instance of substance-induced mood disorder, although she was also believed to have "uncomplicated bereavement," a form of major depression that is a reaction to a loss experience. She was never given the diagnosis of bipolar disorder.

I hope you can see now how important it is to obtain a proper diagnosis and to rule out competitive diagnoses. Knowing the diagnostic criteria for bipolar disorder and understanding how these symptoms manifest themselves, both in you and in others, is empowering. As you'll see later, awareness of the symptoms that you typically experience during mood episodes will go a long way in helping you to prevent these episodes from spiraling out of control.

In the next chapter, I'll discuss the problems people have in adjusting to or coping with the diagnosis of bipolar disorder. Some deny the reality of the disorder and believe that their symptoms are just exaggerations of their personality. Some overcommit to the diagnosis and unnecessarily try to limit their career and personal aspirations, and others reluctantly agree to the diagnosis but continue living their lives as if they were illness free. No one likes to believe that he or she has a psychiatric disorder that requires long-term treatment. Coming to accept the diagnosis is a difficult emotional process.

4

"Is It an Illness or Is It Me?"
Coping with the Diagnosis

In Chapter 3 we discussed the rather dry (though useful) DSM-IV-TR diagnostic criteria. What these criteria do not address or convey is the emotional impact of learning you have bipolar disorder and acknowledging its reality. Most of my patients go through painful struggles in coming to terms with this diagnosis. Initially, they experience anger, fear, sadness, guilt, disappointment, and hopelessness. These are not manic–depressive cycles but rather a healthy process of forming a new sense of who they are, a new self-image that incorporates having biological dysregulations that affect their moods. It may sound like I'm talking about people who have had only one or two manic or depressed episodes and are surprised by the diagnosis, but I've also seen these reactions in people who have been hospitalized for the disorder numerous times.

Why is the process of acceptance so painful? Coming to terms with having the disorder may mean admitting to a new role for yourself in your family, in the workforce, or in your personal relationships. It may require you to make some decisions about restructuring your life and priorities, which may mean viewing yourself differently. For example, Luiz, age 25, gave up his apartment and returned to live with his parents after his hospitalization. He then had to deal with their hypervigilance and increased attempts to control his behavior, which made him feel like he was a child again. Rob, age 38, had been quite successful in his work as a civil engineer. After his bipolar I diagnosis was revealed, he found that people at work seemed afraid of him. He attributed losing his job to the disclosure of his illness. Nancy, age 44, noted that after she learned of her bipolar II diagnosis and told many of her friends about it, at least one "dumped me because I was too 'high maintenance.'"

You can imagine the pain and confusion you might feel when there are such costs to acknowledging the disorder.

What's Unique about Bipolar Disorder?

People who have to live with medical diagnoses such as diabetes or heart disease go through similar emotions in coping with their diagnoses. Nobody likes to believe they have a long-term illness that requires regular treatment. But bipolar disorder has its own particularities. As I mentioned in Chapter 2, bipolar disorder can be difficult to distinguish from the normal ups and downs of human life. You may have always been moody or temperamental and believe that your manic or depressive periods are just exaggerations of your natural moodiness. How do you know what is really your illness and what is your "self" or your personality (your habits, attitudes, and styles of relating to others—the way you are most of the time)? How do you train yourself to know the difference between you when you're well and you when you're ill, and not fool yourself into thinking that changes in mood, energy, or activity are just "how I've always been"?

On a practical level, the ability to recognize these differences between personality traits and disorder symptoms is important so that you and others know when emergency procedures need to be undertaken. On an emotional level, understanding these distinctions can contribute to a more stable sense of who you are. Maureen, for example, knew she had always been extraverted but realized she needed to visit her doctor when she began staying up late to call people—all over the country—to whom she hadn't spoken in years. The requirement of an increased dosage of lithium did not interfere with her appreciation of others.

The reaction of many of my clients upon learning of the diagnosis is disbelief or denial, which is only natural. After all, they have to revise their image of themselves, which is painful and difficult to do. Others, especially those who were diagnosed some time ago, come to believe they have the disorder but continue to lead their lives as if they did not. You can imagine why people would react this way; in fact, you may even recognize these reactions in yourself. Nevertheless, these styles of coping can cause trouble for you, especially if they lead to your refusal to take medications that would help you, or to engaging in high-risk activities (for example, staying up all night, getting drunk frequently) that can worsen your illness.

For example, Antonio, age 35, behaved in self-destructive ways to cope with his confusion and pain. He went off his medications to try to prove to others that he wasn't sick, but then relapsed and ended up back in the psychiatrist's office, with more medication being recommended. Rosa, who had received her diagnosis years ago, often turned to alcohol when she experienced the shame, social stigma, and hopelessness she felt the diagnosis conferred on her.

After they have lived with the disorder for a while, some people begin thinking of themselves as if they were nothing more than a diagnostic label or a set of dysfunctional molecules. They start automatically attributing all of their personal problems to the illness, even those problems that people without bipolar disorder routinely experience. They usually accept the need for medications but unnecessarily limit themselves and avoid taking advantage of opportunities that they actually could handle.

By the end of this chapter you will have a greater sense of the various emotional reactions people have upon learning of the diagnosis. You'll feel empowered knowing that your own emotional reactions are shared by others and that admitting to the diagnosis doesn't mean giving up your hopes and aspirations. The chapter ends with suggestions for coping with the difficult process of coming to terms with the illness.

The Emotional Fallout of the Diagnosis

Most of the people who consult me have been told by someone at some time that they have bipolar disorder, even if they don't believe it themselves. When we actually sit down and begin discussing the disorder, they experience a wide range of emotions, including bewilderment, anxiety, and anger. Some people feel relief: learning that you have a psychiatric disorder that has a name, and that explains a great deal of what has happened to you, can help alleviate your feelings of guilt or self-blame. More often, however, the diagnosis raises more questions than it answers—most of which concern what the future holds for you and those close to you.

When you first learned that you had the disorder, you may have asked yourself questions like the following:

"Why me?"
"Why is this happening now?"
"Am I 'only bipolar' now, or do I still have a separate identity?"
"Where does my identity stop and the disorder begin?"
"Were my prior periods of high energy, creativity, and accomplishment nothing more than signs of an illness?"
"How much mood variability am I 'allowed' before people think I'm getting sick again?"
"How responsible am I for my own behavior?"
"Will I have a normal life and achieve my goals?"

> **Effective prevention:** *Bipolar disorder is something that you have, but it is not who you are.* Knowing this difference can keep you from rejecting the diagnosis or, at the other extreme, giving your life over to the illness.

Even if you've had numerous episodes of bipolar disorder, you may still ask yourself these questions. It's natural to do so, and healthy—to the extent that struggling with these questions helps you clarify your feelings and goals.

If any close family members (for example, your spouse or parents) learned of your diagnosis at the same time as you did, they probably had questions of their own. They may not have voiced these questions to you directly because they understood that hearing their worries might be painful for you and because they didn't wish to cause family conflict. For example, Kyana's parents worried that she would always be tagged as mentally ill and never have a normal life. They worried that they would have to take care of her for the rest of their lives and that their hopes and dreams for her had been dashed. Greg's wife wondered if she had married the wrong man and whether she should leave the relationship. None of these family members raised their worries until they began talking openly about the disorder with Kyana or Greg. On the positive side, learning more about the disorder was comforting to Kyana, Greg, and their families, because they learned together that the prognosis was not as poor as they had feared.

"It's No Big Deal": Rejecting or Underidentifying with the Diagnosis

"I want to go back to the place where I used to live in Miami, back before all this mess started. Who knows? Maybe the apartment I lived in is still available. People liked me there. I had so many friends. I sometimes think if I go back there, I'll find the old me sunning herself under some big old palm tree."
—A 26-year-old woman who had just been hospitalized for her second manic episode

Perhaps you remember the first time someone told you that you had bipolar disorder. Did any of the reactions in the box on page 59 describe how you felt then or now?

Consider the first reaction of rejecting the diagnosis outright. Did you (or do you now) believe that the diagnosis was all just a misunderstanding of your behavior? Did you think others were just trying to rein you in and weren't interested in your private experiences? Did you get confused about whether your medication was meant to treat your mood swings or whether it caused them in the first place? Were you convinced that the diagnosis was wrong and that alternative treatments were the answer?

Carter, age 49, rejected the diagnosis, refused to see his doctor, and refused to take medications. His obstinate stand usually surfaced when he was manic, but he also dug in his heels when he had few or no symptoms of the disorder. He believed that whatever problems arose could be controlled by diet (particularly by limiting his sugar intake) and acupuncture treatments. He argued that his behavior—no matter how dangerous or bizarre it had been—was just being mis-

Common Reactions to Being Told You Have Bipolar Disorder

■ "The diagnosis is wrong: it's just a way for other people to explain away my experiences." [rejecting the diagnosis]

■ "I'm just a moody person." [underidentification with the diagnosis: giving some credence to it but making few, if any, lifestyle adaptations]

■ "My illness is everything, and I have no control over my behavior." [overidentification with the diagnosis: rethinking your life problems and beginning to blame all, or most of them, on the disorder, or unnecessarily limiting your aspirations because of the illness]

understood and misinterpreted. He blamed his behavior on people he thought had provoked him—typically, family members, employers, or romantic partners. During the few times in which he did agree to take medications, he mistakenly concluded that they had caused his illness ("My moods were fine until they gave me Depakote, and now they swing all over the place").

As I discussed in Chapter 3, you will certainly want to explore with your doctor why he or she thinks the diagnosis applies to you, and why other possible diagnoses are being ruled out. Second opinions are often helpful, and there is no substitute for learning as much as you can about the symptoms of the disorder, the purposes of various medications, and self-management strategies. But rejecting the diagnosis is a dangerous stance to take, because, as in Carter's case, it can lead to the rejection of treatments that may be life saving. People who take this stance often go through several episodes and hospitalizations before they admit that anything is wrong, and even then may distrust the diagnosis, the doctors, and the medications.

Now consider the second reaction, what I call underidentifying with the diagnosis. Underidentification is a very common reaction style, and, for many people, is a stage in coming to accept having an illness. It is similar to being in denial, which is not the same thing as rejecting the diagnosis. *Denial* or *thought suppression* refers to the process of avoiding emotionally painful problems by pushing them out of conscious awareness. Being told that you have an illness that will recur and that requires rethinking your life goals is extraordinarily painful. Who wouldn't want to push away their emotional reactions to this news and try to keep living their life as if the diagnosis were not true?

People who learn that they have other medical diagnoses also react by underidentifying. For example, people who have had heart attacks may acknowledge to

New research: In an experiment conducted at Oxford University, we (Miklowitz et al., 2010) asked a group of people with bipolar disorder to unscramble six-word strings into five-word sentences, leaving one word out (example: "am ruining I life my improving"). The sentences could be completed in a negative or a positive manner, as in the example. In one condition of the experiment, in which participants were given a reward bell for every four items they completed, the people with bipolar disorder completed more sentences in the negative direction than people with major depression or healthy persons. We interpreted these findings to mean that, for people with bipolar disorder, reward brings to mind memories of failure in achievement situations and feelings of low self-worth. The illness label may also bring to mind painful memories of lost hopes, disappointments, and dashed expectations. Understandably, these painful memories may make people prone to deny the illness when faced with evidence of it.

others that they need to make lifestyle adaptations yet go on smoking, exercising little or not at all, and sleeping irregularly. People with diabetes or hypertension can also superficially acknowledge their diagnoses but go on eating sugary or salty foods.

Ellen Frank, a professor at the University of Pittsburgh, has termed the emotional issues underlying the denial of bipolar disorder "grieving the lost healthy self" (Frank, 2005). People with bipolar disorder were often very energetic, popular, bright, and creative before they became ill. Then, once their illness is diagnosed and people around them start treating them like a "mental patient," they become resentful and start yearning for who they used to be. They may think that if they go on acting as if nothing has changed, their old self will come back, like a long-lost friend—the way the woman quoted earlier dreamed of finding her old self back in Miami. Underlying these reactions are deep feelings of loss over the dramatic changes the illness has brought.

If you're just now being diagnosed for the first time, it's normal to be in a certain amount of denial. But even if you have had the diagnosis for some time and feel you've accepted its reality, you may be able to recall times when you were in denial about it. When you have been hypomanic or manic, have you found yourself doubting whether the illness was real? Perhaps thinking that the diagnosis has been a mistake all along? Perhaps "testing" the diagnosis by staying out all night, drinking a lot of alcohol, or taking street drugs? Have you found yourself "forgetting" to take your lithium, Depakote, or Seroquel? Have you believed you could take your medications without any supervision (regular doctor's appointments to discuss side effects and monitor your blood levels)? Inconsistency with medication is a big problem among people with bipolar disorder, with more than 50% discontinuing their drug regimen at some time in their lives (Colom et al., 2000). Frequently, when people don't take their medications it is because they are manic, hypomanic, or otherwise in denial about their illness (see Chapter 7).

"If I'm Bipolar, So Is Everybody Else"

"My mother really gets on my case about my medications, about my visits to my doctor, about the men I'm going out with, my job, my sleep—you name it. She's always asking me if I've been drinking. She goes behind my back to try to find out. She's always been critical and disapproving of me. I think she's the one who's bipolar."

—A 29-year-old woman with bipolar II disorder and alcoholism

Sometimes people who deny they have the disorder say it's because they're confused about where normal mood variation ends and bipolar illness begins. Perhaps you've wondered at times whether your emotional reactions to events or situations are really any different from other people's. Have you found yourself thinking or saying, "People around me have it, but they just don't know it yet"? You are most likely to think this way when your relatives or friends become increasingly angry or overcontrolling, accusing you of being sick even when you feel you are in remission and are having fairly ordinary ups and downs.

You may be right that others around you are moody. We do know that bipolar disorder runs in families (see Chapter 5) and that people with bipolar disorder tend to find mates who themselves have mood disorders (called *assortative mating*; Smoller & Finn, 2003). So it's not impossible that others in your family have the disorder or a mild form of it. Of course, if you or I asked them why they're so moody, they might say they're only reacting to your behavior. In turn, you may think that your behavior occurs in reaction to their moods.

Being aware of the moodiness of your close relatives or friends is not necessarily a bad thing. You can learn to avoid doing the things that provoke them and, even better, help them find appropriate sources of help (for example, a support group). Remember that their mood fluctuations may occur because of matters that have nothing to do with you. Chapter 3, which discusses communicating with family members, should help you with some of these issues.

Simply having moods that shift doesn't make one bipolar (recall the discussion of symptom thresholds in making the diagnosis in Chapter 3). But if you find yourself seeing bipolar disorder in everyone else, the reason may be that you don't want to feel alone or isolated. Admitting that you're ill and different from others is stigmatizing and can be quite painful. However, as we'll see later, acknowledging the disorder can also be empowering and doesn't mean that life as you know it has to stop.

The Personality–versus–Disorder Problem

"I feel like everything I do is now somehow connected to my being sick. If I'm happy, it's because I'm manic; if I'm sad, it's because I'm depressed. I don't want to think that every time I have an emotion, every time I get angry at somebody, it's because I'm ill. Some of my feelings are justified. People say I'm a different person every day, but that's me! I've never been a stable person."
      —A 25-year-old woman who had a severe manic episode followed by a
      6-month depression

Having a sense of how your personality, habits, and attitudes differ from your symptoms is an important part of learning to accept the disorder. Most people want to feel that they have a sense of self that is separate from their symptoms and biological vulnerabilities. They especially feel this way if they've been led to believe, by their doctors or by anyone else, that their illness is a "life sentence." Defining yourself in terms of a set of stable personality traits that have been with you through most of your life may make you feel less vulnerable to the kinds of conflicts the young woman just quoted is experiencing.

Another reason to distinguish between your personality and your disorder is that it will help you determine when you are truly beginning a new episode rather than just going through a rough time. For example, if you are extraverted by nature, socializing a great deal in one weekend may be less significant in determining whether you are developing a manic or hypomanic episode than changes in your sleep patterns, increased irritability, or fluctuations in your energy levels. In contrast, if you are habitually an introverted person, increased socializing may be quite useful as a sign of a developing episode.

Bipolar Disorder and Temperament

You may believe—and others who interact with you may believe—that your symptoms of mania are just your exuberant, optimistic, high-energy self; that your depression is just your tendency to slide into pessimism or overreact to disappointments; or that your mixed episodes or rapid cycling reflect your natural moodiness or dark temperament. In fact, there is evidence that people with bipolar disorder have mood swings or *temperamental disturbances* that date way back to childhood. A questionnaire given to members of the National Depressive and Manic–Depressive Association (now known as the Depression and Bipolar Support Alliance) revealed that many people with bipolar disorder had depressive and hypomanic periods even when they were children, well before anyone diagnosed them (Lish et al., 1994).

One of the more creative thinkers in our field, Hagop Akiskal, has an interesting slant on the whole question. He believes that the behaviors, habits, and attitudes we often refer to as a bipolar patient's personality are really mild forms of mood disorder, or the bipolar disorder in its early stages of development. He describes four temperamental disturbances that he believes predispose people to bipolar disorder (see the box on this page) and presents evidence that people with these temperaments, even if they have never had a major depressive, hypomanic, mixed, or manic episode, often have a family history of bipolar disorder and are vulnerable to developing the illness (Akiskal et al., 2006).

Why is it important for you to examine whether one of these temperaments applies to you? Because if you have one of them, you're at risk for a worsening of your disorder if you are not getting proper treatment. For example, if you had dysthymia or cyclothymia in adolescence, you are at risk for developing bipolar depressive episodes earlier rather than later (Hillegers et al., 2005; Lewinsohn et al., 2003). Lithium can be used to treat cyclothymia as well as bipolar disorder. If you had dysthymia or hyperthymia as a child or adolescent, you are at risk for developing hypomanic episodes, especially if you take an antidepressant medication and are not simultaneously taking a mood stabilizer such as lithium (Akiskal et al., 2005; Kwapil et al., 2000). If you have any of the four temperaments, you may still experience mood variability even once you return to your baseline after a manic or depressive episode. The notion is that these temperaments are relatively constant and reflect a biologically based vulnerability to your disorder. They come before the onset of the disorder and remain present even after the worst of the symptoms have ceased.

So, in one sense, when people with bipolar disorder say that they have always been moody, they're right. But the key point is that your moodiness may reflect the changes in the brain underlying the disorder rather than character or personality. What may look like personality traits can really be ongoing symptoms of your disorder that require more aggressive medical or psychological treatment.

Akiskal's Four Temperamental Disturbances

- *Hyperthymic:* chronically cheerful, overly optimistic, exuberant, extraverted, stimulus seeking, overconfident, meddlesome
- *Cyclothymic:* frequent mood shifts from unexplained tearfulness to giddiness, with variable sleeping patterns and changing levels of self-esteem
- *Dysthymic:* chronically sad, tearful, joyless, lacking in energy
- *Depressive mixed:* simultaneously anxious, speedy, irritable, restless, and sad, with fatigue and insomnia

A Self-Administered Checklist

It may be impossible to tell fully what is your personality and what is your disorder, particularly if you've had a number of episodes and you've become accustomed to the wide mood swings and the changes in energy and behavior that go with them. The following exercise may clarify your thinking about these matters. In filling out this exercise, compare your personality traits to the symptoms you have when you get manic or depressed. Under "personality traits," try to think of the way you are most of the time, not just when you're having mood cycles.

Does your personality consist of a group of traits that "hang together" (for example, sociable, optimistic, affectionate, open)? See if you can distinguish the cluster of traits that have described you throughout your life from those that typify the way you feel, think, or behave when you are manic, hypomanic, or depressed. How do you usually relate to other people, and does this change when you get into high or low mood states? When you're racing and charged up, are you really "affectionate and open" or just physical with many different people and talkative across the board? Would people describe you as boisterous, assertive, or energetic even when you're not in a manic episode? Are you pessimistic and withdrawn when you're not feeling depressed?

If you're not sure about whether you have certain personality traits, check with others to see if they would describe you with these trait terms. Frequently, those close to you will have different ideas than you do about what your personality is like and how it differs from your mood disorder symptoms. Of course, you may feel uncomfortable approaching certain close relatives with these questions, especially if you feel these family members have an agenda, such as getting you to take more medication. For now, try to select someone you think is not invested in the outcome of the discussion (that is, whether you conclude that certain behaviors are your illness rather than your personality, or vice versa). A close, trusted friend may be a good choice. Perhaps frame the question like this: "I'm trying to figure out why I've had so many mood changes. I want to know whether I've really changed or whether I've always been like this. Can you help me with a simple exercise?"

"Won't Bipolar Disorder Change My Personality?"

The flip side of this "personality versus disorder" question is whether one or more episodes of mania or depression can actually change your personality or character. This is a very complicated question. There is some research evidence that very painful events can change the fundamental character of a person (the "scar hypothesis"; see Just et al., 2001). Many people, particularly those who have had many bipolar episodes, feel that the disorder and the experiences of hospitalization, medications, psychotherapy, and painful life events have fundamentally changed who they are. People who have just been diagnosed may not worry so much that their personality

What's Me and What's My Illness?

Check as many of the following as apply.

Your personality traits	Your manic or depressive symptoms
_____ Reliable	_____ Euphoric
_____ Conscientious	_____ Grandiose ✓
_____ Dependable	_____ Depressed ✓
_____ Indecisive	_____ Loss of interest ✓
_____ Assertive	_____ Sleeping too much
_____ Open	_____ Sleeping too little
_____ Optimistic	_____ Racing thoughts ✓
_____ Sociable	_____ Full of energy ✓
_____ Withdrawn	_____ Doing too many things
_____ Ambitious	_____ Highly distractible
_____ Aloof	_____ Feeling suicidal ✓
_____ Critical	_____ More easily fatigued
_____ Intellectual	_____ Unable to concentrate ✓
_____ Affectionate	_____ Irritable ✓
_____ Spirited	_____ Feeling worthless ✓
_____ Passive	_____ Taking big or unusual risks
_____ Talkative	_____ Wired
_____ Seeking novelty	_____ Highly anxious ✓

will be changed by the diagnosis. They may worry instead that people will relate to them differently because of it—and that they may start acting differently as a result.

Certainly, a long-standing mood disorder—especially if it has not been treated—can profoundly affect your attitudes, habits, and styles of relating to others. It can also require lifestyle changes that are a lot like changes in personality. But if you were really free of your mood disorder symptoms for a long period of time, would you go back to being the way you were before the illness began?

We really don't know whether there are fundamental changes in a person's character as a result of long-term bipolar illness. It is possible that what look like changes in personality (for example, becoming less sociable, acting more aggressively) following repeated episodes of bipolar disorder are really just *subsyndromal symptoms*—depressive or manic symptoms that never fully disappeared after the last major episode. But no one doubts that the experience of bipolar mood swings is very profound and can change the way you view yourself and those around you.

"I Am My Disorder": Overidentifying as a Coping Style

"I've become very worried about having another episode. I keep thinking that even the smallest thing will push me over the edge—a glass of wine, traveling, eating a rich dessert, even just going to the store. My husband wants me to do more, like go with him to restaurants or shows, but I'm afraid going out will make me manic. I'm now leading a pretty sheltered life, I guess."
—A 58-year-old woman in a depressed phase of bipolar I disorder

Some people deal with the emotional pain of the disorder by giving themselves over to it. They *overidentify* with the illness, viewing all of their problems, emotional reactions, viewpoints, attitudes, and habits as part of their disorder. If your last period of illness was quite traumatic for you (for example, your life or health was threatened, you experienced public shame or humiliation, or you lost a great deal of money or status), you may have become fearful of the disorder's power over you, and placed severe restrictions on your life as a way of warding off future damage. If this coping style does not describe you now, perhaps you can recall periods of time when it did.

There are many reasons for overidentifying with the illness. First, you may have received inaccurate information from your doctors or other mental health sources. You may have been told that your illness is quite grave, that you shouldn't have children, that you can't expect a satisfying career, that you may end up spending a considerable amount of time in hospitals, that your marital problems will worsen, and that there is little you can do to control your raging biochemical imbalances. If you've been given this kind of information, it's not surprising that you would give up control to this affliction that destroys everything—or so you've been told.

Being given this kind of "life sentence" by your doctor may make you start reinterpreting your life in the context of the label. You may start thinking back on normal developmental experiences you had (for example, being upset about breaking up with your high school boyfriend or girlfriend) and labeling them as your first bipolar episode. You may start to think that you can accomplish little in your life, believing, "All I am is bipolar, and I can't change. It's all a brain disease and I can't take responsibility for myself." This way of thinking may make you avoid going back to work, withdraw from social relationships, and rely more and more on the caregiving of your family members.

In case it isn't obvious, I disagree with this way of characterizing bipolar disorder. Many—in fact, most—of my patients are productive people who have successful interpersonal relationships. They have adjusted to the necessity of taking medication, but they don't feel controlled by their illness or its treatments. They have developed strategies for managing their stress levels but don't completely avoid challenging situations either. I have been amazed by how many of my most severely ill clients call me years later to tell me they've gotten married, had kids, and/or started an exciting new job. But without knowing the future, some people "overarm" themselves and go too far in trying to protect themselves from the world.

You may find that you're more likely to underidentify with the disorder when in the manic pole of the illness, whereas you may overidentify with it when experiencing the depressive pole. This is, in part, because depression dampens your motivation to initiate certain activities, like work, socializing, or sexual contact. You may have subtle problems with memory or concentration as well, rendering the world a confusing, blurry place that demands too much. The illness can seem like an incredible burden that erases any hopes for the future. When you feel this way, you may, understandably, begin to merge the illness with your sense of who you are and who you will become.

If you have symptoms of depression, it's important not to take on more than you can handle, and to stick to your guns about what you do and don't feel able to do (even when others want you to do more). But remember also that your depression is likely to go away, with the proper combination of medications, psychotherapy, family and friendship support, and time. So, it's a good idea to set some limited goals for what you can accomplish even while you're depressed, to help you become more energized. Maintaining a certain level of *behavioral activation* can protect you against a worsening mood state (see Chapter 10).

"What Is the Best Way for Me to Think about the Diagnosis?"

Getting into debates with yourself or others about whether your behavior stems from your personality or your disorder can be quite discouraging. You'll find yourself intensely disagreeing with your friends or family members about whether you really have changed or whether you're just being yourself and reacting to circumstances. Alternatively, you may disagree with others who expect you to be "up and rolling" when you feel like you're not back to full capacity. But if underidentifying and overidentifying are both problematic, what is a helpful view? Is there an accurate *and* empowering way to think about the disorder? Keep in mind several "mantras" about the diagnosis of bipolar disorder.

1. *Bipolar disorder is not a life sentence.* As I've discussed, underidentifying and overidentifying are based on painful experiences from the past and understand-

able fears and uncertainties about the future. But having a bipolar illness doesn't mean you have to give up your identity, hopes, and aspirations. Try to think of bipolar disorder in the same way you would think of diabetes or high blood pressure. That is, you have a chronic medical illness that requires you to take medication regularly. Taking medication over the long term markedly reduces the chances that your illness will interfere with your life. There are also certain lifestyle adaptations you will need to make (such as visiting regularly with a psychiatrist or therapist, arranging blood tests, keeping your sleep–wake cycles regulated, moderating your exposure to stress, choosing work that helps you maintain a stable routine). None of these changes, however, requires that you give up your life goals, including having a successful career, maintaining good friendships and family relationships, being physically healthy, having romance, or getting married and having children.

2. *Many creative, productive people have lived with this illness.* Bipolar disorder is one of a very small set of illnesses that may have an upside to it: people who have it are often highly productive and creative. This is because, in part, when you're not actively cycling in and out of episodes of the disorder, your innate mental capabilities, imagination, artistic talents, and personality strengths come to the fore. In her book *Touched with Fire,* Jamison (1993) discusses the link between manic–depression and artistic creativity. In reading her work, you will discover that you are not alone in your struggles. Some of the most influential people in art, literature, business, and politics have had the disorder and have produced work that has had lasting effects on our society.

3. *Try to maintain a healthy sense of who you are and think about how your personality strengths can be drawn on in dealing with the illness.* As you reflect on who you were before you were diagnosed (and after completing the trait checklist in the exercise above), you will probably recall many of your personality strengths. Perhaps you are assertive, sociable, or intellectual. How can you be appropriately assertive in getting proper medical treatment? Can you use your natural sociability to call on your friends, family, and neighbors to help you through rough times? Can you use your natural intellectual inclinations to read up on and learn as much as you can about your illness? Doing so may generate a feeling of continuity between who you used to be and who you are now.

4. *The way you feel right now is not necessarily the way you will feel in 3 months, 6 months, or a year.* You may be feeling bad about your diagnosis and unable to function at the level that you know you're capable of. This rough period may make you feel like you have to give up control to your family, your doctors, and, worst of all, your illness—a prospect that feels highly distasteful. But in all likelihood, with proper treatment, you will return to a state that is close to where you used to be, or that at least is more manageable (see Chapter 6 on medication treatment). In the same way that someone who has had a bad viral flu has to stay in bed for another few days after the worst symptoms have cleared, you may need

a period of convalescence before you can get back to your ordinary routines and functioning.

5. *There are things you can do in addition to taking medications to control the cycling of your mood states.* Coming to terms with the diagnosis of bipolar disorder also means learning certain strategies for mood regulation. Later chapters (8–11) describe these in more detail. Knowing the practical self-management strategies will keep you from feeling victimized by the disorder.

I hope the last chapters have given you a sense of the challenges the disorder can bring to your self-image, and how, when you're challenged in this way, it is natural to want to reinterpret the events that have occurred in ways that feel more acceptable. Your reactions to the illness label are shared by others with the disorder. You may be able to make even more sense of your disorder when you think about the biological imbalances of the brain that create different mood states, and how certain stressful circumstances in your life can trigger these imbalances. Becoming familiar with the causes of bipolar disorder will help assure that you ask for, and get, the right treatments.

Part II

Laying the Foundation
for Effective Treatment

5

Where Bipolar Disorder Comes From
Genetics, Biology, and Stress

Stacy, 38, had two young daughters and worked part time for an accounting firm. She had been diagnosed with bipolar I disorder more than 15 years ago and took divalproex sodium (Depakote) on a regular basis. Although she agreed that she'd had severe mood swings, her interpretations of their causes tended toward the psychological rather than the biological. She often doubted that she had bipolar disorder: she was scientifically trained and felt that the absence of a definitive biological test meant the diagnosis should remain in doubt. Her psychiatrist frequently reminded her of her family history: her uncle had been diagnosed with bipolar illness and alcoholism, and her mother suffered from major periods of depression. But she remained unconvinced and continued to wonder whether she really needed medication. After all, she had been feeling fine for more than a year. She toyed with the idea of discontinuing her divalproex but was talked out of it, time and time again, by her psychiatrist. Over the course of a year, Stacy went through a series of life changes, including divorcing her husband. Other than some mild depression, she made it through the initial marital separation reasonably well. It wasn't until she and her children had to undergo a child custody evaluation that she began to show symptoms of mania. As the evaluation proceeded, she found that calls from her lawyer made her spring into action: She would rush off to the library and copy every legal precedent that was even remotely pertinent to her case, call friends all over the country to ask them to speak to lawyers they knew, and fax numerous documents to her lawyer's and doctor's offices. She often called her estranged husband and screamed threats into the phone. Her lawyer assured her that the divorce and custody agreement would be comfortable for her and her children, but his assurances did little to stop her from working harder and harder and sleeping less and less.

When her psychiatrist suggested to her that she was getting manic, she shrugged and said "probably," adding that she needed to spend every minute preparing for her upcoming court date. As her mania escalated, her doctor convinced her to try an increased dosage of divalproex and to add a major tranquilizer (risperidone/[Risperdal]). She reluctantly agreed to these modifications but still insisted her problems were stress related.

The divorce and custody arrangement were eventually settled out of court (and in Stacy's favor). Perhaps due to the additional medication and the removal of this life stressor, her mania gradually stopped and a major crisis was averted.

Two major questions plague virtually everyone diagnosed with bipolar disorder: "How did I get this?" and "What triggers an episode of mania or depression?" Some people put it more simply: "What's wrong with my brain?"

As you read this chapter, you'll make distinctions between factors that cause the onset of the disorder and factors that affect the course of the disorder once it is manifest. These factors are not necessarily the same. When they are the same, they may carry different weight in the onset than in the course of the disorder. Specifically, the initial cause of the disorder is strongly influenced by genetic factors (having a family history of bipolar disorder or at least depressive illness). In contrast, new episodes that develop after the first one appear to be more heavily influenced by environmental stress, sleep disruption, alcohol and substance abuse, inconsistent drug treatments, and other genetic, biological, or environmental factors.

If you have had the disorder for quite some time, you may have learned that your mood swings have a strong biochemical basis. (There is definitely some validity to that idea, though we now know that what is happening in the brain involves much more than a neurochemical imbalance; more on this later in the chapter.) You may also be aware that bipolar disorder runs in families. You may know several other people in your family tree who have had it or versions of it. If you are learning about bipolar disorder for the first time, you may not have been told that the cycling of the disorder is influenced by disruptions of regulatory mechanisms in the brain. Medications are designed to correct these disruptions, or dysregulations. In either case, it is useful to know about the genetic and biological origins of the disorder, because this knowledge will help you accept the illness and educate others close to you about what you are going through (see also Chapter 13). Also, knowing about the biological bases of your disorder will probably make taking medications feel more reasonable to you if you have any doubts.

But genetics and biology are not going to be the whole story. As Stacy's case reflects, a major life stressor, such as going through a divorce, can serve as a catalyst for the cycling of mood states. Everybody gets mad, sad, or happy, depending on the nature of the things that happen to them. People with bipolar disorder, because of the nature of their biology, can develop extreme moodiness in reaction to events in their environment. We don't know whether stress causes people to have bipolar disorder in the first place, but we're fairly certain that it makes the course of the illness worse in people who already have it.

Vulnerability and Stress

We needn't think of bipolar disorder as "only a brain disease" or "only a psychological problem." It can be both of these things, and each can influence the other. Most professionals think of the cycling of bipolar disorder—and, for that matter, the waxing and waning of most illnesses—as reflecting a complex interplay among:

▪ *genetic vulnerabilities*—inheriting a propensity toward the disorder from one or more blood relatives

▪ *biological agents*—abnormal functioning of brain circuits involving neurotransmitters such as dopamine

▪ *psychological agents*—such as your beliefs about relationships or your expectations about your ability to control things

▪ *stress agents*—either events that bring about changes, whether positive or negative (e.g., transitions in your job or living situation, financial problems, or a new romantic relationship), or more chronic problems (such as ongoing, severe conflicts with your family members; living in close, cramped quarters; or taking care of someone who is severely ill).

Think of it this way: You have underlying biological vulnerabilities with which you were born. Essentially, the strength of the signals transmitted through the spaces between your nerve cells is different from that of people without bipolar disorder. This dysregulation is called *abnormal synaptic plasticity* (Schloesser et al., 2008), and it can have various different effects:

▪ Your brain may be over- or underproducing certain neurotransmitters, such as dopamine, serotonin, norepinephrine, or GABA (gamma-amino-butyric acid).

▪ You might undergo changes in the structure or function of your nerve cell receptors.

▪ You might also experience changes in the functioning or volume of certain brain structures, such as the subgenual prefrontal cortex or the amygdala.

If these disturbances seem alarming, know that most of the time they are dormant and have little effect on your day-to-day functioning, though they still make you more susceptible to experiencing manic or depressive episodes. When stressors reach a certain level, these biological vulnerabilities or predispositions get expressed as the symptoms you're already familiar with—irritable mood, racing thoughts, paralyzing sadness, and sleep disturbance. In other words, your biological predispositions affect your psychological and emotional reactions to stress (and in all likelihood, vice versa). Likewise, when the stress agent is removed (for example, you end a relationship that was causing you grief), your biological dysregulations may become dormant again (as happened for Stacy).

Some psychiatrists and psychologists use a vulnerability–stress model to explain a person's bipolar symptoms. This model requires thinking about the interactions among several levels:

- *molecular factors*—genes that make you susceptible to bipolar disorder or, alternatively, genes that protect you from getting severe mood swings
- *cellular events*—such as how quickly cells grow or die
- *brain systems*—the circuits or nerve pathways involved in mood regulation
- *behavior*—such as personality attributes that make one more likely to encounter stress
- *environmental stressors*—life events that cause sleep deprivation or goal striving, family conflicts, or poverty or other adverse living conditions (Schloesser et al., 2008).

Look at the graph on the facing page. If you were born with a great deal of genetic or biological vulnerability—for example, the disorder is present across multiple past generations of your family or the nerve pathways in your brain related to mood stability become highly dysregulated—a relatively minor stressor, such as a change in your working hours, could be enough to elicit mood symptoms. Less genetic vulnerability (only one extended relative, like an uncle, had bipolar disorder, or a few relatives had depression, but no one was bipolar) could mean bipolar symptoms will be triggered only by a relatively severe stressor, like the death of a parent.

To make matters even more complex, certain genes can predispose you to favor certain environments. Someone who inherited a strong physique, for example, might choose work that built muscle, like construction work. Or a person who is socially withdrawn might choose activities that don't require interacting much with others—forestry, for example. Likewise, as a person with a genetic vulnerability to bipolar disorder, you may be drawn to highly stimulating, creative, and spontaneous or unpredictable activities, like writing and performing music, politics, or stock trading. You may have the energy to perform well in these endeavors most of the time, but then become highly emotionally dysregulated by the constant stress and changes in stimulation associated with these activities. When you become depressed, you may find it impossible to do them anymore.

This chapter provides examples of what is meant by genetic and biological vulnerability and ways to determine whether your family tree puts you at greater or lesser risk. You'll also learn more about the kinds of stressors that have been shown in research to trigger mood cycling. Recognizing that you may be biologically and genetically vulnerable and that certain factors are stressful for you is the first step in learning skills for managing your disorder. By the chapter's end you should have a general idea of how genetics and biology answer the question "How did I get this?"

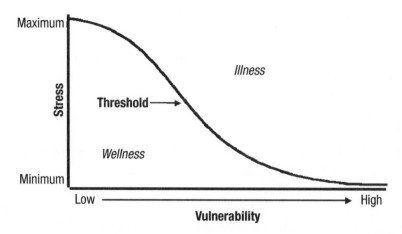

A vulnerability–stress model for understanding periods of illness and wellness. Adapted by permission from Zubin and Spring (1977). Copyright by the American Psychological Association.

and how these factors combine with stress to bring about new episodes of bipolar disorder. Later chapters provide practical suggestions for minimizing the impact of stressful events or circumstances.

"How Did I Get This?": The Role of Genetics

We have known for many years that mood disorders are genetically heritable and run in families. Genetic studies of persons with bipolar disorder (reviewed in the next section) have consistently supported this finding, although no one thinks that genetics provide all the answers.

As I noted in Chapter 3, your family history should be a part of your initial diagnostic evaluation. Stacy, as it turned out, had a mother and an uncle who showed signs of mood disorder, although it was only her uncle who had bipolar disorder. It is not unusual for bipolar disorder to *co-segregate* or be associated in family trees with other kinds of mood disorders, particularly various forms of depression or dysthymia (milder but more chronic depression).

How do we know that bipolar disorder runs in families? Geneticists usually establish that an illness is heritable through family studies and twin studies. If you want to know more about these topics, there are some great reviews (for example, Barnett & Smoller, 2009; Willcutt & Mcqueen, 2010).

Family History Studies

Family history studies examine people who have an illness and then find out who in their family "pedigree" also has the disorder or some form of it (recall from earlier chapters that bipolar disorder can look quite different among different people). We know that when one person has the disorder, often a brother, sister, parent, or aunt or uncle will also have it. We also know that some relatives of people with bipolar disorder will have other mood disorders, such as major depressive disorder or dysthymic disorder. They may also be affected by alcoholism, drug abuse, panic or other anxiety symptoms, or an eating disorder (for example, obesity with binge eating), which, while not mood disorders themselves, are problems that co-occur with and sometimes mask underlying depressive or manic symptoms. The diagram on this page depicts Stacy's family pedigree. The circles represent women, and the squares represent men. Notice that some of her relatives had mood disorders and some did not.

The average rate of mood disorder (major depression, dysthymia, or bipolar disorder) among first-degree relatives of bipolar persons is about 25%. That is, one of every four siblings, parents, and children of a person with bipolar disorder has some kind of mood disorder. On average, about 9% of a person's first-degree relatives have bipolar I or II disorder (compared to about 1–2% of the general population), and about 14% have strictly defined major depression without mania or hypomania. These numbers are averages: some people have many more relatives who have mood disorders and some have fewer. Nonetheless, if you have bipolar disorder, the chances that one of your first-degree relatives has it are about 9–10 times the general population rate.

Twin Studies

Another way to establish heritability is to ask this question: When one identical twin has the disorder, what is the probability (percentage) that the other identical twin also has it? Identical twins, as you probably know, share 100% of their genes.

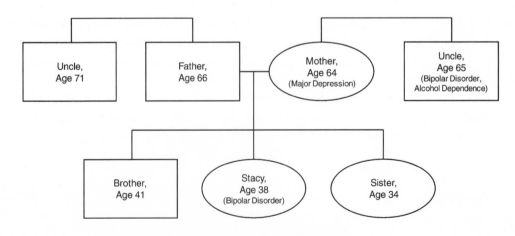

Stacy's family pedigree.

Fraternal twins (from two different eggs) share only about 50% of their genes, just like brothers and sisters. If we think a disorder is heritable, we would expect the identical twin pairs to have higher *concordance* or agreement rates—when one twin is bipolar, the other should be also—than fraternal twin pairs.

The most recent twin studies find that concordance rates for bipolar disorder among identical twins average 48% and between fraternal twins 6% (Barnett & Smoller, 2009; Willcutt & Mcqueen, 2010). Stated another way, when one identical twin has bipolar disorder, there is about a 50% chance that the other identical twin does too. When a fraternal twin has bipolar disorder, there is only about a 1 in 16 chance that his or her twin has it. This means that bipolar disorder has a strong genetic component, but if the illness were entirely genetic, the identical twin rate would be 100%. We know there must be nongenetic, environmental causes as well, and these are discussed later in this chapter.

The conclusion from the various studies is that bipolar disorder is 79–93% heritable, meaning most of the variation in risk for the disorder is due to genes. This makes bipolar disorder more genetic than, for example, medical disorders like breast cancer (Barnett & Smoller, 2009). But knowing these facts may or may not make you feel better about your condition. Some people feel absolved of self-blame upon learning the disorder is inherited, especially if they previously believed or were told that their symptoms of depression or mania were expressions of a character weakness. Other people feel "defective" or fearful that they will pass on bad genes to their children. I will talk about these issues more below, but first let's consider what it is that is actually passed on from generation to generation.

What Exactly Is Inherited?

We know that inheriting bipolar disorder can't be as simple as inheriting brown hair or blue eyes. Too many people with the disorder do not have relatives with mood disorders, or the last time it occurred in the family was several generations ago. This means that the way the disorder is passed on has to be more complicated. It may be that the tendency to become *emotionally dysregulated*—extremely moody—runs in families. It may be that people inherit a mild form of bipolar disorder or perhaps just a moody temperament, but develop the full bipolar condition only in the presence of other predisposing conditions, like these:

- Inheriting genes for bipolar disorder from both sides of the family
- Being "in utero" when the mother contracted a virus and undergoing a difficult, complicated birth
- Taking street drugs when growing up
- Sustaining a head injury
- Surviving highly adverse environmental circumstances

Some people with bipolar disorder experienced highly traumatic sexual, physical, or emotional abuse as children, not necessarily from their parents but often from other relatives, family associates, babysitters, or strangers. Traumatic experiences in childhood strongly contribute to difficulties in regulating one's emotions in adulthood, although we don't think that abuse alone can cause bipolar disorder.

The hypothesis that a person's genetic inheritance or biological vulnerabilities interact with specific environmental conditions to produce bipolar disorder is just that—a hypothesis. To test this hypothesis in a research study, we would have to determine whether children born with a genetic history of bipolar disorder and affected by predisposing environmental conditions are more likely to develop bipolar disorder in adulthood than children with a similar genetic history who have not been affected by these environmental conditions. These long-term studies, which would take many years to complete and are extremely difficult to execute, have not been done.

Current advances in *molecular genetics* allow researchers to examine regions of the chromosomes in an attempt to locate genes for bipolar disorder. Although a number of genes have been found to be associated with bipolar disorder, no single gene provides an adequate explanation. Researchers suspect that many genes—each with a quite small effect—contribute to a genetic vulnerability to the illness. Examples of these "candidate genes" may include:

- genes for brain-derived neurotrophic factor (BDNF), which is involved in the stress response
- genes for the serotonin transporter (SLC6A4) and the NMDA (*N*-methyl-D-aspartate) glutamate receptor
- the monoamine oxidase A (MAOA) gene
- "clock genes" (see the pullout on this page; Barnett & Smoller, 2009)

At this stage, there is a lot we don't know about how bipolar disorder is inherited, but scientists are working very hard to solve the puzzle. Once the genes are located, more accurate diagnoses and better treatments are likely to follow.

"Do I Have a Genetic Vulnerability?": Examining Your Own Pedigree

Before we get into the issue of what the genetic data might mean for your own life, take a look at whether bipolar disorder runs in your family. Are you genetically predisposed to the disorder? To begin this exercise, fill out the form on page 81 to the best of your knowledge. Confine yourself to your own children, your siblings (note in the table if the person is a full sibling or a half sibling), your parents, grandparents, aunts, and uncles. Leave out cousins, nephews, and nieces—the information people have on these relatives tends to be unreliable. Consult your relatives if you want more information. I have filled in the first four lines from Stacy's family as examples.

Next, place a star next to anyone you think may have had (or still has):

1. full bipolar I or bipolar II disorder or even a milder form of bipolar disorder, such as cyclothymia (short depressed periods that alternate with short hypomanic periods)
2. major depressive episodes or long-term periods of milder depression (dysthymia)
3. any other psychiatric problem that is not a mood disorder but that may

New research: We know that bipolar disorder involves changes in circadian rhythms: people with the disorder can have recurrences following a single night's sleep loss. Recent evidence suggests that genes that control our circadian rhythms ("clock genes") may be involved in the risk for bipolar disorder and its recurrences (e.g., Benedetti et al., 2003). For example, laboratory mice with mutations in clock genes behave in ways that resemble the behavior of people with mania (e.g., increases in activity, decreased sleep, reward-seeking behavior). These changes are reversed when mice are given lithium (Roybal et al., 2007).

Collecting Information to Draw Your Pedigree

Richard   Grandfathe   94 oldest Still alive

Name of relative	Relationship to you	Age now (or at death)	How did he/she die?
1. Robert	Step Father	66	Heart attack
2. Isabelle*	Mother Karla	64	(Still alive)
3. Mark	Cort Brother—in-law	41	(Still alive)
4. Valerie	Sister Lynette	34	(Still alive)
5. _____	_____	___	_____
6. _____	_____	___	_____
7. _____	_____	___	_____
8. _____	_____	___	_____
9. _____	_____	___	_____
10. _____	_____	___	_____

* = major depression.

be masking changes in mood (for example, drinking or drug problems, panic attacks, or eating disorders)

Answers to the following questions will give you clues as to your relative's health or illness:

■ How did the relative die (if deceased)? Was it an accident, suicide, or an illness?

■ Was the person ever unable to work for a period of time, or did she constantly switch jobs?

■ Did he jump from one marriage or relationship to another?

■ Are there family stories about the person being drunk, hurting himself or others, or having a "nervous breakdown"?

■ Are there stories about how this relative was a recluse, shutting herself away in a room for days at a time?

■ Did he ever take psychiatric medications? What kind?

■ Was the relative ever in a psychiatric hospital?

Now assemble your information into the pedigree. Again, circles refer to female relatives and squares to males. Fill in the circle or square of any relative you think may have had bipolar disorder. Fill in only half of the circle or square if the person had major depression, dysthymia, cyclothymia, or any of the other problems mentioned that can mask a mood disorder (for example, alcoholism, drug abuse, eating disorders). Put an *S* above anyone who committed suicide. Put a question mark in the circles or squares of any relatives you're not sure about.

Next, examine the pedigree (paying particular attention to the solid and half-solid circles or squares) and ask yourself the following questions: How many of your relatives have bipolar disorder? If none, are there relatives in your family tree who are or were depressed or addicted to alcohol or drugs or had an eating disorder? If so, consider whether these relatives had a hidden depressed or bipolar condition. For example, if the person had bursts of rage even when not drunk, and became withdrawn for periods of time even when "on the wagon," he or she may have had an underlying mood disorder as well as alcoholism.

Disorders like alcoholism or drug abuse tend to affect males more than females, whereas major depressive episodes affect more females than males. Does this pattern help you determine whether the male versus the female relatives in your family tree had psychiatric conditions? Did any relative spend time in a psychiatric hospital or take psychiatric medications for a long period of time? Did anyone commit suicide? Although we cannot know for sure, there is a possibility that a suicidal relative had a mood disorder and/or an alcohol or substance dependence disorder.

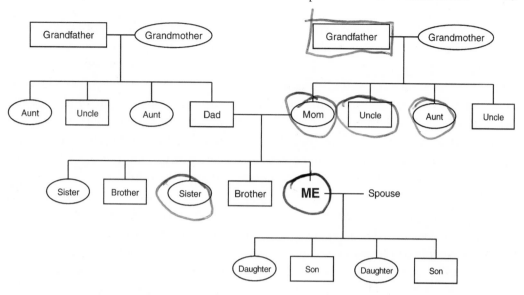

Locating relatives with mood disorders in your family pedigree.

If you have children, you may know whether one or more of them has a psychiatric disorder and can fill in those circles or squares. Of course, your children may not yet have reached an age when the disorder is recognized—bipolar disorder can be diagnosed at any age, but many people develop it in the middle to late teens. Be sure to fill in any psychiatric information relevant to your children's other parent and draw in "tree branches" to any affected or unaffected relatives in his or her family of origin. As you know, it is possible that your children inherited mood disorders from the other side of the family, or from both sides.

"What Does the Genetic Evidence Mean for Me?"

Practical Implications of Genetics

It is not yet possible to assign a number to a person's genetic vulnerability to bipolar disorder. Instead, vulnerability is usually described in general terms like *low, medium,* or *high.* One way of assessing your family tree is to ask whether the number of late-teenage or adult first-degree relatives in your pedigree who have had a mood disorder exceeds the average rate of 25%. If your family tree is dotted with people who have had bipolar disorder or some other mood disorder (more people are affected than unaffected), your vulnerability is high. Likewise, if bipolar disorder or other mood disorders are present in several generations (for example, in your siblings, parents, and grandparents), then your genetic vulnerability is higher than that of a person with bipolar disorder in only one generation. If only one of your first-degree relatives had a mild dysthymic depression and no one had bipolar disorder, your genetic vulnerability is probably on the low end of the continuum.

Now, what do you do with the information if you have concluded that bipolar disorder, or at least depression, runs in your family? Genetic evidence has practical implications for your life. First, the fact that the disorder runs in your family should make you feel less ashamed of having the illness. None of us can control the genes with which we come into this world. As you'll see in later chapters, there are things you can do to control the cycling of your disorder. But getting the disorder in the first place is heavily influenced by your genetic makeup. We don't know how to engineer the environment to prevent the original onset of the disorder. *In other words, it isn't your fault—a fact that your family members may also need to hear* (see Chapter 13). As the father of one young man with bipolar disorder told me, "For a long time we thought he was just a screw-up. He seemed able to screw up everything. But eventually we realized there was an illness and that there was something really wrong with his brain. He had a real problem that had a chemical basis, and it was probably something he got from me or from my side of the family. He wasn't doing all that stuff to hurt us. That's when we came to some understandings as a family."

Having a family history of bipolar disorder may also help confirm your diagnosis if you still have doubts (see also Chapter 3). If bipolar disorder clearly runs in your family, this fact will sway your doctor toward a bipolar diagnosis rather than, say, ADHD, depression, or schizophrenia. A family history of bipolar disorder is not a conclusive piece of evidence, but it provides one piece of the diagnostic puzzle. This is not to say that genetic evidence is the key to why you have mood swings. We believe genetics play a big role in who has bipolar disorder, but we know that genetics alone do not explain when and why your mood swings occur. Even if bipolar disorder runs in your family, you probably feel that your mood swings are a product of more than just your clock genes or some circuits in your brain that have gone haywire. Stacy certainly felt this way. That's why it's very important to think of genetics as providing only a background for problems you may have in regulating your emotions, thinking, and activity levels. It's the same way with high blood pressure: it certainly runs in families, but not everyone in a genetically susceptible family ends up with high blood pressure, and certainly not everyone with a family history of heart disease ends up dying of a heart attack. What people eat, whether they smoke, their weight, their levels of stress, and a whole host of other factors come into play. Again, there is an important distinction to be made between the original causes of the disorder and triggers of episodes.

"What If I Don't Have a Family History of the Disorder?"

You may examine your family pedigree and see no evidence of any mood disorders or other mental illness. This is unusual, but it does happen. The thing to ask yourself is whether you know enough about the people in your pedigree to say that they had no illness. Could the "exhaustion" that your mother describes in her own mother have been depression? If your grandfather is described as "dominating," "angry," or "aggressive," could he have also been manic? If not, could bipolar illness have occurred in someone several generations back?

Usually, your older relatives will know more about your family pedigree than you do, in which case you can enlist their help in filling out your pedigree chart. Your parents, if they are alive, will almost certainly know more about the lives of their parents, siblings, and other relatives. Consider asking your doctor to perform a family history interview with one or more of your relatives, if such an interview was not done as part of your initial evaluation (see Chapter 3).

Nonetheless, you may not be able to identify any relatives in your pedigree who have had mood disorders. We believe there are other triggers for the onset of bipolar disorder, but we aren't certain what these are. It's possible that prolonged drug abuse can bring on bipolar disorder in some people. An injury to the head or a neurological illness such as encephalitis or multiple sclerosis can bring on mood swings that look just like those of bipolar disorder. Perhaps we will find that the onset of bipolar disorder can be attributed in some people to complications that occurred during their birth or to viruses their mothers contracted during pregnancy, as has been found for schizophrenia. As I said above, adverse childhood experiences, such as physical or sexual abuse, may also contribute to the onset of bipolar disorder.

Even if your disorder doesn't have an obvious genetic basis, you may still respond to the medications that are used to treat bipolar disorder (see Chapter 6), just as a headache caused by environmental stress can be alleviated by aspirin. Some studies indicate that if you have a high prevalence of bipolar disorder in your family tree, you may respond better to lithium than if you have a low prevalence (Grof et al., 1993). But the evidence for this is not strong enough to guide our choice of treatments. Given our current state of knowledge, to make drug treatment recommendations your physician will probably place greater emphasis on your current and past symptoms and pattern of mood cycling than on your family history.

"What about Having Children?"

As indicated above, if you have bipolar disorder, your chances of passing it on to your kids average about 9% (14% for major depression). These probabilities are relatively low and are comparable to other psychiatric disorders—the rate is about 13% for schizophrenia, for example. So, the odds are in your favor: in most cases, your children won't develop anything.

Of course, the question of whether to have children goes well beyond statistics. Whether you are a woman or a man, your answer to this question should be based on considerations such as whether you are clinically stable enough to take care of a child, whether you are physically healthy in other ways, and, where applicable, whether you are satisfied with your relationship with your partner. I'll talk more about these concerns in Chapters 12 and 13.

Genes Are Not Destiny

Despite the relatively small chance that bipolar disorder will be passed genetically from parent to child, many people feel doomed by the evidence that they may have those genes. They assume that having the associated genes means they and their children have nothing to look forward to but a lot of mood cycling, doctors, medications, and hospitals. Being genetically prone or vulnerable to a disorder means that, due to your biology, you are more likely to get an illness than someone without the same genetic susceptibility. But being genetically vulnerable does *not* mean that you will necessarily get ill within a certain stretch of time; it does *not* tell you the probability or the timing of your recurrences. It also does *not* mean that there is nothing you can do to control your cycling. High blood pressure, high cholesterol, and diabetes are all heritable, but exercise, diet, and appropriate medications go a long way in controlling these diseases. Likewise, lifestyle management and medications are critical to controlling episodes of bipolar illness (see Chapters 6–10).

Genetics are not destiny for your first-degree relatives either. Illnesses skip generations or can be transmitted in a milder form. Even if you see signs of disturbance that suggest the beginnings of bipolar disorder, there are steps you can take to get your child treatment. I have written about a number of strategies for coping with bipolar disorder in adolescents in *The Bipolar Teen* (Miklowitz & George, 2008). Make sure your child gets a thorough diagnostic evaluation with a psychiatrist or psychologist who specializes in pediatric mood disorders before starting him or her on drugs like Ritalin or Adderall. You should also talk to your child's teachers about what accommodations can be made in your child's educational plans (see sample educational plans at *www.bpkids.org*).

Effective prevention: If you're worried that your children might develop bipolar disorder, be alert for these early warning signs:

- Irritability
- Aggressiveness
- Sleep disturbance
- Suicidal or morbid thinking
- School problems
- Inappropriate sexuality
- Drug or alcohol abuse
- Extreme and rapid mood shifts
- Sadness
- Lethargy
- Withdrawal from others

What Is a Biological Dysregulation?

Stacy had been told that her illness was "probably chemical." She understood that having a biological dysregulation meant that her illness was not fully under her control, but she was unclear what "chemical" meant. Unfortunately, "chemical imbalance" is, we now know, inadequate to describe all of the dysregulation that occurs in the brains of those with bipolar disorder. As mentioned earlier in the chapter, biological dysregulation affects more than neurochemicals. Stacy wanted to know more:

- Was this dysregulation something that could be measured?
- Why was there no blood test or brain scan for detecting it?
- Were the relevant changes in her brain occurring only when she was manic or depressed?
- What were the medications doing to it?
- Were the medications creating a different kind of dysregulation?
- Could these vulnerabilities be corrected by diet?

Stacy became frustrated that her doctor didn't give clear answers to these questions, even though he seemed quite knowledgeable otherwise. She felt that she was being asked to accept a lot of things on faith, and her scientific background made her feel doubtful.

Biological Vulnerabilities: Neural Circuits and Second Messenger Systems

Given that genetic background so strongly influences the onset of bipolar disorder, surely anatomical and/or physiological factors play a role as well. As I discussed in the preceding sections, a biological vulnerability can be dormant and then become activated by a trigger, such as environmental stress or drug abuse. Defining the nature of this biological predisposition is much trickier, however. If you have been told that you have a "biochemical imbalance in the brain," you may feel that this explanation raises as many questions as it answers, as it did for Stacy.

You may find you're more willing to accept the necessity of a medication regimen if you understand what your doctors mean by a biological vulnerability or dysregulation. They are usually referring to something that is part of you even when you're not having any symptoms. To use the blood pressure analogy, people with hypertension always have a vulnerability to an attack of high blood pressure, even when they're doing fine. Their system is such that their blood pressure is above normal even when they are relatively stress free and eating well, and stress causes their blood pressure to rise even higher. Likewise, we think that in bipolar disorder, biological dysregulations are present even when you are feeling well.

In bipolar disorder, biological vulnerabilities may be evoked by stress agents (for example, a sudden change such as loss of a job), alcohol or street drugs, or, for some people, antidepressants (see Chapter 6). When a stressor brings biological vulnerabilities to the foreground, the symptoms of bipolar disorder are more likely to appear.

For a long time, scientists talked about bipolar disorder in terms of the *amount* of certain neurotransmitters: people with the disorder had too little serotonin, too little norepinephrine, or too much dopamine. A major figure in our field, Husseini Manji, encourages us instead to think about the disorder as an "impairment of synaptic and cellular plasticity" (2009, p. 2). This means that people with bipolar disorder have genetically influenced problems with information processing in synapses (the spaces between nerve cells) and circuits (the neuronal connections between one brain structure and others), rather than too much or too little of a certain chemical.

To get technical for a moment, we suspect that people with bipolar disorder have disturbances in *intracellular signaling cascades,* which regulate the neurotransmitter, neuropeptide, and hormonal systems that are central to the limbic system. The limbic system, which includes the amygdala and the hippocampus, regulates emotional states, sleep, and arousal, all of which are strongly affected by the disorder. People with bipolar disorder and major depression also have an abnormal production of hormones (for example, glucocorticoids) by the adrenal glands when they are under stress. Long-term stress and glucocorticoid overproduction may damage or destroy cells in the hippocampus, a brain structure that is centrally involved in memory and conditioned fear reactions (Manji, 2009; Sapolsky, 2000; Schloesser et al., 2008).

New research involving persons with bipolar disorder has also found problems in their *second messenger systems* (also known as *signal transducers*), which are molecules inside brain nerve cells. When one nerve cell fires, it sends neurotransmitters (the "first messengers") to the next nerve cell. Then a second messenger system informs the second nerve cell that the first nerve cell has fired. In other words, second messengers help to determine whether a cell communicates messages to other parts of the same cell and to nearby cells. For example, lithium and divalproex slow down activity of the *protein kinase C signaling cascade,* an important mediator of signals within the cells when their receptors are stimulated by neurotransmitters (Newberg et al., 2008). This exciting research suggests that changes in second messenger systems may constitute one form of biological vulnerability to bipolar disorder—one that may be partially correctable by medications.

The Lack of a Definitive Test

"I've been told for years that there's something wrong with my brain. I just wish there was a blood test or a brain scan or something that I could look at and see my illness. Then I'd be more convinced that I need medications. What if I'm taking all these drugs to treat some chemical deficiency that I don't even have?"

—A 57-year-old man with bipolar I disorder

Despite this promising research, there is no definitive biological or genetic test for the impairments of synaptic and cellular plasticity characteristic of bipolar disorder. Most professionals, patients, and families wish there were, because that would make diagnosis and treatment planning much easier.

The absence of a definitive test makes it easy to forget that you have a biological dysregulation and even easier to believe that you never had one in the first place. Notice that Stacy, who had been free of symptoms for quite some time, started to wonder whether she really had a biological predisposition. It is understandable to ask this question. Could your manic or depressive episodes have been one-time occurrences that were set off by unpleasant life circumstances? Many people start to think, "I had this illness once, but now it's under my control," especially when they've been well for a while. But bipolar symptoms have a way of recurring when you least expect them. We believe this is because genetic and biological vulnerabilities are still present, even when your symptoms are controlled by medications and psychotherapy.

Despite the limitations of our current technologies, I believe we will see some real advances in diagnostic tests for the illness in the next decade. The *neural circuits* (brain pathways) most associated with bipolar symptoms are being mapped through brain-imaging techniques such as functional or structural magnetic resonance imaging (MRI) or positron emission tomography (PET). These scans find evidence that the amygdala—a structure that is central to identifying emotional stimuli, both positive and negative—is both more active and larger in volume in people with bipolar disorder, and areas of the prefrontal cortex may be correspondingly less active and smaller in volume (Chang et al., 2004; Phillips et al., 2008). These are not the only brain structures or circuits involved in bipolar disorder. Nonetheless, neuroimaging is likely to provide more reliable diagnostic tests in the near future.

What Turns a Biological Vulnerability into an Episode?

Learning that you probably have certain inherited biological dysregulations, although perhaps frightening, should help to arm you against recurrences of your illness. Like the diabetic who knows he or she must avoid ice cream, or the person with high blood pressure who must avoid high-salt foods and be sure to exercise, you can exert a degree of control over bipolar disorder by learning to avoid triggers that influence the expression of your biological vulnerabilities. When people who do not have biological dysregulations experience these triggers (for example, they take drugs or alcohol or intentionally subject themselves to high levels of stress), they may experience changes in mood but not to the degree that characterizes a person with bipolar disorder.

Some triggers may directly impinge on a person's biological vulnerabilities and set them off, kind of like lighting a fuse connecting a string of firecrackers. For example, bipolar disorder is believed to be related to diminished functioning of the serotonin system. LSD stimulates the action of serotonin receptors in the brain, which produces other biochemical events that will increase your risk of developing a manic episode. Another example: bipolar disorder has been related to increased sensitivity of the dopamine receptors and changes in the regulation of dopamine "reward pathways." Studies of laboratory animals as well as humans find that amphetamine (speed) stimulates the release and prolongs the activity of dopamine in the brain, which can also result in a state of high arousal, paranoid thinking, irritability, and increases in energy or motor activity.

Alcohol inhibits the activity of your central nervous system (for example, it increases the effects of the inhibitory neurotransmitter GABA on its receptors) and, like caffeine and other substances, interferes with your sleep–wake rhythms. When you stop drinking, your brain circuits become more excitable, much like they do in mania.

Environmental stress can aggravate your biological vulnerabilities, but the mechanisms by which this happens are not well understood by scientists. Some of the stressors that activate bipolar disorder are negative (for example, the loss of a loved one), and some are positive (e.g., an unexpected promotion). Stress cannot be avoided in the same way that alcohol or drugs can be avoided, but knowing what kinds of stress agents will be particularly troublesome will help you know when you are most at risk for recurrences. This awareness will help you plan preventively in the ways that are covered in the next few chapters.

Stress and Bipolar Episodes

Can bipolar disorder be caused by environmental factors, such as a high-conflict marriage, problems with parents, life changes, a difficult job, or abuse as a child? These are extremely important questions. Most scientists in the field doubt that a traumatic event or an emotionally abusive family alone can *cause* bipolar disorder without the contributing influences of genetics and biology. However, we are reasonably certain that stress and trauma affect the course of your illness or increase the chances that you will have a recurrence of mania or depression. Your level of stress may also affect how long it takes you to get over an episode. That is, the level and type of stress you experience are risk factors that help determine whether you will get better or worse within a certain time frame. Clinicians are interested in knowing about the role of stress in your life because it can help them in treatment planning, such as deciding what type of therapy to recommend to you.

What kinds of environmental stress are particularly influential? Encountering a major life change—whether positive or negative—increases your likelihood of having a manic or depressive recurrence. Stacy's divorce had relatively little immediate effect on her mood state, but the child custody evaluation played a major role in her manic episode. Other kinds of stress include sleep–wake cycle disruptions and conflicts with significant others. I'll be talking about each of these and giving examples. I'll also talk about some of the current thinking about mechanisms by which biological vulnerabilities might be affected by stress.

Life Changes

Changes are a part of life, and sometimes they are quite welcome. Some of them are positive and some quite negative. Examples of positive life changes include getting married, having a child, buying a new house, making a large sum of money from an investment, or getting a job promotion. Negative life changes include the death of a loved one, the loss of a relationship, the loss of a job, a car accident, or the development of a medical illness in yourself or another family member. Stress can come in the form of conflicts or unpleasant interactions with people you know well, particularly your family.

Manic and depressive episodes often follow major life changes, both positive and negative. Sheri Johnson, a psychology professor at the University of California, Berkeley, has written extensively about the role of life events in bipolar disorder (for example, Johnson, 2005a). She points out that it is not always clear whether life events are a cause or an effect of the mood episode.

Patrick, age 36, provides an illustration. When he was cycling into mania, he would become overconfident and frequently tell off his employers. He often lost jobs as a result. When discussing his history, he would argue that his pattern was to lose jobs and *then* become manic—when the reality was probably the other way around. But even when considering only events that couldn't have been brought about by the illness itself (for example, the death of a parent or losing one's job at a plant that closed down), researchers find that life events play a role in the onset of manic and depressive episodes.

All of us are emotionally affected by stress, but not everyone has the severe mood swings that people with bipolar disorder have when under stress. Are these people somehow more sensitive to life events? Johnson and her colleagues (2008) point out that the kinds of events that precede manic episodes are often goal- or achievement-oriented. Examples of these kinds of events include job promotions, new romantic relationships, financial investments, and athletic successes. She and her colleagues think that these kinds of events activate a circuit in the brain known as the *behavioral activation system*, which regulates the activity of the brain when stimuli indicating reward are present (for example, investments that signal the possibility of great financial gain). One theory is that the prefrontal cortex, which is important in foresight, planning, and emotional control, becomes underactive and fails to "dampen down" the activity of the amygdala or other brain structures when these structures become activated by a reward opportunity.

In contrast, other kinds of events cause people to shut down and withdraw, as they do when they get depressed. These events, which usually involve loss, grief, or rejection, may activate a different set of neural circuits, called the *behavioral inhibition system*. This system motivates the person to avoid stimuli that signal punishment. For example, the loss of a relationship may make a person withdraw from others as a way of avoiding further rejection.

The behavioral activation and inhibition systems of people with bipolar disorder probably involve abnormal dopamine and serotonin activity in brain structures involved in reward processing, such as the amygdala, nucleus accumbens, and ventral tegmentum. People with bipolar disorder might therefore be more biologically sensitive to events that are goal-oriented or that involve loss/rejection. Johnson's hypothesis is an intriguing one, and she has supported it in her research by showing that, among people with bipolar I disorder, manic episodes are often preceded by events that stimulate goal-directedness (Johnson, 2005b; Johnson et al., 2008).

Stressful Events: Examining Your History

Have stressful events played a role in your previous episodes? If you have had more than one clear-cut episode, you may find the following exercise useful. Fill out the dates of three or more of your previous manic/hypomanic or depressive episodes and see if you can determine whether life events occurred before (or during) any or all of them. If your previous episodes have been mainly mixed, indicate this in the second column of the table so that you can keep them separate when evaluating the exercise. Currently, we don't know whether mixed episodes have different environmental stress triggers than manic or depressive episodes.

Include major events (for example, a move to a new state, new romantic relationships or relationship breakups, car accidents, job changes, unexpected financial problems, deaths in the family) as well as events that, by comparison, are less severe

What Role Has Stress Played in Your Illness?

Approximate date of episode (or your age at the time)	Type of episode (manic, hypomanic, depressed, mixed)	Stressful events (describe)
_____	_____	_____
_____	_____	_____
_____	_____	_____
_____	_____	_____

or disruptive (for example, buying a new pet, getting the flu, taking a vacation, changing your job hours). Include both positive and negative life events.

Try to take a somewhat removed stance when examining the role of life stress in your own illness. Are particular types of events consistently related to your episodes? Has an event involving loss or grief ever preceded one or more of your depressive episodes? How many of your prior manic or mixed episodes were related to romantic relationships, even if the event was positive (such as finding a new partner)? Do events that involve achievement (for example, an increase in your work assignments) often precede your manic or hypomanic episodes? How many of these events might have resulted in changes in when or how much you slept? More generally, do these events occur independently of your mood disorder? Or does your manic or depressive behavior play a significant role in causing these events?

Don't be disappointed if you have difficulty answering these questions. Many people with bipolar disorder have trouble recalling when their episodes started and ended and when certain stressful events occurred, and it can be especially hard to tell whether your episodes caused them. If you are having trouble, try consulting a family member or a doctor who has seen you through several episodes. Go through the exercise together and see if he or she can help jog your memory about when certain events occurred, whether these events came before or after an episode, and what type of mood episode you had.

The temporal relationship between a life event and a resulting mood state can be quite complicated. For example, 27-year-old Annie became mildly depressed after she broke up with her live-in girlfriend but did not develop a full bipolar depression. However, when her physician started her on an antidepressant, she developed a mixed episode. In this case, the environmental stressor (the relationship ending) was related to the outcome (the mixed episode) only because she started a new medication.

Discovering a linkage between life events and your mood disorder episodes does not mean that you are somehow at fault for causing your own illness. Many life events are unavoidable. Some of these events can be more likely to occur when you get manic or depressed, but that still doesn't mean you are fully in control of their occurrence. For example, you may have lost certain jobs once your mood cycled into irritability or depression, but that doesn't mean you should have been able to control these mood states or their effects on others, particularly without having any tools to do so.

The Role of the Sleep–Wake Cycle

We've already talked about one set of mechanisms by which stress can affect bipolar symptoms—the behavioral activation and inhibition systems. Another mechanism is sleep. If you remember back to your first episode or any subsequent episodes, you will probably agree that sleep played some role in them. Perhaps it is simply that when you were manic you slept less, and when you were depressed you slept more. But changes in sleeping and waking are important in another way. Researchers believe that people with bipolar disorder are very sensitive to even minor changes in sleep–wake rhythms, such as when they go to bed, when they actually fall asleep, and when they wake up (Frank, 2005). If so, events that change your sleep–wake cycle will also affect your mood.

Stacy became quite manic when she began the child custody proceedings, possibly because the preparations were stressful and forced her to stay up later at night. Darryl, age 24, became manic shortly after his graduate school finals, during which he had stayed up later and later. Losing even a single night's sleep can precipitate a manic episode in people with bipolar disorder who have otherwise been stable (Malkoff-Schwartz et al. 1998). In parallel, sleep deprivation can improve the mood of a person with depression, although only briefly (Harvey, 2008).

What Affects Our Sleep–Wake Regularity?: Social Zeitgebers and Zeitstorers

Unless you speak German, you've probably never heard these terms before—nor had I until I started reading about the *social rhythm stability hypothesis* of Cindy Ehlers and her associates at the University of Pittsburgh (Ehlers et al., 1993). This theory helps us understand why life events might affect the mood cycles of people with bipolar disorder.

Ehlers's theory states that the core problem in bipolar disorder is one of instability. Usually, people maintain regular patterns of daily activity and social stimulation, such as when they go to bed, when they get up and go to work, how many people they ordinarily socialize with, or where they go after work. These *social rhythms* are important in maintaining our *circadian rhythms,* which are the more biologically driven cycles such as when you actually fall asleep, the production of hormones like melatonin (which is produced when you are approaching sleep), or your pattern of rapid-eye-movement activity during sleep.

Social rhythms stay stable, in part, because of *social zeitgebers,* which are persons or events that function as an external time clock to regulate your habits. Your dog can be a social zeitgeber if he or she needs to be walked at a certain time of the morning. If you have a spouse, he or she almost certainly plays a role in organizing your eating and sleeping schedules and probably affects how much stimulation you have from other people during the day. If you were to split up with your spouse, or even if he or she were to go away on a business trip for a period of time, your daily and nightly routines would be disrupted. Your job also keeps you on a regular routine.

In contrast, a *social zeitstorer* (time disturber) is a person or a social demand that throws everything off balance. When you start a new relationship, your patterns of sleeping, waking, and socializing change. The same thing will happen if you have a baby. In these cases, the new romantic partner or your baby is a zeitstorer.

If you take on employment that has constantly shifting work hours or requires that you travel across different time zones, your social and circadian rhythms will be disrupted considerably.

What does all of this mean for a person with bipolar disorder? Events that bring about changes in social rhythms, either by introducing zeitstorers or removing zeitgebers, alter circadian rhythms. You are particularly vulnerable to a manic episode after you have experienced a social-rhythm-disrupting life event. Let me give you some examples.

Debra, a 36-year-old woman with bipolar II disorder, lived with her husband, Barry. During a therapy session with the couple, Debra complained that Barry had changed the schedule for feeding their two cats. He had begun feeding them both in the morning instead of the evening, and as a result one or both of the cats were coming into the couple's room in the middle of the night, crying for food. Debra wanted to feed the cats before she and Barry went to bed, but he refused, saying it would make the cats overweight. After three consecutive nights of poor sleep, she became irritable, experienced mental confusion at work, and developed racing thoughts. This was the first time I had heard of a manic episode being induced by a crying cat.

Barry finally agreed to the new evening feeding schedule, which alleviated the problem with the cats. As Debra got back on a regular sleep–wake cycle and experienced several nights of restorative sleep, her hypomania started to settle down. In Debra's case, a major episode was averted by reestablishing routines that had been disrupted by a relatively minor event.

Miriam, a 47-year-old woman with bipolar I disorder, reported that she developed manic or mixed symptoms the morning or afternoon after drinking alcohol, even if she drank only small quantities. It wasn't entirely clear to me why a small amount of alcohol would make her manic until I considered her sleep cycle: alcohol was acting as a disruptive zeitstorer. She had much more difficulty falling asleep after drinking. Once she stopped drinking (or limited herself to one beer, usually consumed early in an evening), she had less trouble sleeping and fewer shifts in her mood states.

In Chapter 8, "Tips to Help You Manage Moods and Improve Your Daily Life," I'll tell you about a method for keeping your social routines regulated even when events conspire to change them (the social rhythm stability method). This self-monitoring technique can help you keep your mood and sleep–wake cycles stable.

Conflicts with Significant Others

"I started writing a blog about my moods and what was going on with me. Each night, I described what I felt like and what had happened that day. It wasn't of

much interest to anyone but me, but I was surprised to find that each 'up and down' went along with something involving my family. I always knew this to be true on some level, but it was so obvious once I wrote it down.

"Sometimes my mood would drop because of something stupid, like an annoying phone call from my mother about forgetting someone's birthday. Other times it was more serious, like when my brother's wife said she didn't want me to babysit my nieces anymore because she didn't trust me not to be crazy. And then if something good happened—like my stepmom compliment- ing my cooking or my dad telling me he liked my writing—I could feel my mood escalating. Every time I had some interaction with my family, anything involving emotion, I would get stressed out and my mood would change."

—A 32-year-old woman with bipolar II disorder

So far, we've talked about single life events and changes in your routine. The other major type of stress has to do with your ongoing relationships. Chapter 13 is devoted to dealing with family members, so I'll give it only brief mention here. There is no evidence that disturbances in family relationships (for example, poor parenting when you were a child) are a primary cause of bipolar disorder, but high-intensity, high-conflict family or marital situations can increase your likelihood of having a recurrence of bipolar disorder once you have it.

I conducted my dissertation research on this topic at UCLA with my former mentor, Michael Goldstein (Miklowitz et al., 1988). In this study, we worked with young adults who were hospitalized, usually for their first manic episode, and who were planning to live with their parents after hospital discharge. We examined the level of conflict between these patients and their parents while the patients were in the hospital and once they got out. Not surprisingly, those who returned to high- conflict, high-intensity families were more likely to have manic and depressive recur- rences within 9 months after their discharge than those who returned to low-conflict families. Though all of the people in our study were hospitalized, many people with bipolar disorder never enter a hospital. Nevertheless, other researchers have found similar associations between family relationships and the outcome of bipolar disor- der, whether or not the patients had been hospitalized (for a review, see Miklowitz, 2004).

We don't know exactly why conflict-ridden family environments make bipolar people more recurrence prone (though it makes sense), but we do know that fam- ily environments affect the course of many other psychiatric disorders, including schizophrenia, depression, alcoholism, and eating disorders. We also suspect that it is not only conflicts with family members or a spouse that can affect the cycling of your disorder but also conflicts with other significant people in your life, such as your employer, coworkers, or friends. In Stacy's case, her conflicts with her ex- husband may have played a role in her escalating mania. Had she been able to sit down with him and work things out with civility, her chances of staying stable might have been better. But she really didn't have that option.

For now, let's simply recognize that family and interpersonal conflicts can be risk factors in the course of your illness. Begin thinking about what role family or marital conflict has played in your disorder. Do your episodes typically coincide with significant family or marital arguments? Do these conflicts come before the episode, after the episode has begun, or is it impossible to tell? Many of my clients say that the family conflicts came before their episodes; others say that the conflicts arise once they've become manic, mixed, or depressed—but also make it harder to get better. Some report that family conflicts that have been there all along get worse when they become ill or that buried issues come out in their dealings with family members. When you are becoming ill, it can be difficult to "edit" the things you want to say to your family members, and these family members may have similar difficulties in communicating with you (see Chapter 13).

When thinking through these issues, try to avoid blaming others for their role in your illness—in most cases family members are trying their best to be helpful and often don't know what to do or say. As you'll see in Chapter 13, there are good and bad ways to deal with your family members regarding issues surrounding your disorder. Managing your family relationships is an important element of maintaining wellness.

▪

Bipolar disorder does not have clear-cut causes, but we know enough to say that it involves biological dysregulations that are partly under genetic control. These biological vulnerabilities can be set off by various kinds of stressors, conflicts, or life changes, whether positive or negative. Stacy's experiences with life stress, family conflict, and sleep–wake disturbances may mirror some of your own.

Medications are designed to correct the underlying biological vulnerabilities. The next chapter describes the available medications, what we think they do, their side effects, and the role of psychotherapy as an adjunctive treatment. Later chapters describe lifestyle management techniques. Usually these techniques are recommended alongside medications as a way of improving your ability to cope with stress. As you read on, try to think of biology and environment as interacting with each other—you'll have an easier time making choices about treatments if you can keep these multiple causes of bipolar disorder in mind.

6

What Medications and Psychotherapy Can Do for You

We have known for a long time that medication is the first-line treatment for bipolar disorder. We know that people with bipolar disorder remain well longer if they take medication regularly. But we also know that medication requires careful monitoring by you and your physician and sometimes demands that you deal with unpleasant side effects. Fortunately, ongoing research continues to produce treatments that are both increasingly effective and more easily tolerated, as well as new ways to minimize the side effects that still exist.

People have strong feelings about taking mood-stabilizing medications and sometimes don't take them even when they would clearly benefit—often because they lack information about the medications and their side effects. This chapter's overview of the medications used to treat bipolar disorder will allow you to take on a much more powerful role in dealing with your disorder. Knowing what these medications do, which side effects are common and which are rare, and how you can deal with them, as well as what the most recent research tells us about the track record of these medications, will help you plan your medication regimen with your doctor and manage it over time. The different medications in your regimen will make more sense if you think of each of them as belonging to a certain class of drugs (for example, antidepressants, mood stabilizers) and having a unique purpose (such as improving sleep). Because it is so important to take medications consistently, I've devoted Chapter 7 to exploring the factors that can stand in the way of your sticking with a medication regimen even when it has proven beneficial to you.

I strongly believe that people with bipolar disorder do best when they are taking medications and simultaneously working with a therapist. In study after study, we find that people who take medications and get therapy for their bipolar disorder do better than those who only take medications (Miklowitz, 2008a). Although psychotherapy is not a substitute for medications, there are things you can accomplish in therapy that won't be accomplished by medications. There are also things that medications can do for you that therapy won't. For this reason I discuss the role of psychotherapy as an adjunct to medications in this chapter.

What Will You Gain from Learning about the Latest Research Findings?

Knowing the facts about your medications and psychotherapy—including what the latest studies say about their effectiveness and side effects—is a crucial foundation for staying with a treatment regimen. You'll feel more confident about the medications you take and the psychotherapy sessions you attend if you know about the research that has been conducted on these strategies.

Medications have to be validated through randomized controlled trials (RCTs) before they can obtain a U.S. Food and Drug Administration (FDA) indication for use in bipolar or other conditions. In most RCTs, a coin is flipped and people receive the medication or a placebo (an inert tablet like a sugar pill), and neither they nor their doctor knows which they have received. To receive an FDA indication, the medication has to work better in alleviating depressive or manic symptoms than a placebo and not cause unacceptable side effects. These effects have to be observed in multiple studies conducted by different groups of investigators. Sometimes medications are tested as singular treatments for mania or depression (*monotherapy studies*) and sometimes as adjuncts to other drugs in *combination therapy* studies.

Psychotherapies can also be evaluated in RCTs, such as when we compare the illness outcomes of people who are assigned randomly to receive cognitive therapy and medication or medication alone. Psychotherapies do not undergo the same FDA certification process that drugs do, although some scientifically oriented clinical psychologists think they should (Baker et al., 2008). I agree with their position, although evidence that one psychotherapy is more effective than another for a specific condition is often lacking.

What Medications Can Do for You

You'll recall from earlier chapters that bipolar disorder follows a relapse/remission course. Research by Michael Gitlin and his colleagues at UCLA found that a person who has had a manic or depressive episode has a 60% chance of having another one within 2 years and a 73% chance over an average of 4–5 years (Gitlin et al., 1995). A 13-year follow-up of patients with bipolar disorder found that they had depression, mania, mixed episodes, or cycling for almost half the weeks of their lives (Judd et al., 2002). In the Systematic Treatment Enhancement Program for Bipolar Disorder (STEP-BD), a follow-up study of 1,469 people with bipolar disorder, 416 (49%) experienced recurrences over the next 2 years, with more than twice as many developing depressive episodes as manic, hypomanic, or mixed episodes (Perlis et al., 2006).

The good news is that virtually everyone suffering from the disorder finds that medication makes recurrences less likely. One review of studies in the 1970s through the 1990s concluded that lithium reduces rates of hospitalization by 82% (Tondo et al., 2001). Across a number of studies, the average relapse rate on lithium is 34% over periods of treatment ranging from 5 months to 40 months. The relapse rate is 81% on placebo (Goodwin & Jamison, 2007).

> **Effective prevention:** Lithium decreases the chances that a person with bipolar disorder will think about or commit suicide. But it is not only the drug that makes the difference; it is also the regular contact and collaboration with a caring professional.

Even more important, long-term treatment with mood-stabilizing medications (notably lithium) decreases the chances that a person with bipolar disorder will commit suicide (Baldessarini et al., 2003). One only has to read autobiographical accounts of people with bipolar or depressive disorders to know the positive impact that medication has had on their lives, including the reduction in suicidal thoughts, impulses, and attempts (for example, Jamison, 2000a; Solomon, 2002; Wurtzel, 1994). Sadly, many people who commit suicide had little or no access to psychiatric treatment. They did not receive the appropriate medications or psychiatric care, or their illnesses were not even detected by mental health professionals in the first place. Not surprisingly, regular contact with a caring mental health professional who *collaborates* with you on your health care will increase your feelings of hopefulness (Morris et al., 2005).

Acute versus Preventative Treatment

For the purposes of medication treatment, think of your disorder as having an *acute phase* (during which the goal of medication is to treat an existing illness episode) and a *maintenance phase* (when the goal is to prevent future episodes). The medications you take during the two phases may be different. Your daily regimen during the acute phase is likely to involve more medications at higher dosages than your regimen during the maintenance phase.

The acute phase involves bringing you down from a severe manic high or up from a depressive low. Acute-phase treatment is usually done on an intensive outpatient basis through regular psychiatry appointments, or in some cases through inpatient hospitalization. On average, the acute phase of treatment lasts up to 3 months, although nowadays in the United States less than a week of this (if any) is spent in the hospital. The length of the acute phase may be shorter or longer, depending on your response to the medications.

In contrast, the maintenance phase involves keeping you well and preventing you from developing more severe symptoms. This is also called *prophylactic (preventative) treatment.* The maintenance phase does not have a prescribed length, although some doctors say that at least 6 months of stable medication is necessary after the acute phase to help prevent recurrences of the disorder. As you'll see in Chapter 7, many people take their medications during the acute phase but mistakenly want to stop them during the maintenance phase, thinking they no longer need them. Often the result is that they have rapid recurrences of the disorder, even though they were better at the point when they discontinued the medications.

The two graphs on page 102 show how acute and maintenance treatment works. Two patterns are described in each: one in which a person with bipolar disorder takes medications (solid line) and one in which he or she does not (dotted line). In the first figure, Albert, a 32-year-old with bipolar I disorder, developed a severe manic episode. Just before the mania would have crested, he began taking two medications, lithium and quetiapine (Seroquel), an antipsychotic drug. The dotted line shows what would likely have happened if he hadn't taken medications at that point.

The second figure shows what the longer-term course of Albert's illness looked like with medications and what it would have looked like without them. Notice that medications do not eliminate Albert's mood cycling, but they do slow it down and prevent full recurrences. The periods of wellness are longer, his episodes are shorter and less severe, and his symptoms between episodes are milder.

When your symptoms are well controlled, as was the case for Albert, you can expect to be more in control of your life and have an easier time pursuing your goals. Having more control increases the chances that you'll be able to function better at work and in your family and social life.

Do I Have to Take Medication Forever?

This is a question many people with bipolar illness ask. It is an understandable and very important question, but one we really don't know how to answer. As you know from Chapter 5, bipolar disorder is related to underlying biological vulnerabilities involving the activity of brain neurotransmitters and their associated intracellular signaling systems. These vulnerabilities are inherited in many cases. We also believe that medications help correct biological disruptions in some of the ways described below. For this reason, most people with bipolar disorder must take medications indefinitely, especially if the diagnosis seems certain, if they have had more than one major episode, and if they have a family history of bipolar illness. Much like diabe-

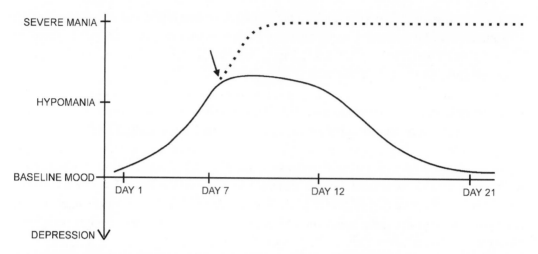

The effects of medications on Albert's acute manic episode. The arrow indicates the point at which Albert began taking lithium and Seroquel. The dotted line indicates what might have happened to his mood had he not taken these medications.

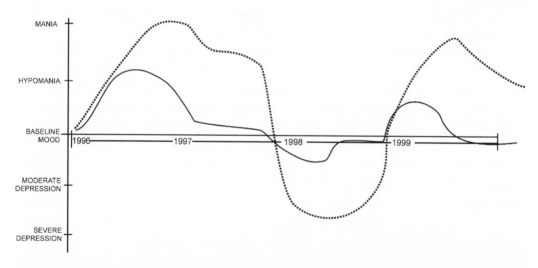

Albert's longer-term mood cycling as it would appear on appropriate medications (solid lines) and off medications (dotted lines).

tes or high blood pressure, bipolar disorder involves biological vulnerabilities that require long-term treatment.

There are exceptions to this rule, such as if a woman wants to become pregnant (certain mood stabilizers can increase the risk to the fetus of central nervous system defects). I'll be talking about pregnancy in some detail in Chapter 12. You may also have to stop your medications if you develop a medical condition that prevents you

> **In the best-case scenario, a medication regimen should do three things for you:**
>
> 1. Control and help resolve an episode that has already developed
>
> 2. Delay future episodes and minimize the severity of those that do occur
>
> 3. Reduce the severity of the symptoms you experience between episodes

from taking mood stabilizers (for example, certain diseases of the liver or kidney). Fortunately, your mood-stabilizing medications are not addictive or habit forming: you will not crave them when they are withdrawn.

If you have had only one episode, your doctor may recommend that you take medicines for 1 year and then reassess your need for them. But that recommendation will vary from doctor to doctor and will depend on how stable your mood remains over the year. It's a good idea to ask your doctor how long he or she expects you to be taking medicines.

Needless to say, accepting a long-term medication regimen is a very significant decision. I'll say more about the emotional significance of taking medications in Chapter 7. For now, let's focus on the mechanics of medications: which ones you are likely to be prescribed, in what dosages, their effectiveness as shown in research studies, their likely side effects, and how long they take to have an effect.

What Is a Mood Stabilizer?

Mood stabilizers are usually given during the acute phase and continued during the maintenance phase of treatment. To be defined as a mood stabilizer, a medication has to be effective in (1) treating acute manic, mixed, and/or depressive episodes of bipolar disorder without causing a switch to the opposite pole of the illness or rapid cycling (i.e., rapidly alternating between poles; see Chapter 3) and (2) preventing future episodes from occurring. As you'll soon see, antidepressants like fluoxetine (Prozac) are not considered mood stabilizers, because they impact only depression, not mania, and because they can cause rapid cycling if given alone.

Note that medications have at least two names: a generic name that reflects their chemistry (which I'll give first) followed by a specific brand name created by the pharmaceutical company that developed the generic drug for commercial use (given in parentheses). Doctors and pharmacies usually refer to drugs by their brand name. The main mood stabilizers in use today are *lithium carbonate* and the *anti-convulsants*, typically *divalproex sodium* or *valproate* (e.g., Depakote, Depakene), *lamotrigine* (Lamictal), or the older agent *carbamazepine* (Tegretol). Certain of the atypical antipsychotic medications, such as *quetiapine* (Seroquel), *aripiprazole* (Abilify), and *olanzapine* (Zyprexa), also qualify as mood stabilizers.

Your mood-stabilizing medications are likely to change over time, both in type and in dosage. The need to change medications doesn't mean you're getting worse. No single medication works to alleviate bipolar symptoms over a person's entire life span. It's also likely that you'll be treated with more than one mood-stabilizing medication or atypical antipsychotic agent at some point or perhaps even on an ongoing basis (for example, lithium and divalproex together). Many people with bipolar disorder experience an additive therapeutic benefit from taking more than one mood stabilizer or atypical. Perhaps this is because agents like lithium and divalproex have different but complementary effects on brain mechanisms, such as the protein kinase C signaling pathway (Schloesser et al., 2007; see Chapter 5).

Taking more than one medication doesn't mean that you are sicker than the next person with bipolar disorder—it just may mean that your unique physiology doesn't respond as well as that person's to an individual compound. People vary in their response to medications in part because of their patterns of symptoms, such as whether they have pure manic highs versus mixed episodes, or rapid cycling versus infrequent and distinctive episodes.

Types of Mood Stabilizers

Lithium Carbonate

The most well-known mood stabilizer is lithium, which is dispensed under brand names like Eskalith, Lithobid, Lithonate, and Cibalith-S. Lithium was the first medication proven to stabilize mood in bipolar disorder and also to prevent manic or depressive episodes from returning. Although various forms of lithium bromide were used during the late 1800s to quell agitation or overexcitement, the discovery of lithium as a treatment for bipolar disorder is usually attributed to John Cade (1949; see the box on page 105).

Lithium is usually given in 300- or 450-milligram (mg) tablets, and people usually take between one and eight of these per day (300–2,400 mg). Some people take their lithium in divided doses, several times a day, and some only once. This is one of the decisions you and your doctor can make when trying to figure out how best to control your side effects. A correct dosage is one that brings your blood level into a *therapeutic range*. The therapeutic range your doctor targets for you during treatment of your acute episode may be higher than the one he or she targets during your ongoing maintenance treatment, which is usually between 0.8 and 1.2 millequivalents per liter (a chemical measure of lithium concentration in the blood). Children with bipolar disorder or persons over the age of 65 can often be maintained on lower dosages of lithium.

The Discovery of Lithium

Lithium has been known to have mood-calming properties since at least A.D. 200, when a Greek doctor named Galen used it in baths for people with mental illness. Various lithium bromide compounds were marketed to the public in the 1800s, but were found to be highly toxic. The soft drink 7Up used to have lithium in it.

John Cade was an Australian physician who theorized that there were toxic compounds in the urine of patients with what was then called manic–depressive illness. He happened upon lithium by accident. His experiment involved injecting uric acid mixed with lithium into the bloodstream of guinea pigs. Injection with lithium calmed the animals down and made them less active. Cade then thought to try lithium with a human guinea pig, one of his most severely ill manic patients, a 51-year-old man. The patient responded very well and for the first time was able to function outside of a hospital. This story of scientific serendipity is tempered somewhat by the fact that this patient took himself off the medication, against medical advice, 6 months later, perhaps foreshadowing the wide-ranging problem of medication nonadherence among people treated for bipolar disorder. Nonetheless, lithium came into general use in the 1960s and has been used regularly in the United States since 1970, to the great benefit of many people with the illness.

How well does lithium work? About 60–70% of people with bipolar disorder show a remission of their manic symptoms when treated with lithium (Goldberg, 2000). Lithium reduces rates of hospitalization by 82%, but patients still have an average of about one manic or depressive episode per year when taking lithium (Tondo et al., 2001). In seven placebo-controlled trials that lasted between 1 and 2 years each, lithium was associated with a 22.5% relapse rate, compared to 50% on a placebo (Coryell, 2009). A meta-analysis (a "study of studies") of maintenance trials of long-term lithium usage, which included 770 participants, concluded that lithium was effective in preventing manic relapses but was only marginally better than placebo in preventing depressive relapses (Geddes et al., 2004).

Despite its apparent lower effectiveness in treating depression, lithium is the only single treatment for bipolar disorder that has been found to reduce the risk of sui-

Effective treatment: Don't give up on lithium if you don't feel its benefits right away. It will probably take at least a week and often a few weeks before you start seeing improvement in your manic or depressive symptoms. In fact, when taking it for the first time, you might feel a slight elevation in mood for the first week or so.

cide or suicidal behaviors. In a study of 21,000 patients by Dr. Frederick Goodwin and colleagues at George Washington University, people with bipolar disorder who were taking lithium were less likely to attempt or complete suicide, and less likely to require hospitalization for suicide attempts, than people taking either divalproex or carbamazepine (Goodwin et al., 2003). So, on balance, lithium is still the first choice for bipolar I depressive or manic episodes.

How Do You Know Whether You'll Respond to Lithium?

A lot of studies have tried to predict who will respond to lithium, with inconclusive results. The box below lists the symptoms and course patterns that tend to go along with a good response to lithium. Knowing about these factors may help you understand why your doctor is recommending lithium versus an anticonvulsant, alone or in combination. In general, the more your illness reflects the textbook description of bipolar disorder (euphoric, grandiose, manic highs followed by deep depressions, combined with a family history of bipolar disorder in one or more of your first-degree relatives), the more likely you are to respond positively to lithium. If your disorder is atypical (for example, you have irritability and dysphoric, sad

---

Which Mood Stabilizer Is Likely to Work Better for You?

Predictors of a good response to lithium:

- "Pure" euphoric or elevated manic highs
- Mood cycling marked by manias followed by depressions, followed by normal mood
- High prevalence of bipolar disorder in the family tree
- A good response to lithium previously
- Fewer, rather than more, previous episodes of illness
- Clear-cut episodes with relatively symptom-free intervals in between

Predictors of a poor response to lithium:

- Rapid cycling
- Irritability, hostility, and dysphoria accompanying manic episodes
- Co-occurring substance or alcohol abuse
- Mania symptoms that occur after a neurological illness or brain injury

Sources: Bowden (2009); Calabrese et al. (1996); Coryell (2009); Grof et al. (1993); McDonald (2000).

mood rather than euphoric mania), some doctors will recommend an anticonvulsant instead of (or in addition to) lithium. We used to think that rapid cycling or mixed episodes were better treated with anticonvulsants than lithium, but the latest data do not support this conclusion (Coryell, 2009).

How Lithium Works

We don't know exactly why lithium is effective in controlling manic and (to a lesser extent) depressive episodes, but we suspect it has effects on the underlying biological vulnerabilities discussed in Chapter 5. As explained there, lithium appears to affect pathways that determine whether chemical messages are sent successfully from the brain to other parts of the body or from one part of the brain to another.

Even more intriguing is the possibility that by increasing some proteins and enzymes in the brain and inhibiting others, lithium slows down or even stops the process of cell death in various brain structures. Those structures include parts of the limbic system, which is central to emotional processing and higher-order control over lower parts of the brain. Lithium may improve the structural stability of cells and even cause new cells to grow or proliferate (Machado-Vieira et al., 2009). As a result, people who take lithium may have increased gray-matter volumes. One study found that people with bipolar disorder taking lithium or valproate had larger volumes of gray matter in a certain part of the prefrontal cortex than people with bipolar disorder who hadn't taken these medicines (Drevets, 2001). This would mean that mood stabilizers do not cause long-term brain damage, as many people fear. Instead, these drugs reverse some of the damage caused by the illness.

Side Effects of Lithium

When you take any medication, it's important to know the possible side effects so that changes in your body will not come as a surprise to you, and you'll know to report them to your doctor. All mood-stabilizing agents have some side effects. In fact, be skeptical of "natural" or "homeopathic" mood remedies that presumably have no adverse effects. There is no evidence that any natural substance is both free of side effects and effective as a mood stabilizer or antidepressant. For example, hypericum (St. John's wort) can cause high blood pressure and headaches.

Your doctor will usually include any side effects you report as an important source of information for planning your treatment. Side effects can often be controlled in some of the ways described below. In Chapter 7 you'll find a side-effect recording sheet that will help you communicate with your doctor about complications associated with your medications.

People with bipolar illness have some predictable side effects with lithium, but their severity will vary a great deal from person to person. Common side effects of lithium include thirst, retaining water, frequent urination, fatigue, diarrhea, or a metallic taste in the mouth. More troublesome side effects include weight gain, mental sluggishness or problems with memory, shaky hands, development or flare-up of skin conditions (such as acne or psoriasis), or stomach discomfort or pain. Some people also develop hypothyroidism, a condition in which the thyroid gland does not produce enough hormone. Kidney functioning (i.e., the ability of the kidney to concentrate urine) can also be affected if lithium is taken over a long period of time.

The side effects of lithium can be related to the dosage you take. Many doctors adopt the "start low, go slow" approach, in which you start the medication at a low dosage and gradually increase to the therapeutic dosage as a way of keeping your side effects in check. If you are already taking a certain dosage of lithium but have unpleasant side effects, your doctor may decide to reduce your dosage, although this carries the risk of making the medication less effective for you. In other words, treatment with lithium can be a bit of a balancing act in which you and your doctor collaborate to find the blood level that stabilizes your mood (for example, keeps you episode free for at least a year) but also allows you to function with the fewest possible annoying side effects (for example, not having to deal with slowed-down thinking).

Other side effects require more creative solutions: frequent urination, for example, can be reduced by taking lithium once during the day instead of several times a day; thirst can be controlled by drinking more water, chewing on ice chips, or using sugarless cough drops. Stomach irritation can be helped by taking lithium after a full meal, or even switching to an extended-release formulation to reduce gastrointestinal symptoms. In other cases, your side effects may require additional medications, such as thyroid supplements (for example, levothyroxine [Synthroid]) or beta-blockers for hand tremors (for example, propranolol [Inderal]). Kidney functioning is usually monitored during lithium treatment through a variety of blood tests (for example, testing your creatinine level).

> **Effective treatment:** If you are taking lithium, make sure your doctor is monitoring your creatinine levels, which should be below 1.4.

Lithium Blood Tests and Toxicity

People who take lithium must have their blood drawn regularly to make sure they are getting the proper dosage. If you are starting lithium for the first time and are being stabilized from a manic or depressive episode, you will probably have to get your blood tested every week or two for the first 1 or 2 months of treatment, then every month for about 3 months. If all has gone well up to that point, your doctor will probably recommend you get it tested every 3 months or so. The purpose is to make sure you have the proper level of lithium in your bloodstream. Generally, your physician will check your blood level 10–14 hours after your last lithium dosage.

Having your blood tested regularly helps prevent *lithium toxicity,* in which your body accumulates lithium at very high levels. The signs of toxicity include problems with balance and coordination, severe diarrhea, abdominal discomfort, blurry vision, slurring of speech, extreme shakiness of the hands, severe nausea or vomiting, and mental confusion or disorientation. *Because this toxic state is extremely dangerous and even potentially deadly, it is important to know the signs (and inform your close relatives as well) so that you can get in to see your doctor as soon as possible, have your blood level checked, and, in most cases of toxicity, have your lithium adjusted or stopped.*

Your lithium blood levels can increase in reaction to dehydration or from taking over-the-counter medications such as ibuprofen. Your levels can also be too low or even nontherapeutic, especially if you are getting an inadequate dosage or have been taking the medication inconsistently. It is helpful to know these facts and to become familiar with the blood-level scale so that you can become an active participant in your lithium treatment. Ask your doctor which blood level he or she is targeting for you, so that you'll know when your levels are getting too low or too high. If you decide to see another doctor, he or she will want to know what therapeutic blood levels you are currently maintaining and which levels have been problematic for you in the past.

Effective treatment: If you are over age 60, you may be more sensitive to the side effects of lithium, and you can become toxic at blood levels that are usually considered therapeutic. If lithium is new to you, it may be best to start at lower dosages such as 150 mg twice a day. Certain diseases that are common in aging, such as kidney disease, may rule out using lithium (Thase, 2010).

You may find blood testing difficult: no one likes to be stuck with a needle, and having one's blood tested can remind you of being ill. But it is a very important aspect of your care. If you find it particularly unpleasant, discuss it with your doctor. He or she may choose to put you on a mood stabilizer that requires less frequent blood testing.

Divalproex Sodium (Depakote)

Divalproex sodium, which is also called *valproate* or *valproic acid,* is an anticonvulsant that has been used for decades to treat epilepsy and other seizure disorders. Many anticonvulsant drugs have mood-stabilizing properties. Divalproex is a fatty acid that is similar to other compounds found in animal fats and vegetable oils. It probably works in several ways, including reducing activity of the protein kinase C pathway and enhancing the action of the inhibitory neurotransmitter GABA (Manji et al., 2003).

Divalproex has come into wide use as both an acute and a long-term preventative agent. In fact, rightly or wrongly, it has replaced lithium as a first-choice therapy in the United States, probably due more to drug company marketing than research evidence (Thase, 2006).

Divalproex appears to be most effective as a treatment for acute manic episodes or mixed manic episodes. A meta-analysis of randomized trials found that divalproex had a 151% advantage over placebo in terms of improvement from mania; carbamazepine had a 200% advantage and lithium had 189% (Smith et al., 2007). Some but not all investigators find that divalproex may be better than lithium in controlling mixed episodes. Divalproex also can help alleviate bipolar depression, although the evidence base is less impressive than for mania (Bowden, 2009). Unlike lithium, it does not seem to help prevent suicide.

It is not clear whether divalproex can prevent future episodes of depression or mania. A large-scale study organized by researchers at Oxford University (see the sidebar) found that by itself divalproex was no more effective than placebo in preventing relapses, although it was effective in combination with lithium.

There are at least three reasons why your physician might give you divalproex rather than lithium. First, if you have mixed episodes, it may be more effective for you. Second, it seems to work a bit more quickly, even within as few as 3–5 days after the onset of a major manic episode. In contrast to lithium, your dosage can usually be raised rather rapidly without severe side effects. Third, there is evidence that people have less severe side effects with divalproex than with lithium. These advantages must be weighed against the greater abundance of supportive research on lithium, particularly as a preventative agent and in the treatment of people who feel suicidal.

People usually take divalproex in 250- to 500-mg tablets and typically take from 1,500 mg to 3,000 mg per day. Three times a day is a common dosing pattern. As with lithium, regular blood tests can tell you and your doctor whether you are getting the proper dosage of divalproex. Your doctor will probably want you to have a therapeutic serum level between 45 and 125 micrograms per milliliter (the measure used to indicate divalproex concentration in the blood). Some doctors use the beginning dose of 25 mg per kilogram of body weight a day (so, for example, if you weigh 130 pounds, you would start on about 1,500 mg).

New research: In the Oxford BALANCE trial, Oxford University researchers John Geddes and Guy Goodwin compared lithium, divalproex, and a combination of both in the maintenance treatment of 330 patients with bipolar I disorder in clinics all over the world (Geddes et al., 2010). They followed patients for 2 years. They found that both the combination of lithium and divalproex and lithium alone delayed relapses for longer than divalproex alone. The combination did not do substantially better than lithium by itself. This evidence suggests that, given a choice of lithium or divalproex, you may be better off (on average) choosing lithium. If, however, you are already taking divalproex alone, you may benefit from adding lithium to it.

Side Effects of Divalproex

Because divalproex is broken down by the liver, you can develop an elevation in liver enzymes, which in rare instances can lead to liver inflammation. Divalproex can also affect the production of blood platelets. For this reason, your doctor should conduct liver enzyme tests and blood platelet counts at regular intervals. When you start taking divalproex, you may feel nauseous, sleepy, or sedated, or have indigestion; and you may have a hand tremor (as can occur with lithium). These side effects usually disappear relatively soon. Some people also develop hair loss or hair thinning. More worrisome is significant weight gain, which can contribute to other medical problems (for example, high blood pressure, heart disease, or diabetes). Women may risk other complications when taking divalproex; these are discussed in Chapter 12.

Generally, your doctor will treat side effects by changing the schedule of your pills or adjusting your dosage (for example, dropping the dosage may help you feel less sedated). New formulations of divalproex help people who are very sensitive to the side effects of the 500-mg tablets. Depakote 125-mg sprinkles—a popular alternative for many adults and children—can be put on food to reduce stomach irritation. There is also an extended-release 500-mg tablet (Depakote ER) that may be less likely to cause stomach distress or significant weight gain.

Effective solution: Your doctor may recommend certain drugs as adjuncts to divalproex to resolve side effects: ranitidine (Zantac) for nausea, metformin (Glucophage) for weight gain, or vitamins containing selenium and zinc for hair loss.

Anticonvulsants like divalproex and carbamazepine often interact with other medications, meaning that side effects or medical complications can occur when these drugs are used together with other drugs. For this reason, you should be sure to tell your physician, especially if he or she is new to you, about any other drugs you are taking for any other medical conditions.

Lamotrigine (Lamictal)

"My partner, Beth, swears by Lamictal. She gets really down and can't get back up again, and it's the only thing that helps her. But it didn't help me, so I stopped taking it. My depressions are more like these periods of being mopey and all 'poor me' and stuff, but I still go to work, feed the cats, and once in a while drag myself to the gym. I think I do better when I stay active."
—A 29-year-old woman with bipolar II disorder

Lamotrigine (Lamictal), another anticonvulsant used in the treatment of epilepsy, is being used more and more for people with bipolar depression. It has become fairly popular in the last 10 years because of its mild side-effect profile and its ability to prevent depressive episodes without causing a switch into mania or hypomania. A meta-analysis of five randomized trials found that it has modest effects on the acute treatment of bipolar depression (Geddes et al., 2009). As illustrated by the young woman quoted above, it is most effective for people who have more severe bipolar depression when they start treatment (for example, intensely sad mood that rarely lifts, nightly sleep disturbance, severe problems with inertia) and less effective with people whose depressions are milder (i.e., feeling tearful and sad but still able to function with extra effort).

Lamotrigine is somewhat better than lithium in protecting people against depressive relapses, but not as good as lithium in preventing manic relapses. Lamotrigine is often recommended as an adjunct to lithium for stabilizing depression or preventing recurrences. It also seems to be effective for people with rapid cycling bipolar II disorder, which is characterized by frequent episodes of depression that never fully remit (Calabrese et al., 2000). Sometimes it is prescribed, usually in combination with other drugs, when people with manic or mixed episodes don't respond well to other medications. It is not a particularly good treatment for mania by itself.

Lamotrigine is easier to take than lithium or valproate because it is less likely to cause serious weight gain, tremors, or other unpleasant side effects. Typically, the side effects are temporary and include problems with physical coordination, dizziness, vision, nausea, vomiting, and headaches (Malhi et al., 2009). Nonetheless, there are some concerns about this drug because 5–10% of people who use it develop a benign skin rash within 2 to 8 weeks of beginning treatment. This typically mild rash can, in rare instances (about 1 in 1,000), lead to more serious skin conditions such as Stevens–Johnson syndrome, a potentially life-threatening condition involving a blistering or burning of the skin tissue or lining of the mucous membranes, often accompanied by fever. Rashes are more likely when doctors increase the dosage of lamotrigine too quickly or combine it with divalproex. Only a small proportion of rashes develop into Stevens–Johnson syndrome, but doctors are usually conservative and stop prescribing lamotrigine at the first indication of a rash.

Your doctor can try to prevent rashes by increasing your dosage very slowly to bring you up to a therapeutic level. Generally, doctors recommend starting at 25 mg per day and then gradually increasing the dosage for the first 4–6 weeks until you are getting some therapeutic benefit.

Carbamazepine (Tegretol)

Carbamazepine (Tegretol, Carbatrol, or Atretol), an anticonvulsant, was quite popular as a treatment in the 1980s, especially when used in combination with lithium. It appears to be comparable to lithium in controlling mania and an effective adjunct to lithium in treating rapid cycling (Denicoff et al., 1997). But it can be difficult to find the appropriate dose with carbamazepine, and difficult side effects can occur, some of which don't occur with lithium, lamotrigine, or divalproex. As a result it is being used less and less. Nonetheless, some doctors will recommend car-bamazepine if you have a difficult time with the side effects of other anticonvulsants or if you don't respond to those medications.

About as many people with bipolar disorder (two-thirds) respond to carbam-azepine as to lithium when they are in a manic episode. Like divalproex, carbam-azepine seems to work well for people with mixed episodes, rapid cycling, or psy-chotic manias. Among people who don't respond to lithium, about one-third will respond to carbamazepine within a month. Although it seems to work better for manic symptoms than depressive symptoms, about one in three people who have not benefited from other treatments for depression will respond well to carbamazepine (Post et al., 1998).

Your doctor will probably start you on a dosage of 200–400 mg per day and increase it by 200 mg (one tablet) every 2–4 days. Typical dosages are between 400 mg and 1,600 mg per day, given in 200-mg tablets. As with lithium or divalproex, your physician will probably start low and go slowly upward to minimize your side effects. Typical blood levels for people who take carbamazepine are between 4 and 12 micrograms per milliliter. Because the liver breaks down carbamazepine more quickly over time, your doctor may have to increase your dosage after the first 4 to 6 weeks of treatment—and periodically thereafter—to maintain a therapeutic level.

The most common side effects are sedation, nausea, and mild memory impair-ment (for example, difficulty finding words). These side effects are usually related to the dose you take and often disappear after a few weeks or months of treatment. Some people experience blurry vision, constipation, or loss of muscle coordination. There is less of a problem with weight gain on carbamazepine, which is why some people prefer it. Usually your doctor will treat side effects by adjusting your dos-age.

People taking carbamazepine, even more often than for divalproex, can develop a mild elevation in liver enzymes, which can be identified through regular liver func-tion tests. Your doctor will probably discontinue your carbamazepine if you develop signs of hepatitis, such as feeling sluggish or experiencing stomach pain or other gastrointestinal problems. From 10 to 15% of people develop skin rashes. As with lamotrigine, this side effect should be reported to your doctor immediately because it can progress to Stevens–Johnson syndrome.

The most serious side effect of carbamazepine—although quite rare (affect-ing about 1 in 100,000)—is a bone marrow reaction called *agranulocytosis,* which involves a dramatic drop in white blood cells. Fever, infection, sore throat, sores in your mouth, and easy bruising or bleeding are all signs to report to your doctor (Ketter et al., 1998), though none of these side effects is, by itself, reason to rule out carbamazepine at the outset. Agranulocytosis can be prevented if your doctor regu-larly monitors your blood count.

A new medication that is chemically related to carbamazepine, called oxcarba-zepine (Trileptal), came on the scene about 10 years ago but is already starting to fall out of favor. The controlled-trial research on oxcarbazepine is inconclusive. It does not appear to work as well as other anticonvulsants, such as divalproex, in treating bipolar disorder (Rosa et al., 2009). Its side effects include fatigue and a possible decrease in sodium levels, but it is easier to take than carbamazepine and does not carry the same risk of liver or blood dysfunction.

The table on the facing page summarizes some of the information you've just read. You may want to refer to it from time to time, to see if your side effects for any given medication are consistent with those listed and if your dosages and blood levels are within the expected range.

Atypical Antipsychotics

"What a great medication. There's no question that it improved my mood. Too bad it made me blow up like a balloon."
> —A 44-year-old woman with bipolar II disorder, upon discontinuing the antipsychotic olanzapine (Zyprexa)

Increasingly, people are being treated with atypical ("second-generation") antipsychotics instead of or in addition to mood stabilizers. The notion of taking an antipsychotic medication is scary to many people because they equate the use of these drugs with having severe delusions, hallucinations, and even schizophrenia. The fact that many doctors refer to them as "major tranquilizers" doesn't help much. Antipsychotic medications are not to be taken lightly, but they have broader applicability than just the treatment of schizophrenia. In fact, several of the second-generation antipsychotics have strong mood-stabilizing properties.

Unfortunately, most of the atypicals cause weight gain, metabolic disturbances, shakiness or stiffness, daytime sleepiness, and sedation (Tohen & Vieta, 2009). Some of these side effects can be controlled or at least contained.

What Is an "Atypical" Antipsychotic?

Twenty years ago, doctors were recommending a traditional line of antipsychotics that you may have heard about, such as chlorpromazine (Thorazine) and haloperidol (Haldol). These drugs have severe long-term side effects, including a serious movement disorder called *tardive dyskinesia*. The newer, atypical antipsychotics have less severe side effects and appear to be less likely to cause tardive dyskinesia. The newer drugs include olanzapine (Zyprexa), quetiapine (Seroquel), risperidone (Risperdal), aripiprazole (Abilify), and ziprasidone (Zeldox, Geodon). Many of these atypical antipsychotics qualify as mood stabilizers—they control acute episodes, decrease the vulnerability to future episodes, and do not worsen the course of the illness.

Common Mood-Stabilizing Medications

Drug	Dosage	Blood level	Common side effects
Lithium	300–2,400 mg per day	0.8–1.2 mEq/L	• Weight gain • Fatigue, sedation • Stomach irritation, diarrhea • Thirst and frequent urination • Metallic taste in mouth • Hand tremor • Thyroid dysfunction • Acne or psoriasis • Mental sluggishness or memory problems • Kidney clearance problems
Divalproex sodium (Depakote)	1,500–3,000 mg per day	45–125 mcg/ml	• Nausea, stomach pain • Fatigue, sedation • Hand tremor • Hair loss, curlier hair • Dizziness • Headaches • Weight gain • Elevated liver enzymes • Drop in platelet count
Lamotrigine (Lamictal)	200–400 mg per day	—	• Skin rashes • Dry mouth • Nausea, vomiting • Dizziness • Headaches • Sleepiness or insomnia
Carbamazepine (Tegretol)	400–1,600 mg per day	4–12 mcg/ml	• Fatigue, sedation • Nausea, stomach pain • Mild memory impairment • Constipation • Dizziness, lightheadedness • Blurred vision • Rash • Problems with physical coordination, unsteadiness • Elevated liver enzymes • Drop in white blood cell count

Note. mEq/L, millequivalents per liter; mcg/ml, micrograms per milliliter.

Antipsychotics are used in bipolar disorder for several purposes. First, some people with bipolar disorder do have severe disturbances in thinking and perception (psychosis) that are not fully controlled by the traditional mood stabilizers. For example, during the period in which they are escalating into mania or during the manic episode itself, they may hear their name being called or music being played (even though no one else is around), see movement out of the corner of their eye (even though nothing is there), or believe they are being followed. These symptoms can be alleviated by antipsychotic medicines.

Second, antipsychotic drugs, particularly the second-generation antipsychotics, have antimanic and sometimes antidepressive properties, either alone or in combination with lithium or the anticonvulsants. A meta-analysis of 24 studies found that atypicals were significantly better than placebo in treating mania and were just as effective as mood stabilizers like lithium, valproate, or carbamazepine (Scherk et al., 2007). The most effective treatment for mania was found to be the combination of an atypical antipsychotic and a mood stabilizer (for example, olanzapine or quetiapine plus divalproex).

Atypical antipsychotics are sometimes substituted for traditional mood stabilizers when people haven't done well on the latter. They work fairly rapidly in stabilizing acute manic or mixed episodes and are sometimes recommended for rapid cycling, severe anxiety, or sleep problems.

Effective prevention: To head off the side effects of an atypical antipsychotic, your doctor should regularly monitor you for weight gain and metabolic disturbances (glucose, triglycerides, lipid levels). Also, tell your doctor if you think you might be developing any unusual movements, such as twitching, tics, stiffness, or smacking your lips. These movement problems may be more easily detected by those around you.

If these medications are recommended to you, it doesn't necessarily mean that your illness is getting worse or that you are psychotic. It may mean that your profile of symptoms (for example, agitation, thinking disturbances, restlessness, rapid cycling) will respond better to these medications than to mood stabilizers alone.

Often, antipsychotic medications are given for a period of time and then discontinued gradually once a person has stabilized.

Which Atypical Should You Take?

It is unclear whether you should choose certain atypicals over others, although the medications differ in their side-effect profiles. The most well-studied is *olanzapine,* which has particularly strong effects on mania, mixed states, and rapid cycling and is FDA approved for the treatment of mania. Its efficacy in preventing manic or mixed-episode recurrences appears to be comparable to or better than that of lithium or divalproex and it can also augment the effects of lithium or divalproex when they are combined (Tohen et al., 2002, 2005). Unfortunately, olanzapine causes significant weight gain in many people.

Many doctors prefer to prescribe *quetiapine* over olanzapine because it appears to have a milder side-effect profile. In fact, some believe that quetiapine has the best record of *any* medication for treating both depression and mania in bipolar disorder. It has recently been FDA approved for the acute treatment of depression in bipolar I and II disorder. Several randomized trials have found that quetiapine may help prevent recurrences of depression when combined with lithium or divalproex (Thase, 2010). Moreover, quetiapine is useful even among patients with rapid cycling or comorbid anxiety disorders and does not appear to cause

> **Effective solution:** About 50% of people will gain significant weight within the first 6–8 weeks of taking an atypical antipsychotic. If you opt to stay on these medications, you may want to consult a dietician to keep your weight in check or ask your doctor about weight-control drugs.

a switch into mania. Nonetheless, quetiapine is also associated with weight gain and sedation, as well as high blood cholesterol and triglycerides, all of which can put you at risk for developing diabetes.

Two other atypicals—*risperidone* and *aripiprazole*—clearly have antimanic properties and are often recommended as adjuncts to mood stabilizers if a person has manic or psychotic symptoms that do not resolve with a single medication. Both appear to be weak antidepressants, although aripiprazole may be more useful when added to lithium or divalproex for depression. Both can cause symptoms like tremor, restlessness or jitteriness, or rigidity of the muscles. Risperidone can also elevate your levels of the hormone prolactin, which is important for women to know and is discussed in full in Chapter 12.

Finally, some doctors recommend *ziprasidone,* usually as an add-on agent rather than as a primary treatment of mania or mixed episodes. Its evidence base is weak, although it works better than placebo in alleviating mania. Side effects for ziprasidone include motor coordination symptoms, sleepiness, dizziness, and agitation, but it may be less likely to cause weight gain (Thase, 2010; Tohen & Vieta, 2009).

In the coming years, you may hear about the mood-stabilizing effects of other anticonvulsants and atypical antipsychotic agents, such as zonisamide (Zonegran), paliperidone (Invega), amisulpride (Solian), zotepine (Nipolept), or asenapine (Saphris). There are not enough studies yet to determine whether these medications will be more or less effective than the existing medications.

Antidepressants

Because mood stabilizers are generally more effective in preventing the manic pole than the depressive pole of the illness, your doctor may discuss with you the option of combining your mood stabilizer with an antidepressant drug. *Antidepressants are usually recommended only in combination with mood stabilizers or atypical antipsychotic medications, not by themselves.* These agents can be effective in alleviating the sometimes incapacitating symptoms of bipolar depression, such as sadness, loss of interests, insomnia, fatigue, and suicidal feelings.

In recent years there has been considerable controversy about whether antidepressants should be used at all in bipolar disorder, for the reasons given below (Sachs et al., 2007; Schneck et al., 2008). Nonetheless, given the suffering and impairment caused by bipolar depressions, most clinicians believe they should be kept as an option, especially if you have not responded to mood stabilizers or atypicals like lithium, lamotrigine, or quetiapine.

Some antidepressants are more effective than others, and some have more easily tolerated side effects. You have probably heard a lot about the antidepressants called *selective serotonin reuptake inhibitors* (SSRIs). These include fluoxetine (Prozac), sertraline (Zoloft), paroxetine (Paxil), fluvoxamine (Luvox), citalopram (Celexa), and escitalopram (Lexapro). "Novel antidepressants" are also available, including bupropion (Wellbutrin), duloxetine (Cymbalta), venlafaxine (Effexor), trazodone (Desyrel), and mirtazapine (Remeron). Still another class, called the *monoamine oxidase inhibitors* (MAOIs), include tranylcypromine (Parnate) and phenelzine (Nardil). Finally, some doctors still prescribe the old line of antidepressants called the *tricyclics,* including imipramine (Tofranil), amitriptyline (Elavil), nortriptyline (Pamelor), and desipramine (Norpramin).

There has been some alarmism, particularly in the United States, about the use of antidepressants for individuals with bipolar depression. One concern is that they cause people to become suicidal (see sidebar). Another is that antidepressants can bring on hypomanic, manic, or mixed states and cause rapid cycling. My read of the literature is that antidepressants can indeed cause mania or rapid cycling, but mainly when given alone, without an accompanying mood stabilizer or atypical antipsychotic. There is not much evidence that these drugs make people worse if given alongside traditional treatments for bipolar disorder. Antidepressant-induced mania usually occurs when people are misdiagnosed as having depression (without mania) and then learn that they have bipolar disorder when an antidepressant—taken alone—causes their first manic episode.

The other question is whether antidepressants really add anything. The research is not entirely consistent in answering this question. One large-scale randomized trial study found that people with bipolar depression recovered just as quickly on the combination of mood stabilizers and placebo as on the combination of mood stabilizers and antidepressants (paroxetine or bupropion) (Sachs et al., 2007). A smaller study, but one that followed people longer, found that those who responded well to the combination of a mood stabilizer and an antidepressant—and who had not become manic on antidepressants—were better off staying with this regimen than stopping the antidepressant (Altshuler et al., 2003). A third study found that

Effective prevention: Do antidepressants make people suicidal? The FDA has mandated that a "black box" warning be put on the package inserts of antidepressants about the increased risk of suicidal thinking and behavior among children during the first few weeks of antidepressant treatment. The risks are not large (4% of children developed suicidal thoughts, threatened suicide, or attempted self-injury, compared to 2% on placebo). Although the risk seems confined largely to children, you should be aware of new feelings of restlessness, irritability, anxiety, pessimistic thinking, or aggressive impulses when you start an antidepressant. You may need to stop taking it if these feelings persist.

the antidepressant venlafaxine was particularly helpful in alleviating depression in people with bipolar II disorder (Amsterdam et al., 2010). These very different studies did converge in one finding: there was no evidence that antidepressants caused mania or rapid cycling as long as they were combined with mood stabilizers.

If your doctor has recommended an antidepressant with an atypical antipsychotic, consider a single-capsule formulation that combines the two medications: the *olanzapine–fluoxetine combination* (OFC), which contains Zyprexa and Prozac and goes by the trade name *Symbyax*. The FDA has approved OFC for the treatment of bipolar I depression. The rationale for its use is that both agents have antidepressant properties, but the olanzapine will keep the fluoxetine from bringing about a manic switch. OFC is significantly better at treating bipolar depression than olanzapine alone, and both are better than placebo (Tohen et al., 2003). Another study found that OFC worked faster than lamotrigine in alleviating bipolar depression without causing more manic symptoms; nonetheless, other side effects (e.g., weight gain, sedation) were milder with lamotrigine (Brown et al., 2006).

Will You Do Well on an Antidepressant?

Given the potential risks of taking antidepressants, what guidelines can we offer to determine whether an antidepressant is right for you? University of Pennsylvania psychiatrist Michael Thase, who has been studying antidepressants for years, recommends taking adjunctive antidepressants if the conditions in the sidebar (right) are met (Thase, 2010).

Effective treatment: Consider long-term adjunctive treatment with an antidepressant if your illness has been dominated by depression, you have no history of becoming manic or hypomanic when taking antidepressants, and you have done reasonably well on antidepressants before. Reexamine the effectiveness and side effects of your medication regimen at least every 6 to 12 months.

You may be a candidate for adjunctive antidepressants if you have gone for at least 1–2 months with a severe depression that has not responded well to mood stabilizers alone and you have severe depressive symptoms with few or no accompanying manic or hypomanic symptoms (e.g., a decreased need for sleep, racing thoughts), or are having severe suicidal impulses (Dubovsky & Buzan, 1999). If you do take antidepressants, you'll have to be monitored carefully and probably will need to see your doctor and your therapist more often.

Which Antidepressant Should You Take?

Some antidepressants appear safer than others in terms of their likelihood of provoking manic or rapid cycling states. Some experts recommend that when people with bipolar disorder have severe depressions, it's often best to start with the drug bupropion, which has a lower incidence of sexual side effects and weight gain than some of the other agents (Thase, 2010). The SSRIs (for example, paroxetine or escitalopram) appear to be the treatment of choice if you have significant anxiety symptoms. Venlafaxine, while effective for some people, may be the most likely to cause manic switch (Post et al., 2006).

If you have not responded well to these medications or have had bad side effects, your doctor may recommend an MAOI. Many people do quite well on MAOIs, but they are difficult to take in that they require you to avoid foods that are high in the amino acid tyramine (for example, aged cheeses, sausage, chianti wines). The tricyclics are usually recommended last because of their side effects and are usually avoided altogether in people who have experienced mania or hypomania while on antidepressants.

About one in three people develop sexual side effects on SSRIs or MAOIs. These can include a lower sex drive and, if you are male, ejaculatory delay (difficulty reaching orgasm). If these side effects become significant, your doctor may recommend a different antidepressant or advise you to take breaks from the medication. For some people, sexual side effects are reason enough to stop taking the antidepressant, but as with any side effect, you should discuss this with your physician before discontinuing the drug. Going off an antidepressant quickly has been known to increase a person's risk of developing mania or rapid cycling. Other side effects of antidepressants can include weight gain, insomnia, headaches, and daytime sedation.

Thyroid Supplements, Benzodiazepines, and Other Options

One welcome advance in the past few years has been the increased availability of alternatives to traditional mood stabilizers, atypical antipsychotics, or antidepressants. These alternatives are used mostly in combination with the traditional mood stabilizers to create a stronger response (in terms of mood stability), rather than substituting for them. None of these newer medications has the proven track record of the standard mood stabilizers. But you may want to discuss them with your doctor if the other bipolar medications are either causing unpleasant side effects or not stabilizing your moods sufficiently or if you're having cognitive (e.g., memory) problems.

It's not unusual for doctors to recommend *thyroid medications,* usually under the name levothyroxine sodium (Synthroid, Levoxyl, Levothroid). People with bipolar disorder often have hypothyroidism, and certain mood stabilizers, such as lithium, tend to suppress thyroid hormones. This is useful to know if you're feeling fatigued or slowed down on lithium—a thyroid supplement may help bring you back to a normal energy level. Having a normal thyroid level may also increase the chances that you'll respond to an antidepressant.

You may benefit from thyroid supplements even if you have a normal thyroid test result, because they can be helpful in treating depression or rapid cycling. Discuss this option with your doctor, particularly if you are a woman (see Chapter 12).

Many people with bipolar disorder also take one of the *benzodiazepines,* a class of drug that may calm you down, help manage anxiety or panic symptoms, and help with sleep. Remember Valium? Drugs like diazepam (Valium) and alprazolam (Xanax) were prescribed quite readily in the 1970s as a way of managing stress and tension. Other drugs in this class include clonazepam (Klonopin) and lorazepam (Ativan). These drugs need to be taken with caution, because unlike the other drugs discussed so far, the benzodiazepines are highly addictive. People may need higher and higher dosages over time to get the same effects (tolerance) and can have withdrawal symptoms when stopping them—including seizures. But if you're having considerable problems getting to sleep or staying asleep at night, or if you feel chronically anxious during the day, these medications may help you. Your doctor may also recommend a benzodiazepine instead of an atypical antipsychotic to help quell your manic or mixed symptoms.

Topiramate (Topamax) is an anticonvulsant that may be helpful in alleviating the manic side of the illness, at least when combined with other mood stabilizers, but possibly even by itself. It may be useful for people with rapid cycling. Unlike most other mood stabilizers, it can cause weight loss rather than weight gain. For this reason, many people want to substitute it for lithium or divalproex, but the research does not justify this substitution. This drug has side effects in some people, such as blurred vision or eye pain, concentration or memory problems (for example, trouble finding words), tingling feelings in the hands or face, fatigue, feeling slowed down, tremors, nausea, and dizziness (Chengappa et al., 1999).

Two drugs come under the category of *neuroenhancers. Pramipexole* is a drug that increases the availability of dopamine, and that is often used in the treatment of dopamine-related conditions like Parkinson's disease. It may improve cognitive functioning in some people with bipolar disorder. In one small trial pramipexole, when combined with mood stabilizers, alleviated depressive symptoms among people who had not done well on antidepressants (Goldberg et al., 2004). It appears to have a mild side-effect profile, although any drug that increases dopamine carries the risk of mania or psychosis.

Modafinil, otherwise known as Provigil, is a wakefulness drug that appears to have antidepressant benefits for bipolar I patients, as well as cognitive benefits such as improved recall or verbal fluency. It is not clear that it works as well for bipolar II (Frye et al., 2007). Unfortunately, modafinil is very expensive (up to $13 per tablet), and most insurance companies do not cover it.

One popular alternative is the *omega-3 fatty acid plan* (fish oil). In an early randomized trial, fish oil did better than placebo tablets in prolonging periods of wellness among people with bipolar disorder who were also getting mood stabilizers (Stoll et al., 1999). Many people were excited by this study because fish oil is a natural, over-the-counter substance that seems to have few side effects. Subsequent studies of omega-3 have not really panned out, although it may have some weak effects on depression (Kraguljac et al., 2009). It may be an option for milder forms of depression or perhaps in conjunction with a mood stabilizer or atypical antipsychotic.

There is also a class of drugs known as *calcium channel blockers.* Although these are used mainly for the treatment of heart diseases and blood pressure, they may also have mood-stabilizing properties. These drugs include verapamil (Calan, Isoptin), nimodipine (Nimotop), and other agents. They are sometimes recommended for treatment-resistant mania, but only rarely, given their questionable efficacy.

More research is needed on all of these medications. Right now, they are recommended mainly as add-ons to traditional mood stabilizers or as alternatives for people who can't tolerate the side effects of any of the first-line medication choices.

Electroconvulsive Therapy: What Is and Isn't True about It?

Josh, a 35-year-old man with bipolar I disorder, was hospitalized for a manic episode and then returned home on a combination of lithium and risperidone. Shortly after his discharge he swung into a severe depression, which was characterized by sleeping most of the day, suicidal thoughts, low energy, mental slowness, and loss of interest in his family and work. He began to have unusual thoughts, such as fearing that his body was rotting. His physician was unwilling to give him an antidepressant because he'd had several bad reactions to antidepressants before, including periods of rapid cycling and mixed symptoms. Increasing his dosage of lithium did not help his depression and gave him more side effects—and "more to be depressed about" (his words).

Josh eventually asked to be admitted to the hospital again. Although he had been quite frightened of electroconvulsive therapy (ECT) the first time he had it, this time he asked for it, thinking it was the only option that would help. He was started on a course of ECT three times a week. He responded to this treatment within 3 weeks and was discharged from the hospital, his depression largely lifted. He felt brighter, mentally sharper, and more able to engage with his wife and children. His suicidal thoughts had diminished.

ECT, or what is often disparagingly labeled "shock treatment," is one of the more powerful treatment options available for people with bipolar disorder and other severe forms of depression. ECT works quickly and efficiently. It is mainly an acute treatment, and one of the most effective methods we have for pulling someone out of a severe depression or mixed episode. ECT can also be used to bring a person down from a manic high, although it is rarely used for that purpose, given the rapid effects of medications such as the atypical antipsychotics.

What happens during ECT? Typically, first you stop taking your regular medications, including lithium or anticonvulsants. Once these drugs are washed out of your system (which can take a week or two), an appointment is scheduled. During this session, you are given a general anesthetic (for example, sodium pentathol) and another medication (succinylcholine) to help relax your muscles and prevent a full body seizure. These drugs will make you unconscious while you are undergoing the treatment. The doctor then administers an electrical pulse that creates a mild seizure in your brain. The theory behind ECT is that this pulse and the resulting seizure "jump-start" the brain's production of neurotransmitters.

Usually, between 4 and 12 treatments are needed, or up to three times a week for about 1 month. Because ECT is generally not considered a maintenance (preventative) treatment, you will usually continue with your mood stabilizer, antidepressant, or antipsychotic regimen after the course of ECT is over.

Because of the difficult and turbulent history of ECT, people with bipolar disorder and their family members often don't want to consider it even in the most dire of circumstances. This is unfortunate because ECT is life saving in many cases. It can pull people out of serious depressions that might otherwise have resulted in suicide.

"Won't ECT Destroy My Memory?"

Many physicians recommend ECT only reluctantly because one of its side effects is a loss of memory. The memory loss is usually most noticeable for events that occurred during the treatment itself (that is, during the 4 weeks or so when the treatments were given). But some people also forget events that occurred prior to the ECT procedure. This probably occurs because ECT can affect the transfer of information usually held in short-term memory (the kind of memory that encodes and holds information in your mind for a brief period of time, such as when you first hear people's names and phone numbers) to long-term memory storage. A recent study found that patients who had received ECT did not perform as well on verbal learning and memory tests as those who had never received ECT, but it was not clear whether these effects were permanent (MacQueen et al., 2007).

It is not clear that memories are lost for good. In fact, memories for events that occurred before the ECT may come back several months after the treatment (Mondimore, 1999). It appears that about two-thirds of people who receive ECT experience problems in memory functioning, but the problems seem to be temporary and usually disappear with time.

Nowadays, ECT is a safe and effective treatment that is fairly routine in its administration. It can be done on an outpatient basis. Because of its side effects and high economic cost, it is typically considered when a person has not responded adequately to mood stabilizers or antidepressants and is incapacitated by depression, psychosis, or suicidality. Although it may sound surprising, it is considered a safe option for women who are pregnant and severely depressed or manic. Most mood stabilizers and antidepressants carry some risk of harm to the unborn baby, but ECT does not when administered under standard medical conditions.

ECT will not be done against your wishes. Like any psychiatric treatment, receiving ECT is based on a joint decision between you and your doctor.

New Electrical Stimulation Techniques

An alternative to ECT, called *rapid transcranial magnetic stimulation* (*rTMS*), is a simpler and less invasive way to stimulate the cerebral cortex. It is a reasonably good antidepressant, does not require you to have general anesthesia, and has few side effects (O'Reardon et al., 2007). But it does not appear to be as effective as ECT for depressed people who have not responded well to antidepressant medications. It has not been studied adequately in people with bipolar disorder.

There are two new treatments that are starting to gain traction for people with treatment-resistant depression or rapid cycling: *vagal nerve stimulation* (VNS) and *deep brain stimulation* (DBS). If you opt for VNS, there will be a stimulator device (about the size of a wristwatch) implanted under your skin that sends electric signals to your left vagal nerve (located in your neck). One small study (Marangell et al., 2008) found that people with rapid cycling bipolar disorder that had not responded well to other treatments showed an improvement in depressive symptoms over 1 year. Like all treatments, VNS has side effects, including a decrease in your respiratory flow during sleep and a high risk of sleep apnea (an intermittent closing of the throat while sleeping). Others report snoring, changes in their voice, coughing, and sore throat.

DBS is an even newer method that is not yet clinically available in the United States, except in a few specialty centers. It involves the surgical implantation of a "brain pacemaker," which, as the name implies, sends electrical impulses to various parts of the brain believed to be important in depression. One is the subgenual cingulate, a small area of the prefrontal cortex (Mayberg et al., 2005); another is the nucleus accumbens, which helps regulate the brain's responses to reward (Schlaepfer et al., 2008). A few small studies have found that people with depression who have not responded to other treatments improve with DBS and have no side effects other than some soreness from the surgery. There are no published studies on DBS and bipolar disorder as of yet, but we are likely to see some in the next decade.

Light Treatment

You may have noticed that your moods vary considerably with the season of the year. Some people do have seasonal bipolar disorders, which usually means they have mania or hypomania in the spring or summer and depression in the fall or winter. It may be that changes in exposure to light during the different seasons mediate changes in people's mood states. Sitting in front of full-spectrum bright white lights for half an hour to 2 hours per day can improve mood and serve as an alternative to traditional antidepressant medications for some (Terman & Terman, 1999). But like the antidepressants, light treatment can lead to switches into mania or hypomania or interfere with your sleep. Its recommended use in bipolar depression is not clear because no systematic, controlled studies have been done among people with bipolar disorder taking mood stabilizers. Nonetheless, if you think your depressions have seasonal triggers, discuss this alternative with your physician.

What Psychotherapy Can Do for You

> "I cannot imagine leading a normal life without both taking lithium and having had the benefits of psychotherapy ... ineffably, psychotherapy heals. It makes some sense of the confusion, reins in the terrifying thoughts and feelings, returns some control and hope and possibility of learning from it all. ... It is where I have believed—or have learned to believe—that I might someday be able to contend with all of this. No pill can help me deal with the problem of not wanting to take pills; likewise, no amount of psychotherapy alone can prevent my manias and depressions. I need both."
>
> —Jamison (1995, pp. 88–89)

Many doctors will recommend that you combine your medical treatment with some form of psychotherapy. For example, Clarence, a 19-year-old man who had been hospitalized during a manic episode (see more details in Chapter 7), came to some important decisions about his illness and his need for medication as a result of psychotherapy. He originally refused all medications, but through the support of his therapist he eventually agreed to a trial of lithium. In turn, his combination of psychotherapy and lithium helped him recover from a relatively intractable illness.

Learning to accept medication is only one reason to seek psychotherapy. Like

Jamison, many people with bipolar disorder say that therapy is an essential part of their recovery from episodes, on a par with medications. Psychotherapy can't cure you of bipolar disorder, nor is it a substitute for medications. Nonetheless, psychotherapy can help you learn to recognize the triggers for your mood swings and what to do about them. If you can afford it (or your insurance covers some part of it) and if you can find a good therapist in your community who knows about bipolar disorder, I would highly recommend that you pursue it. In my experience, most people are satisfied with weekly hourlong visits to an individual, couple, family, or group therapist.

Why Try Psychotherapy?

There are several compelling reasons to seek psychotherapy (see the box below). A major reason is to get some guidance in managing your disorder. You may want to discuss the role of stressful events in eliciting your mood cycling, why you feel "set off" by certain interactions with your spouse or other family members, your difficulties accepting the illness or its stigma, or your ambivalence about medications. You may wish to discuss the impact that your illness is having on your work life, social life, or family relationships, or how to talk about it with other people. These are all good reasons to seek therapy to help you cope with and manage your mood disorder.

You may also wish to try therapy to address long-standing personal problems that may be unrelated to your disorder or that seem to continue whether your mood is stable or not. These issues are probably not being addressed in your medication

---

The Objectives of Psychotherapy for Persons with Bipolar Disorder

▦ To help you make sense of your current or past episodes of illness

▦ To discuss long-term planning, given your vulnerability to future episodes

▦ To help you accept and adapt to a long-term medication regimen

▦ To identify and develop strategies for coping with stress or mood cycles

▦ To improve your functioning in school or the workplace

▦ To deal with the social stigma of the disorder

▦ To deal with comorbid disorders like alcohol abuse or other addictive behaviors

▦ To improve family or marital/romantic relationships

sessions with your psychiatrist. For example, many people with bipolar disorder have had very traumatic experiences of physical or sexual abuse (Post & Leverich, 2006). Some people with bipolar disorder feel that they've never had a successful romantic relationship or job experience. Some feel chronically suicidal, even when they are not in an episode of depression. Some experienced painful childhood losses (for example, the suicide of a parent) and need to make sense of their feelings of abandonment and rejection. Even if these psychological issues are not a primary cause of your bipolar disorder, they may become more salient to you when your mood cycles. Gaining insight into the nature of these conflicts and developing skills for coping with them have the potential to make you less vulnerable to new mood episodes.

Hannah, a 27-year-old woman with bipolar II disorder, also suffered from obsessive–compulsive symptoms, which had become bad enough that she had quit her job as a court reporter. She was bothered by intrusive thoughts that she might stab her husband, Carl, also age 27. These thoughts were especially disturbing to her because "I deeply love him … he's the best thing that's ever happened to me, maybe the only really good thing." When she had these violent thoughts, she often cycled into depressive, suicidal episodes. She was consistent in taking her regimen of divalproex and sertraline (an SSRI antidepressant), but her thoughts caused her significant distress. Carl was aware of her impulses but said he wasn't worried about them. She had never acted on them, and "besides, I'd rather she had fantasies about killing me than somebody off the street."

During a course of interpersonally oriented therapy (see next section), Hannah came to realize that she was quite angry at her husband for what she termed his "treating me like his little doll." She recounted how her various attempts at independence were met with vitriolic tirades from Carl, in which he would reassert his dominance over her. In one particularly emotional session she realized that her violent thoughts usually appeared within a few hours of having a frustrating confrontation with Carl regarding her desire to get a job or go back to school. Later in therapy, she became more comfortable with the idea that she had legitimate reasons to be angry with Carl and decided to work on her assertiveness skills in her interactions with him. Whereas Carl continued to oppose her working full time, he did finally agree to support her applying for a part-time job at a health club and enrolling in an evening course. Her violent thoughts gradually receded.

Hannah's problems with her husband did not stem directly from her bipolar disorder, although they contributed to her cycling patterns. Notice that her improvement stemmed from two factors: her *insight* into the reasons behind her violent thoughts and her *decision to do something differently* in her relationship. Most therapists nowadays believe that psychotherapy is most effective when people combine insight with learning the needed skills for changing their thinking patterns or behaviors.

Choosing the Right Therapy

Like medications, psychotherapy comes in different sizes, shapes, and dosages. Depending on your community, you may be able to locate professionals who practice individual therapy from a number of different theoretical viewpoints. You may also have access to family therapy, couple therapy, or self-help groups. If you live in a rural area or a small town, you may be limited to the orientation and type of practice available in your immediate locale.

Almost all therapy goes better if you're with a therapist you respect and trust, with whom you have a good relationship, and who you feel genuinely cares about you. *But it is also important to find a therapist who understands the syndrome of bipolar disorder.* Avoid being in the position of educating your therapist about your bipolar symptoms or having him or her label your behavior as "acting out" or "low self-esteem" when the real issues have to do with unresolved manic or depressive symptoms. Good questions to ask your intended therapist include whether he or she (1) works regularly with persons with bipolar disorder, (2) will integrate his or her knowledge of the disorder into the treatment, and in what ways, (3) places importance on understanding the illness and its effects on your relationships, (4) will communicate regularly with the physician who is managing your medications and develop an integrated treatment plan, and (5) will focus on the present as well as the past. You also should ask how long your therapy is likely to last, although your therapist may not be able to give you a precise answer. It is reasonable to expect weekly or biweekly sessions for about 6 months to a year after an illness episode, with an agreement to evaluate your progress from time to time.

Avoid agreeing to open-ended, long-term contracts with no clearly articulated goals. Avoid therapy approaches in which all disorders—whether bipolar disorder, depression, anxiety problems, or substance/alcohol abuse—are ascribed to traumatic "repressed memories" (that is, memories of negative childhood experiences that are buried and presumably must be uncovered). Despite the fact that these treatments have been around for some time, they are largely unproven by research and have not been evaluated systematically in bipolar disorder. What's more, they tend to downplay or even deny the importance of the biological and genetic origins of the disorder and the need for medications. This is not to say that examining painful childhood events will not help you, but it should be done in the context of a therapy that acknowledges the biological bases of your disorder, educates you about how to cope with it, and deals with your present as well as past difficulties.

You may find different kinds of individual psychotherapy available in your community. Their assumptions and purposes are discussed in the following pages, as well as the research evidence for their effectiveness in stabilizing the cycles of your bipolar disorder when combined with medications.

Individual Psychotherapy

Individual therapy is most often recommended once you have started to recover from an episode of bipolar disorder, so it is considered a maintenance rather than an acute episode treatment. When you are beginning to stabilize on your medications, you may still have significant mood symptoms, disturbances in your thinking patterns, and behavior patterns that can interfere with your long-term stability. Consider finding a psychotherapist who can work with you in a *cognitive-behavioral* or an *interpersonal* framework. These are the two types of individual therapy that have the most research support in terms of improving the course of bipolar disorder when given alongside medications (Miklowitz & Scott, 2009).

Cognitive-behavioral therapy (CBT), a treatment designed by Aaron Beck, is perhaps the most well-established psychotherapy for depression. The few published studies of CBT in bipolar disorder find that people who receive CBT while also taking medications are less depressed and have fewer days of depression than those who take medications only (Miklowitz & Scott, 2009). A therapist who specializes in CBT will encourage you to identify and evaluate patterns of negative thinking about yourself, your world, and your future. By keeping a daily thought record (see Chapter 10), you can learn to identify your assumptions about certain critical events, particularly any self-defeating statements—"hot cognitions"—that arise spontaneously in reaction to these events (for example, "I lost my job because I'm just not capable of holding one"). Your CBT therapist will encourage you to recognize the impact of such assumptions on your mood states and to conduct "experiments" in your day-to-day life to determine whether your assumptions are valid. As therapy proceeds, he or she will encourage you to consider more adaptive and balanced interpretations of events and record these new cognitions on your thought record (for example, "Maybe I lost this job because I was still recovering from my depression and couldn't function at the level I know I'm capable of" or "This last job taught me that I need to work in an environment that will allow me to stay stable and still use my skills").

CBT may also be useful if you have a comorbid condition such as panic disorder, social phobia, or obsessive–compulsive disorder. CBT treatments such as prolonged exposure to feared stimuli, breathing retraining, relaxation, and mindfulness meditation have the best record in treating anxiety conditions. Chapter 10 offers a more thorough discussion of the CBT approach and a selection of cognitive restructuring exercises you can try out on your own.

A second individual approach is *interpersonal therapy*. This therapy is geared toward helping you understand the role that your illness is playing in your close relationships or work life and in turn how your relationships and work life are affecting your bipolar disorder. Interpersonal therapists encourage you to focus on a particular interpersonal problem in your life and consider how it relates to your mood disorder. For example, some people develop a manic or depressive episode after a loss or grief experience (e.g., the death of a parent); some after a life transition such as losing a job or a relationship breakup; some after significant disputes with family members or partners; and some after a series of ongoing problems in maintaining relationships with other people. Interpersonal therapy focuses on your habits in close relationships and how to alter them to help stabilize your mood.

A form of interpersonal therapy called *interpersonal and social rhythm therapy* (IPSRT; Frank, 2005) includes a new element: monitoring your sleep–wake rhythms, patterns of daily activity, and levels of daily social stimulation (for example, the amount of high- versus low-intensity contact you have with friends or family members). This method is discussed more in Chapter 8 (in particular, see the self-rated Social Rhythm Metric). Working with a therapist who specializes in this interpersonal model may be quite helpful to you in implementing sleep–wake and other strategies for stabilizing social rhythms. In one carefully designed study, IPSRT was shown to delay recurrences of bipolar disorder and increase the stability of daily routines and sleep–wake cycles (Frank et al., 2005).

Family and Couple Therapy

Sometimes bipolar disorder is best treated in a family or couple context. The advantage of therapy with your close relatives is that they can be educated about your disorder and taught coping skills for managing stress at the same time as you. People with bipolar disorder often have high levels of family or relationship conflict or tension (see Chapter 5). Family treatments can provide ways of improving your communication with your spouse, parents, or kids (see the communication strategies described in Chapter 13).

The family/couple approach that I developed with Michael Goldstein of UCLA, called *family-focused therapy* (FFT), is a 9-month-long psychoeducational therapy. In FFT, people with bipolar disorder and their spouses or parents are acquainted with useful information about the disorder—its symptoms, causes, prognosis, and treatment. In contrast to psychoeducational programs that focus on learning facts, people in FFT discuss their feelings and beliefs about the disorder, what coping strategies have and haven't worked, and how best to cope now and in the future. Later stages of FFT focus on family or couple communication and problem-solving strategies, including how to listen, negotiate, and solve conflicts. (To learn more about this therapy, see *Bipolar Disorder: A Family-Focused Treatment Approach* [Miklowitz, 2008b]). In four different randomized trials we have found that people with bipolar disorder who get medications and take part in FFT do better over the 1 to 2 years after an episode than those who get medications and supportive individual therapy or case management (Miklowitz & Scott, 2009).

Cognitive, interpersonal, and family educational treatments may be hard to find in your community, but look for them anyway. Several national organizations have therapist locator Web listings. Check out the website for the Association for Behavioral and Cognitive Therapies (*www.abct.org*; go to the "Find a Therapist" link), the Beck Institute for Cognitive Therapy and Research (*www.beckinstitute.org*), the American Association for Marriage and Family Therapy (*www.therapistlocator.net/index.asp*), or the American Psychological Association (*locator.apa.org*). Interpersonal therapists are hard to find (for some reason, there are a lot of them in Iowa), but try searching under the Interpersonal Psychotherapy Institute (*www.uihealthcare.com/depts/interpersonalpsychotherapyinstitute/mapoffaculty.html*).

Self-Help Groups

Many people benefit from educational support groups (Bauer et al., 2009; Colom et al., 2003). In groups, people with bipolar disorder get together and discuss feelings, attitudes, and experiences related to the disorder; sometimes the groups are educational and skill oriented (my recommendation) and sometimes free form (which can be hit or miss). Many people feel that others with bipolar disorder are the only ones who can truly understand them and give them viable solutions. People in bipolar support groups talk about medications they've tried and which have worked, which therapies they've had, how they have dealt with problems in the work, family, or social setting, and what they do to prevent themselves from getting ill again. Of the more than 2,000 respondents to the National Depression and Manic–Depressive Association (now called the Depression and Bipolar Support Alliance) Support Group Compliance Survey (Lewis, 2000)—all of whom had been active in local support groups—95% said that their group experience helped them become more willing to take medications, communicate with their doctors, and cope with side effects. I used to run a support group for people with bipolar disorder and was continually impressed with how effective the members were at helping each other.

Sometimes these groups have leaders who are mental health professionals, and sometimes they are leaderless and include only people with the disorder ("mutual support groups"). Not everyone feels comfortable in a group setting, however. If you have doubts, try going for one session and see if you can relate to the other people in the group. Can you imagine feeling supported and understood by them when talking about your own problems? Do they seem to have had the kinds of life difficulties or illness management problems you've had? To see if there are groups available in your community, try calling the local mental health center in your city or town, local psychiatrists who specialize in mood disorders, or the phone numbers listed in the next paragraph.

Family Support Groups

Your spouse or parents may also want to attend a support group. They may benefit from a group in which they can confide in other relatives of persons with bipolar disorder. Good options for your relatives include the Depression and Bipolar Support Alliance (800-826-3632; *www.dbsalliance.org*), the National Alliance on Mental Illness (800-950-NAMI; *www.nami.org*), and the Child and Adolescent Bipolar Foundation (847-492-8519; *www.bpkids.org*). These organizations usually provide informative lectures, group discussions, educational materials, and referrals to local support groups for relatives.

Try not to be anxious about your spouse's or your parent's desire to join such a group. You may fear that these groups will be composed of angry relatives who will badmouth you and encourage your relatives to give up and leave. In my experience, this is not the case. Rather, these groups provide useful information and support and help relatives feel less isolated in their attempts to understand and cope with bipolar disorder. Sometimes your relative may have his or her own mood problems to discuss. If you are uncomfortable, ask your relative to take you along. In most cases, these groups are open to persons with the disorder as well as their relatives. And, usually, they're free.

───────

As you can see, there are numerous treatments for bipolar disorder. None of these treatments is perfect, but many can effectively treat your acute symptoms and, in all likelihood, even out the course of your illness over time. Adding psychotherapy or support groups to your medication regimen helps ensure that you, the person, are treated, not just your disorder, and that you develop strategies for coping with stress.

You and your doctor may need to experiment with a number of different medication and therapy options before you find a combination that is effective and also minimizes your side effects. This trial-and-error process may be frustrating at times. But there is every reason to be hopeful that, with time, you will find a regimen that is optimal for you. Of course, committing to a long-term program of medications is an important personal decision. You may have significant doubts about whether you should take any of these medications, even if you are suffering from mood swings that interfere with your functioning. These reactions are understandable. But when people with bipolar disorder stop taking medications, particularly if they do so abruptly, they often end up relapsing and worse off than they were before they stopped. To hear more about how people have resolved this dilemma, read on: Chapter 7 is devoted to the issues involved in coming to accept a long-term program of medications.

7

Coming to Terms with Your Medications

Accusing me of mania, my elder sister's voice has an odd manic quality. "Are you taking your medicine?" A low controlled mania, the kind of control in furious questions addressed to children, such as "Will you get down from there?" ...

As if by going off lithium I could erase the past, could prove it had never happened, could triumph over and contradict my diagnoses; this way I would be right and they would be wrong. It had always been the other way; they were right and I was wrong. Of course I had only to take the lithium in order to be accepted back ... on lithium I would be "all right." ... But I am never all right, just in remission. If I could win this gamble. ...

—KATE MILLET, *The Looney Bin Trip* (1990, p. 32)

The nature of bipolar disorder is such that even when you feel better, you still have an underlying biological predisposition to the illness. This predisposition requires you to take medication even when you're feeling well. Often, though, when you feel better, you will be tempted to stop your medication, because you won't see the need for it. That's an understandable reaction. Unfortunately, stopping your medications against medical advice—and sometimes even just taking inadequate dosages or missing dosages regularly—puts you at a much higher risk of having a recurrence of your bipolar disorder. In my experience, people are most likely to consider stopping their medications once they have recovered from a manic or depressive episode. During this phase they may feel good or even hypomanic, but are more in control of their moods than during the height of their illness. Taking medication feels like spoiling a good party. These reactions are especially true of younger people who have had only a few episodes. Inconsistency with medication sometimes stems from feelings of youthful invulnerability or just plain denial of the disorder. But I have also worked with middle-aged and older adults who have had many, many bipolar episodes and still doubt that they need medication, even if they do acknowledge having the disorder. Understandably, they want to know what life would be like without the pills. They may also be worried about the long-term effects of medications on their kidneys or metabolic systems.

In the last chapter, I discussed the various drug treatments available to people with bipolar disorder. In this chapter, let's consider the various reasons that people with bipolar disorder give for discontinuing their drug regimens. Many of these reasons have been offered by my own clients, including those who have been stable for quite some time but question whether the medication is really working. Sometimes the issues surrounding inconsistency or *nonconcordance* are related to feelings or beliefs about the disorder, such as disagreeing with the diagnosis or missing the pleasure of the high periods. Inconsistency can also be a response to unpleasant side effects (for example, weight gain on divalproex), difficulty relating to a particular physician, or dislike of having one's blood drawn. Sometimes people just forget to take their medicine. People also go off medications because of practical matters like prescriptions that lapse (and difficulties getting a new one) and the high costs of paying for medications (for example, see Keck et al., 1997; Lewis, 2000).

In this chapter, I offer some tips for making medications feel more acceptable to you if you're having doubts, as well as ideas for discussing side effects with your physician, so that you can get the greatest possible benefit (and the least possible pain) from treatment. You may recognize your own experiences in the illustrations of issues that people commonly struggle with when trying to accept a long-term program of medications.

What Is Medication Concordance?

Concordance with medication is "a congruence between the plan made with the physician and the plan carried out by the patient" (Sachs, 2000). *Nonconcordance* means that you have not followed the physician's recommendations in taking your medications or have stopped altogether, against his or her advice. But people can become nonconcordant in any number of ways. For example, some people take their medications correctly for several weeks and then stop all of them abruptly. Some stop only one medication in a "cocktail" of medications: they are on lithium, divalproex, and quetiapine and decide to discontinue everything but the divalproex (and sometimes even take a higher dosage of this medication than prescribed). Other people drop their dosages or take medications intermittently (for example, take only half of their recommended olanzapine tablets, miss their evening dosages, skip Saturday nights). For others, nonconcordance takes the form of substituting unproven remedies (for example, medicinal herbs like St. John's wort or omega-3 fatty acids) for mood stabilizers, or trying to use alcohol or marijuana to control their mood states.

Why the term *concordance*? Many alternative terms have been proposed in the medical literature, the most common of which are *adherence* and *compliance*. In my experience, persons with bipolar disorder don't usually like either of those terms. *Nonadherence* feels either critical or judgmental or is associated in the mind with tape or glue (one patient asked, "What am I? A Post-It note?"). It implies that the person with the disorder is unwilling or unable to stick to an agreed-on program. Even worse is the term *noncompliance,* which implies a paternalistic stance: the client with bipolar disorder is *not going along with* what others insist that he or she must do.

I prefer the term *concordance* because it underlines the importance of the alliance between the physician and the person with bipolar disorder. Stopping medications or taking them inconsistently can often be attributed, in part, to the physician, who may not have articulated the purposes of the various medications in the regimen, may not have alerted you to the possible side effects, or may not have been understanding or respectful, or communicated a sense of caring for your individuality.

How Common Is Nonconcordance?

Frequently, people with bipolar disorder discontinue their medications. Estimates vary, but the consensus seems to be that more than half of those with bipolar disorder quit taking their medications at some point in their lives (Colom et al., 2005). A study by Stephen Strakowski and colleagues at the University of Cincinnati College of Medicine (1998) found that 59% of patients with mood disorder were "partially nonadherent" (took medications inconsistently) or "fully nonadherent" (quit taking them altogether) during the year after their first hospitalized episode. You are more likely to be nonconcordant if you are male; younger rather than older; had an early age of illness onset (i.e., teen or preteen years); have rapid cycling of episodes; have been hospitalized recently; are prone to alcohol or substance abuse disorders or comorbid anxiety disorders; and lack a supportive family structure, a spouse, or friends to rely on (Goodwin & Jamison, 2007; Perlis et al., 2010).

Not all medications are associated with the same rate of nonconcordance. For example, Roger Weiss and colleagues (1998) found that only 21% of people with bipolar disorder who were taking lithium were consistent with it all the time. The rate was 50% among people taking divalproex (Depakote), possibly because its side effects are easier to tolerate. In the Systematic Treatment Enhancement Program for Bipolar Disorder, in which people were taking a variety of mood stabilizers and atypical antipsychotics in many different outpatient settings, the rate of consistency was over 75% (Perlis et al., 2010).

People with bipolar disorder are not the only ones who have trouble accepting a long-term program of medication. Those with diabetes, heart disease, hypertension, glaucoma, or any other chronic medical condition that requires ongoing pharmaco-therapy are up against the same challenge you are. People are even inconsistent with taking antibiotics and birth control pills! You're not alone in this type of struggle.

What Are the Consequences of Nonconcordance?

People with bipolar disorder are often told to take medications without being given compelling reasons for doing so or a full understanding of what might happen if they don't. *The main reason that stopping your medications is inadvisable is that it is associated with a high risk of recurrence.* It also greatly increases the risk of suicide. In fact, not taking medications as prescribed is the greatest single factor contributing to when and how often people with bipolar disorder have recurrences (Colom et al., 2000). As Jamison (1995) explains in *An Unquiet Mind*: "That I owed my life to pills was not, however, obvious to me for a long time; my lack of judgment about the necessity to take lithium proved to be an exceedingly costly one" (p. 89).

When medications are discontinued very abruptly (which is usually the case), the chances of relapsing—or of committing suicide—are higher than when medica-tions are discontinued slowly (Suppes et al., 2000; Tondo & Baldessarini, 2000). It will take a while before your medication reaches a stable blood level if you stop suddenly and then restart. If you take medicines inconsistently, you can also end up with inadequate blood levels that lead to the same negative results.

Many people want to go on "drug holidays," thinking that if they get worse, they can always go back on the drug and return to normal—just like that. Because the consequences of discontinuing medications are not always immediate (that is, you can temporarily feel better after stopping your medications), you may feel that you are in the clear and can go on living your life without them. Unfortunately, your good feelings can be due to the hypomania that often develops shortly after medication is withdrawn. This hypomania is often the first stage in the evolution of a serious manic episode.

If you go off a drug such as lithium and then have a relapse of your illness, there is a very real possibility that you won't respond as well when you resume taking it. In fact, starting and stopping medications can lead to a pattern of continuous cycling in which illness episodes beget other illness episodes, and the periods of feeling well between periods of illness get shorter and shorter (the "kindling effect"; Post & Leverich, 2006). On the positive side, getting medical treatment early in the course of your disorder (that is, when it is first diagnosed) and staying with it can prevent these patterns of continuous cycling.

Why Do People Stop Taking Their Medications—and Why Should You Resist Doing So?

Ethan, a 19-year-old man, had his first manic episode while a student at a state university. He became belligerent, inappropriately sexual, giddy, and grandiose, claiming that his artwork and writing were soon to make him millions. His thoughts raced and he became hyperverbal. He was given lithium and an antipsychotic medication while an inpatient at the university's hospital. He showed a partial response but was still hypomanic when he returned to his parents' house after dropping out of school. He abruptly stopped his medications without telling his parents. He sank into a deep depression, marked by insomnia, lethargy, slowed thinking, suicidality, and thoughts such as "I suck ... I don't deserve to live ... I've done nothing for anyone in this universe." He eventually agreed to see a therapist, rather than a psychiatrist, under the proviso that "whoever he is needs to know that I'm philosophically and spiritually opposed to medications of any sort."

Ethan did not rule out the possibility that he had bipolar disorder. He made it clear, however, that the therapist should address Ethan's individual struggles with identity, sexuality, moral values, and family relationships, rather than treating him as a "manic–depressive case." The therapist spent a number of sessions developing an alliance with Ethan and helping him understand the onset of the depression from two standpoints: its psychosocial triggers (events in college, such as rejection by his girlfriend) and its biological and genetic bases, including a history of suicide and bipolar disorder in his maternal grandfather. The therapist did not challenge the idea that Ethan's depression was "existential and spiritual" but gradually introduced the notion that it might have a chemical basis as well. His father and stepmother were brought in for conjoint educational sessions where the treatment options were discussed and Ethan explained his position. Over the next 2 months, Ethan's mood improved somewhat, but he remained moderately depressed and complained of insomnia.

After he and Ethan had developed a solid alliance, the therapist reintroduced the idea of trying lithium. Ethan agreed to try it again for an agreed-upon interval (3 months). The therapist referred Ethan to a psychiatrist who took time to develop a rapport with him and listen to his story. The psychiatrist recommended he try lithium at 1,200 mg. Ethan responded quickly: his depression lifted, his suicidal thoughts disappeared, and his sleep improved.

After 6 months of twice-weekly individual plus family therapy, and regular maintenance lithium treatment, he decided to return to college. Despite initially planning to discontinue it "as soon as I'm on my own," he remained on lithium once back in college, where his treatment was managed by a doctor at the student health service. Contact with the therapist several years later revealed that his mood disorder was stable, he remained in school, and he was still taking lithium.

Accepting a program of pharmacotherapy to treat bipolar disorder is a long-term commitment and thus a very important personal decision. Naturally you will have questions. If you have just been diagnosed with bipolar disorder or are at an early point in its course, questions about committing to a medication regimen may be particularly salient for you, as they were for Ethan. But you may have strong feelings about medications even if you have been taking mood stabilizers for a long time. In this section, I discuss some of the reasons people stop taking their medications, and some counterarguments to consider if you find yourself agreeing with these reasons.

"I Miss My High Periods"

"Does a fish know when it's wet? Hypomania felt good to me. I felt like I was finally getting there in my life. It didn't feel at all like there was anything wrong to me, it felt great, and I'd been feeling bad for so long. So I went off my medication, and then I started getting higher and higher. People told me to go back on, but it felt patronizing. I resented their lack of recognition that I was accomplishing things. I told them, 'You don't understand, you've got me in a box, you're sticking me in one of your categories.' But then I cycled into a depression and got suicidal. I went back to my doc and—wouldn't you know it?—back on lithium."

> —A 38-year-old man with bipolar I disorder, reviewing his most recent mood cycle

The high periods of bipolar disorder, especially if they are accompanied by euphoria and grandiosity, feel quite good. When in this state you feel productive, driven, on top of things, cheerful, and invulnerable. Who wouldn't enjoy this state, and why spoil it with pills?

One of my clients compared mania to being in love. When people fall in love, it can resemble mania: you feel giddy, happy, and driven, and you sleep less; you feel more confident, attractive, and sexual; you want to talk to more people and do more things. My client said, "If you were in love, and someone came along with a tablet that would cure you of the feeling, where would you tell that person to go?"

Not everyone experiences mania as a happy state. It can also be a wired, pressured, irritable state. But even when people experience mania negatively, they resent the idea that their moods are under the control of a substance. As I've said in earlier chapters, no one likes the feeling of being under the control of another person or thing, and in my experience people with bipolar disorder are particularly sensitive to this issue. They often have a love–hate relationship with their moods: they hate the fact that their moods fluctuate so wildly, and particularly resent the lows, but mood variations are also central to who they are and how they experience life.

There is no mincing words about it: mood stabilizers do take away the high periods. When people take lithium or any of the other mood stabilizers or an atypical antipsychotic, their moods become more stable. Some people complain that they are too stable. Stability puts you in the driver's seat and gives you actual control over your fate rather than the illusion of control that mania gives you. *But stability also means giving up the intensity of the roller-coaster ride that bipolar disorder provides.* In other words, taking medicines can mean increased stability at the cost of the exciting, positive features of the disorder.

Nonetheless, the excitement and drama of the high periods often bring debilitating depressions in their wake. The 38-year-old man just quoted experienced an almost immediate crash after his mania crested. This is also true if you have the bipolar II form of the disorder: even if your hypomania is not particularly destructive in itself, preventing hypomanic episodes can help prevent the severe depressions that often follow (see Chapter 9).

"I Feel Fine Now, So Why Do I Need Medicine?"

Many people with bipolar disorder realize that they need medications when they're cycling into an episode, but don't see the need for prophylaxis—the use of medications when they're healthy to *prevent* future episodes. When their manic or depressive episode has resolved, they wonder, "Why should I keep taking medications and dealing with the side effects?" Some people think of mood stabilizers in the same way they might think of painkillers: You take them only when you're hurting, and you stop taking them once the pain disappears. It's the same logic people (like me) use when they're on diets. Once they have met their initial goal of losing, say, 15 pounds, they see no reason to continue dieting, even though continuing to diet is the key to weight maintenance.

This confusion is understandable, but remember one of the key points in Chapters 5 and 6: people with bipolar disorder have underlying biological predispositions that require them to take medicine on an ongoing basis for preventative purposes. There is no guarantee that you'll be free of episodes even if you do take mood stabilizers or antipsychotics. But the chances that you'll remain well over long periods and have less severe episodes are greatly improved.

"Medications Take Away My Creativity"

One of the most fascinating aspects of bipolar disorder is its association with artistic creativity. Many famous artists, writers, poets, and musicians probably had bipolar disorder or a variant of it. Examples may include Sylvia Plath, Anne Sexton, Robert Lowell, Ernest Hemingway, Delmore Schwartz, Vincent van Gogh, and Ludwig van Beethoven. Jamison (1993) has written extensively about this issue in her book *Touched with Fire: Manic–Depressive Illness and the Artistic Temperament.* I can also recommend a thorough review of the studies in this area by University of Iowa psychiatrist Nancy Andreasen (2008).

The link with creativity can put the person with bipolar disorder in a bind. What if you pride yourself on your writing, artistic talent, or musical ability and fear that taking medicines will destroy your creative output? If having mood swings can improve the quality of your art by investing it with emotion and passion, why take these away? Does mood-stabilizing medication actually interfere with creativity? Not many research studies have been done, and most are case studies that have examined a select group of artistic people to observe what effect lithium had on their work. None of these studies on creativity involve people on anticonvulsants or atypical antipsychotics, so we don't know if those medications are better or worse.

Do people with bipolar disorder become more creative when they stop their medications? The literature does not provide a clear answer to this question, at least where lithium is concerned. Shaw and colleagues (1986) found that people with bipolar disorder did better in "associational processing" (producing a creative stream of ideas) when they were off lithium than on it. Kocsis and associates (1993) tested 46 people with bipolar disorder who were on long-term lithium treatment. They found that patients' scores on memory, associative productivity, and motor speed (finger tapping) improved once they went off lithium. The people who improved the most on these measures were those who had the highest levels of lithium in their bloodstream before going off the drug, suggesting that higher dosages may lead to more interference with mental functioning.

> **Effective treatment:** Most professionals believe that people with bipolar disorder do better in their art, music, or writing when they're in remission from their disorder, or perhaps slightly hypomanic but not fully manic or depressed.

What do these findings mean for people who have artistic talent? First, lithium can have effects on your cognitive or motor performance, but it isn't at all certain that it interferes with your creativity. In fact, the opposite may be true. Among eminent writers, the bipolar II form of the disorder (depression with hypomania) is more common than the full bipolar disorder, suggesting that milder manic states may be more clearly linked to creativity than full manic states (Carreno & Goodnick, 1998). If you have bipolar I disorder, reducing severe manic symptoms with medications may enhance your creativity (Andreasen, 2008). In this sense, medication may even be helpful to your work if it successfully controls your more severely manic swings.

If you do think that your lithium or your anticonvulsant is affecting your creativity, talk to your doctor about reducing the dosage before you decide to go off it. Perhaps he or she will think it's safe for you to experiment with a lower dosage, especially if you have been stable for a while.

"Medications Give Me Unacceptable Side Effects"

As discussed in Chapter 6, all of the major mood stabilizers, antipsychotics, and antidepressants have side effects, which can range from the mild (for example, thirst on lithium) to the severe (toxic reactions, kidney clearance problems, rapid cycling, agranulocytosis). In many cases, medication side effects are transient and will disappear or at least become milder after you've been on the medication for a while. Other side effects are not so easy to ignore and can be continuous.

Many people go off their medicines because they find the side effects too unpleasant and disruptive. This is also true when people are prescribed medications for traditional medical conditions. Blood pressure medications, for example, can make people fatigued. Allergy medications can make people feel sleepy or "dried up." Even natural or herbal substances have side effects. For example, St. John's wort, once touted as an alternative antidepressant, can give you stomachaches, make you sun sensitive, and, if not taken alongside a mood stabilizer, cause switches into mania (Nierenberg et al., 1999).

Taking a medication is a cost–benefit decision. There are clearly benefits to mood stabilizers and atypicals. But they also have costs, including side effects and actual financial outlays (see the self-rated cost–benefit exercise at the end of this chapter). Most people with bipolar disorder, if able to weigh the costs and benefits objectively, come down on the side of continuing to take their medications, especially if they've been through some painful mood disorder episodes. But that doesn't mean you should have to live with terrible medication side effects as a trade-off for health and mood stability.

Effective treatment: Managing your side effects should be a collaborative process between you and your physician.

First, don't try to adjust your medications on your own. Instead, keep a record of which side effects you experience each day, and tell your physician about them. The exercise on page 142 will help you organize your thoughts about which side effects you experience from which medications. Copy the completed record, bring it to your next medication visit, and go over it with your doctor.

Ask your physician what can be done to control your side effects. Many can be managed with a simple dosage adjustment (for example, dropping the number of lithium tablets so that you feel less sluggish mentally) or by taking your pills in different dosing patterns. For example, if you take lithium in one dose rather than several, you may have less need to urinate frequently. If you take the extended-release form of divalproex (Depakote ER), you may have less gastrointestinal distress. Other side effects can be controlled with additional side-effect medications. For example, hand tremors or migraine headaches can be helped by adding a beta-blocker, propranolol (Inderal), to your medication regimen. The hair thinning associated with divalproex can sometimes be managed with zinc or selenium supplements.

Your doctor may also decide to switch you to another medication entirely. For example, if you have problems with memory or motivation on lithium, he or she may switch you to divalproex, which is less likely to produce these side effects (Malhi et al., 2009). If you have problems with weight gain on divalproex, then lamotrigine, carbamazepine, or one of the more weight-neutral atypical antipsychotics (ziprasi-

Keeping Track of Your Side Effects

Date/day of week	Medications taken	Dosage	Side effects experienced*

Weight at beginning of week _193_   End of week _190_

9-16-2014

Examples: dry mouth, urinating frequently, rash, acne, stomachaches, insomnia, headaches, fatigue, hair loss, problems with concentration, hand tremor. If you're not sure which medication causes which side effect, simply list each side effect you experience and put a question mark (?) next to each one.

done, aripiprazole) may be alternatives for you. New drugs for bipolar disorder are being developed all the time, and it may be that easily tolerated medications that work just as well as lithium, divalproex, or lamotrigine will eventually become available.

The decision to switch medications will not be made solely on the basis of your side effects, of course. Hopefully, this decision will come out of a discussion between you and your physician concerning the pros and cons of certain medications from the vantage point of effectiveness versus adverse effects.

You may feel angry at your doctor if you feel he or she should have alerted you ahead of time to the side effects you're experiencing. Your anger is understandable, but keep in mind that he or she may not be able to predict your particular profile of adverse effects ahead of time. If you are feeling angry, discuss this with your doctor rather than not showing up for your next session. There is little he or she can do to help you if you aren't coming in on a regular basis.

> **Effective solution:** Side effects represent a problem for which there are solutions other than simply stopping your medicines. Informing your doctor on a regular basis about your side effects will help the doctor consider and discuss with you the alternatives to your treatment plan.

"Taking Medications Is a Sign of Personal Weakness, Sickness, and Lack of Control"

"For me, it's all about control. I have always had trouble with authority figures, and medication feels like just one more authority figure. Someone comes along and says, 'Here, just take this salt and you'll feel better and be like the rest of us.' I think it's garbage, and it makes me realize the person doesn't know me very well. I can handle things by myself just fine, thank you."
—A 19-year-old man shortly after his hospitalization for mania

Many people feel that taking medicines is a sign of personal weakness. It feels like admitting that you're sick, defective, or mentally ill. Certainly, taking medications daily can remind you of your troubles and make you resent the illness even more than you do already. But many people take this perspective further and claim that they can get along without medications just by exerting self-control. If you are in a hypomanic phase, you're particularly likely to feel this way. Unfortunately, bipolar disorder cannot be controlled by sheer willpower. Neither can other biologically based illnesses.

There are many ways to think about control. In some people's minds, control is about not needing help from anyone or anything. For others, control means availing yourself of opportunities to further your life goals. It is true that taking a medicine now means giving up a certain amount of control in the short run. But taking care of yourself in this way can also give you more control in the long run. Achieving mood stability on an ongoing basis translates into a greater likelihood of staying out of the hospital, not having to schedule so many doctor visits, saving money on additional treatments, being able to plan ahead for things you want to do, enjoying better family and romantic relationships, and leading a more productive work life. In other words, *taking medications can give you the kind of control you crave, rather than eliminating it. Not taking medications, in contrast, can mean giving up control if it leads to becoming ill again.*

Later chapters discuss self-management strategies such as sleep–wake monitoring, mood charting, cognitive restructuring, and coping with family stress. Implementing these behavioral strategies can contribute to your feeling of control over your fate. But these strategies will work much better if you are being simultaneously protected by medications.

"Medication Carries a Stigma in Our Society"

Bipolar disorder carries much of the stigma that all forms of mental illness carry, and taking medication can become a proxy for this stigma. You may worry about what employers, friends, and romantic partners will think if they know you're on mood stabilizers.

This is not an easy issue, and it is a very real concern for many people. There may be jobs you can't take because of being on medication (for example, a job that requires fine motor control over your hands). Employers' reactions upon learning of an employee's disorder have been known to range from complete sympathy to finding ways to fire the person (although such discrimination is illegal, as discussed in Chapter 13). But the situation is improving. My impression, especially over the last 20 years, has been that our society is becoming more and more understanding of the biological bases of psychiatric disorders and the need for psychiatric medications. More and more writers, movie celebrities, and public figures are admitting to being on mood stabilizers and antidepressants. Few people would reflexively dump a potential romantic partner or employee simply because that person admits to taking mood stabilizers or antidepressants.

Of course, you are not obliged to tell your employer or other significant people in your life about your mood disorder or its treatments. You may also want to be selective in what you tell them. As I discuss in Chapter 13, there are constructive ways to educate others about your need for medications so that the stigma is minimized.

"The Medications Don't Work"

Some people with bipolar disorder complain that their medication is just not effective. They wonder why they should take one or more mood stabilizers when they don't feel that the medication is really controlling their symptoms, but they still have to deal with the side effects.

The reality is that your bipolar disorder is only partially controllable by medicines (see Chapter 6). But almost everyone with the disorder does better on medication than off it. You will continue to experience mood fluctuations on mood stabilizers, but if you examine the course of your illness carefully, you'll probably find that there has been some improvement. Keeping a mood chart (Chapter 8) will help you determine how your medicines are affecting your sleep and moods in a relatively objective way.

A question to ask yourself is "Is my medication truly ineffective, or does it just not work as well as I would like it to?" Depending on your answer, you may want to discuss the matter with your doctor. It is possible—especially if you are trying mood stabilizers for the first time—that you are not improving as much as you could, and you should not hesitate to tell your doctor if that is what you believe. He or she may agree with you and suggest a different mood stabilizer or various adjunctive medications to enhance your current regimen (Chapter 6).

Try to be objective about whether there has been any improvement. Ask relatives for their opinions about the impact of the medication on your functioning. They may have seen effects that you aren't aware of (for example, being less easily provoked to anger, smiling more often, being less irritated by changes in your environment, seeming like your old self). Sometimes the benefits aren't as straightforward as mood stability. For example, Neil, age 18, did not think that his quetiapine had any effect on his moods. He did believe, however, that he was getting along better with his parents and friends since starting it.

"My Problems Are Psychological, Not Biological"

If you feel that your problems are only of a psychological origin (for example, related to childhood trauma or disturbed family relationships, problems relating to authority figures), then it may not be obvious to you what role medication has in your treatment. You may feel that your underlying vulnerabilities have more to do with a negative view of yourself than to biological or genetic factors.

Take another look at Chapter 5, in which I talk about the vulnerability–stress model. Psychological stress, such as interpersonal or family conflicts or loss experiences, can interact with a person's biological and psychological vulnerabilities (for example, a low opinion of your intellect or your abilities). This is one of the reasons we recommend medications and psychotherapy *in combination*, rather than as substitutes for each other. Remember, your problems needn't be biological *or* psychological. They can be both.

Medications may actually make your psychotherapy more successful. Most psychotherapists say that they can't accomplish much when a person with bipolar disorder is in a severely depressed, manic, or mixed state. If medicines make your mood stable, or at least stable enough that you can make it to regular appointments and carry through on homework assignments, you'll benefit a great deal more from the psychotherapy. You'll be able to deal more productively with the underlying issues that may be contributing to your unhappiness or distress.

"Taking Medications Means I'm Giving in to My Parents (or My Spouse)"

"I'm a product of what I learned from my parents, but I've also learned things from other people, in college, after college, in various work situations, in relationships, and from the hard knocks of life. If I go on lithium, it can't be their decision. Whether I go back on it, when I go back, how much I go back on it, and who will be my doctor are all things I've got to decide by myself. If they make the decision for me, even if I agree with it, I won't be able to follow through."

—A 23-year-old woman with bipolar I disorder

As this woman says, and as Kate Millet says in the quote at the beginning of this chapter, taking medications can mean feeling like you're giving in to your family's demands. If you are a young adult and live with your parents, you can quickly get tired of hearing them nag you to take your pills, interpret your emotional responses to everyday things as signs that you need more medicine, or remind you that you're the sick one in the family. You may believe that others in the family also have the disorder and that they should be the ones taking medicines, not you.

Most people want independence from their parents. Taking medications can feel like giving up your independence: Swallowing pills, seeing doctors, and getting your blood level tested may feel like you are under your parents' thumb. The reality is that taking medications, while perhaps initially reflecting your acquiescence to your parents' plans, greatly increases your chances of independence from them later. If your mood is stable, there is a greater chance that you'll be able to function away from home. But it's hard to take this long-term view when taking pills makes you feel like you're a child again.

If you're married or partnered, you may have the same feelings about your spouse. Your spouse may be taking a hard line with you; some of my clients' spouses have even threatened to leave if their partner didn't remain consistent in taking his or her medications. Your spouse's insistence that you take your pills can make the option feel all the more unappealing to you.

How do people resolve this dilemma? Many of my clients have eventually come around to realizing the necessity of mood stabilizers not only for their own mood stability but also for their relationships with their family members. But it is important that you feel the decision to take the medicine is largely your own.

Perhaps even more important, try to make a distinction between the way you feel about your medicine and the way everyone else seems to feel about it. Do you

> **Effective solution:** Chapter 13 gives you some tips on how to communicate with family members on problems related to your illness, including how to negotiate the sometimes volatile issue of taking medications.

think the medication helps you, even if it's less than you'd like? Does taking medicine have to mean feeling like a child? If so, what do we make of the many successful people who have had this illness and taken mood stabilizers? Many of my clients have reported feeling better about taking medicines once they began to view drug treatment as important for maintaining their health status and furthering their personal life goals. Some have made the transition from engaging in power struggles with their parents or spouse to taking more responsibility for managing their own drug treatment (for example, keeping to the regular dosing schedule so that reminders from others become unnecessary, monitoring their side effects, arranging their own doctor visits and blood tests). This transition helped them feel that medications were less of a threat to their independence and sense of identity.

"I Can't Remember to Take My Medications"

This is a very real problem and one that physicians often underestimate. In fact, one factor that predisposes people with bipolar disorder to nonconcordance is having to remember a greater number of medication dosages (Keck et al., 1997). Sometimes people forget whether they have taken a morning or an afternoon dosage, and then end up taking an extra dose in the evening, which can increase their chances of getting too much of a medication. Others mistakenly remember taking a tablet they haven't actually taken.

If you are using alcohol or street drugs regularly, including marijuana, you're going to have particular problems remembering to take your pills as prescribed. This is probably one of the reasons that substance abuse is so highly correlated with medication nonconcordance. If you are able to get your substance use problem under control (see Chapter 8), you'll have a much easier time remembering to take your medications. Also, the medications will almost certainly be more effective!

If you are having trouble remembering to take your tablets, ask your physician whether you can be given the medication in its least complex dosing pattern. Some medications, including lithium, can be taken all in one dosage. Sometimes the

> **Effective solution:** If you have trouble remembering to take your medications, try one of these devices:
>
> - pill boxes that divide up the day's doses
> - key chains with an attached container that holds one day's pills
> - alarms on cell phones or watches
> - Post-It notes next to your toothbrush or breakfast cereal

regimen can be simplified to morning and evening dosages only. Don't be ashamed of forgetting—it's a more common problem than you think.

Some people try to time their dosages around events that will "cue" them, like meals, or their morning or bedtime routines. Others keep spare pills in their desk drawers at work in case they forget to bring them. Still others acquaint their spouse with the medication routines and ask for reminders. If you are comfortable with your spouse taking this role, it may be helpful to you in staying on schedule.

In Chapter 8, on maintaining wellness, you'll be introduced to the daily self-rated mood chart. On the chart you'll see places to record the number of tablets of each medication you've taken. Keeping a daily mood chart will not only remind you to take your medicines but will also help you see the relation between your medication consistency and the stability of your mood states. One of my clients related the following: "Breakfast and medications were always connected for me. But then when I got my new job, I forgot to eat breakfast and also missed my morning medication dose—I took it to work with me and would completely forget about it. When my mood started dropping and I started keeping a mood chart, I discovered I wasn't taking my morning dose as frequently as I thought I was. Keeping track made me more conscious of remembering my morning dose and also helped me make breakfast more of a priority."

Summarizing the Pros and Cons of Medications: A Self-Rated Chart

After you've thought through some of the issues just discussed, it may be useful to summarize the costs and benefits of medications in your own terms. The exercise on pages 149–151 will help you organize your thinking about pros and cons and about things you can do to make medications feel more acceptable to you. You may want to copy this page and take it with you to your doctor's office—it can provide a format for discussing issues of concern to you. It may also be helpful to review this list if you have the impulse to discontinue your medications, to remind yourself of your reasons for taking them in the first place and the other alternatives available to you.

Try to individualize this exercise as much as possible: you may know of advantages and disadvantages of the medications that I have not listed here. Your family members may be able to help you identify the costs and benefits of your medicines.

■■

The decision to commit to a long-term program of medication is a very difficult one. As you can see from this chapter, people with bipolar disorder struggle with many practical and emotional issues when coming to terms with their need for medication. You are not alone in your struggles to accept the disorder and its required treatments.

The Pros and Cons of Taking Medications

REASONS TO TAKE MOOD MEDICATIONS

(*Examples:* helps control my manic symptoms, helps with my depressed mood, improves my sleep, makes me better able to focus, decreases my anxiety, improves the way I relate to other people, decreases my conflict with family members, improves my energy level, makes me feel more confident, helps me concentrate better at work, keeps me from spending too much money, helps me avoid traffic tickets)

1.

2.

3.

4.

5.

(*cont.*)

DISADVANTAGES OF MOOD MEDICATIONS

(*Examples:* side effects [give specifics], miss my high periods, cost of medications and psychiatry visits, dislike having my moods controlled, dislike my doctor, dislike making medical appointments, feel less sexual or less creative, medications carry a stigma, medications aren't that effective)

1.

2.

3.

4.

5.

(*cont.*)

THINGS I CAN DO TO IMPROVE THE SITUATION

(*Examples*: discuss side effects with physician, consider other medications or dosing strategies, take more responsibility for my own regimen, change my doctor, change my insurance plan, educate others about my disorder, create reminders to take my tablets, cut down my use of alcohol or drugs)

1.

2.

3.

4.

5.

New drugs for bipolar disorder are being developed and tested all the time. In all likelihood, some will prove successful and others will come into vogue for a while and then disappear. But there is good reason to believe that you will find a medication regimen that will work for you over the long term and won't require you to tolerate debilitating side effects.

Above all, remember the meaning of the term *concordance:* a collaborative process between you and your physician. It is very important to communicate your concerns to your physician and see if anything can be done to adjust your regimen so that it is maximally effective as well as more easily tolerated. Most physicians are open to this kind of communication and even welcome it, particularly if you talk to them before you decide to stop on your own or make your own decisions about changing your dosages. The exercises in this chapter can help you organize information about your drug treatment so that you can work with your physician more efficiently within the limited blocks of time that managed care allows.

Fortunately, managing bipolar disorder is not just about taking medications. In addition, there are self-management strategies you can use during periods of wellness (Chapter 8), when experiencing the beginning signs of mania (Chapter 9), and when depressed or suicidal (Chapters 10 and 11). Try to think of medication as one element in a collection of strategies for managing your disorder.

Part III

Practical Strategies for Staying Well

8

Tips to Help You Manage Moods and Improve Your Daily Life

Amy, age 33, had a 6-year history of bipolar disorder. Three years after being diagnosed, she began a period of rapid cycling that seemed to be provoked, in part, by an on-again, off-again relationship with her boyfriend. When she abruptly relocated out of state due to his business, her rapid cycling intensified. She obtained part-time work in her new city and sought psychiatric treatment. Her psychiatrist gave her a combination of lithium and divalproex (Depakote), which helped even out her cycles, but she still experienced unpleasant ups and downs. Her sleep was quite variable from night to night.

Her psychiatrist suggested that she supplement her medication treatment with therapy from a psychologist with whom she (the psychiatrist) worked. The psychologist encouraged Amy to start a mood chart, in which she kept track of her moods on a daily basis, the number of hours of sleep she had each night, her medications, and any events that she found stressful, whether positive or negative. At first she found this assignment to be a hassle. She told her therapist that it took time and she didn't like being reminded of her illness so frequently. Her therapist acknowledged the discomfort of the assignment but reminded her that tracking her moods was a first step toward gaining more control over them. After some discussion she agreed to try it but made no commitment to keeping the chart on a regular basis. Amy and her therapist began examining her charts during their weekly meetings. Over a period of several months, they began to identify certain behavioral patterns associated with Amy's mood swings. For example, Amy learned that her mixed mood states often began with a rejection by her boyfriend (such as being ignored or slighted by him in the company of others). Rather than directly confronting him about these experiences, she would usually go out drinking with her female friends that night or the next night. Her sleep would then become more disturbed, and her mood would take on an irritable, anxious quality. Her mood would usually stabilize once she had reestablished a regular bedtime and wake time.

She asked her friends whether they would feel any differently about her if she went out with them but didn't drink. None seemed particularly bothered by this. Although she did not stop drinking entirely, Amy did find that limiting her alcohol intake helped her sleep better, which in turn made her feel less irritable, anxious, and depressed the next day. She made clear to her therapist that she had no intention of giving up her "outrageous side." But with time, she has become more consistent with these lifestyle changes, pleasantly surprised by the beneficial effects they've had on her mood stability.

What can you do to maximize your intervals of wellness and minimize the time you spend ill? Many people go for long periods of time without having significant symptoms, but virtually everyone with the disorder has recurrences of their illness at some point. Research studies are telling us that the people who do the best over time are those who not only take their medications regularly and see their doctors but also successfully implement self-management strategies.

What does it mean to manage bipolar disorder successfully? In Chapter 5 we talked about the risk factors in bipolar disorder (things that make your illness worse). There are also protective factors: things that keep you well when you are vulnerable to mood swings. You are already familiar with some of these protective factors from earlier chapters—for example, consistency with your medications and having social supports.

In essence, maintaining wellness means minimizing the risk factors and maximizing the protective factors (see the table on page 157). Sometimes risk and protective factors are simply opposite sides of the same coin. For example, sleep deprivation is a risk factor, whereas staying on a regular sleep–wake rhythm is a protective factor. In other cases, protection involves introducing a new element into your daily life, such as keeping a mood chart.

Minimizing risk and maximizing protection will almost certainly improve the course of your illness and quality of life. But doing so can be difficult. It can require giving up things that you have come to depend on (for example, drinking alcohol to relax, staying up late at night). It will probably be impossible for you to avoid every risk factor and take full advantage of every protective factor in the table. For example, some people can scrupulously maintain their medication regimen and have learned to avoid alcohol but find it impossible to prevent sleep disruption.

> **Effective prevention:** *Know yourself.* If you know your strengths and limitations well, you may be able to decide which risk factors you can and cannot realistically avoid and which self-management strategies are possible to implement within your current lifestyle.

Risk and Protective Factors in Bipolar Disorder

Risk factors that increase your chances of becoming ill	
Risk factors	Examples
Stressful life changes	Loss of a job, gaining or losing a new relationship, birth of a child
Alcohol and drug abuse	Drinking binges; experimenting with cocaine, LSD, or Ecstasy; excessive marijuana use
Sleep deprivation	Changing time zones, cramming for exams, sudden changes in sleep–wake habits
Family distress or other interpersonal conflicts	High levels of criticism from a parent, spouse, or partner; provocative or hostile interchanges with family members or coworkers
Inconsistency with medications	Suddenly stopping your mood stabilizers; regularly missing one or more dosages

Protective factors that help keep you from becoming ill	
Protective factors	Examples
Observing and monitoring your own moods and fluctuation triggers	Keeping a daily mood chart or social rhythm chart
Maintaining regular daily and nightly routines	Going to bed and waking up at the same time; having a predictable social schedule
Relying on social and family supports	Clear communication with relatives; asking your significant others for help in emergencies
Engaging in regular medical and psychosocial treatment	Staying on a consistent medication regimen, obtaining psychotherapy, attending support groups

Others can keep relatively consistent daily and nightly routines but find it difficult to regulate their exposure to family stress or other interpersonal conflicts.

This chapter will acquaint you with practical self-management strategies that fall into four broad categories:

■ Tracking your mood with a daily chart

■ Maintaining regular routines and sleep–wake cycles

■ Avoiding alcohol and other mood-altering substances

■ Developing and maintaining social supports

The strategies you'll learn will be of most help when you are feeling well or experiencing only mild mood swings. They can also help protect you from more severe bipolar episodes. Throughout the chapter, I'll show you how other people with bipolar disorder have used these strategies in their daily lives and how they have avoided some of the pitfalls associated with implementing them. Chapters 9, 10, and 11 give you tools to use when you want to stop a developing manic, depressive, or suicidal episode from spiraling beyond your control.

Maintaining Wellness Tip No. 1: Keeping a Mood Chart

If you've been seeing a psychiatrist for a long time, you're probably familiar with some form of mood chart. If this is your first episode, your psychiatrist or therapist may not have introduced this assignment yet. A mood chart is simply a daily diary of your mood states, with dates indicating when these moods start and stop. The chart can also incorporate information about your sleep, medications, and life stressors.

Why should you keep a mood chart? First, becoming aware of even subtle changes in your mood and activity levels will help you recognize if you are having a mood disorder relapse and determine whether you should contact your doctor to see if a change in medication would be helpful. Many people with bipolar disorder have been able to catch their episodes early by observing the minor fluctuations on their mood charts, which often herald the onset of major manic, mixed, or depressive episodes. A picture is worth a thousand words!

Second, your doctor will find the chart useful, in that he or she will be able to see how well your medications are working or, alternatively, know when they are making you feel worse (such as when antidepressants bring about rapid cycling). He or she may also want to monitor symptoms other than mania or depression, such as your anxiety, sleep disturbance, or irritability.

Third, you can use your mood chart information to identify environmental triggers of your mood cycling, which can then lead to stress management strategies to lessen the impact of these triggers. With time and practice, many of my clients have become effective at identifying triggers, such as the onset of their menstrual cycle, arguments with particular family members, or work stress. Amy, for example, came to recognize through mood charting that conflicts with her boyfriend were a trigger for her mood cycling. She also found that her usual strategy for coping with distress—going out drinking—was contributing to her irritable mood states for several days later. This realization did not stop her from drinking altogether, but it did make her weigh the pros and cons of alcohol as a means of self-medicating her emotions.

The chart on page 159 was used in the National Institute of Mental Health (NIMH) Systematic Treatment Enhancement Program for Bipolar Disorder (Sachs et al., 2003). There is a blank version of this chart at the end of the book that you can copy for your own use, or you can download it from *www.manicdepressive.org*. The website also contains instructions for filling out the chart, which are provided below as well. Each chart allows you to track your moods for up to one month. So, if you have started the chart in the middle of the month, continue to use the same sheet until the middle of the next month and then begin a new sheet. In other words,

Mood Chart

Name Amy

TREATMENTS
(Enter number of tablets taken each day)

Month/Year August 2010

MOOD
Rate with 2 marks each day to indicate best and worst (if applicable)

0 = none
1 = mild
2 = moderate
3 = severe

___ mg	Antipsychotic ___ mg	___ mg	Antidepressant ___ mg	Anticonvulsant Depakote 1000mg	Benzodiazepine ___ mg	Lithium 1200mg	Verbal Therapy	Daily Notes	Irritability	Anxiety (circled)	Hours Slept Last Night	Depressed: Severe – Significant Impairment NOT ABLE TO WORK	Depressed: Mod. – Significant Impairment ABLE TO WORK	Depressed: Mild – Without significant impairment	WNL: MOOD NOT DEFINITELY ELEVATED OR DEPRESSED. NO SYMPTOMS. Circle date to indicate menses	Elevated: Mild – Without significant impairment	Elevated: Mod. – Significant Impairment ABLE TO WORK	Elevated: Severe – Significant Impairment NOT ABLE TO WORK	Psychotic Symptoms Strange Ideas, Hallucinations
				(4)		4		argument with Dad	1	1	7			×	1				
				4		4			1	1	6			×	2				
				4		4	√		0	0	8				× 3				
				4		4			0	0	6				× 4				
				4		4			0	0	6				× 5				
				4		4			0	0	6				× 6				
				4		4			0	0	6				× 7				
				4		4			0	0	6				× 8				
				4		4		boyfriend was rejecting	2	1	10			×	9				
				2		2		concert, stayed out until 3am	0	1	5				10		×		
				2		2			0	0	3				11		×		
				4		4			1	0	6				12	×			
				4		4			0	0	5				13	×			
				4		4	√		0	0	6				14	×			
				4		4			0	0	6				15	×			
				4		4		dog got sick, went to hospital	2	(2)	4			×	16	×			
				4		4			1	(2)	6			×	17	×			
				4		4			1	(2)	6			×	18	×			
				4		4			1	(2)	6			×	19	×			
				4		4			1	(2)	6			×	20	×			
				4		4	√	dog out of hospital	1	0	7			×	21				
				4		4			1	0	7			×	(22)				
				4		4			1	0	7			×	(23)				
				4		4			1	0	7			×	(24)				
				4		4			1	0	6			×	(25)				
				4		4			1	0	6			×	(26)				
				4		4			1	0	6			×	27				
				4		4	√		0	0	6				28				
				4		4			0	0	6				29				
				4		4		friend's wedding	1	0	5			×	30	×			
				4		4		cooking most of the day	1	0	5			×		×			
								Weight: 127											

Note. WNL = Within normal limits. Adapted by permission of Gary Sachs, MD (Copyright 1993).

Amy's Self-Rated Mood Chart.

"day 1" need not be the first of the month. It could be the 10th, and day 10 could be the 20th.

People with bipolar disorder find this to be a user-friendly method of recording the cycling of their moods over time, even though it looks intimidating at first. Once you get used to it, you can usually fill it out in a few minutes each day. I usually suggest that people keep the chart on an indefinite basis, but if this seems daunting, try it for a month or two to see if it proves useful. After that, you may decide to chart your moods in a different way (or your doctor may have another chart for you to use).

For now, let's consider Amy's mood chart, which she completed during a month in which she experienced significant mood fluctuations. Her "X" marks indicate her mood states on any given day. Notice that on some days she has made two ratings, one for mania and one for depression (her mixed mood states).

Amy identified some of the factors that contributed to her mood swings, including life events such as the illness of her dog. Her mood had been relatively stable (note the absence of peaks between the argument with her dad and the rejecting event with her boyfriend), but then she stayed out late at a concert and experienced a hypomanic period. By day 16 of the month, she'd had seven consecutive nights of poor sleep and began to experience mixed mood symptoms. Her medication was not changed during this interval, but she had been inconsistent with her regimen during days 10 and 11. So she identified four things that may have correlated with her mood shifts during this particular month: events involving her pet, problems with her boyfriend, sleep deprivation, and medication inconsistencies.

We don't know for sure whether these variables would have affected Amy's moods during a different month. This is one of the reasons it is important to keep the chart on an ongoing basis—to determine whether you have a predictable set *of mood triggers* (for example, arguments with family members, final exams, changing time zones, a specific pattern of sleep deprivation). Identifying mood triggers is an important step in gaining control over your moods, which you'll learn more about in this and subsequent chapters.

Step 1: Rating Your Mood Each Day

The first step in learning to fill out a mood chart is to become familiar with a numerical scale that corresponds to various levels of mood disturbance. The box on pages 161–162 gives you guidelines for making judgments about your daily mood, using a scale from −3 (severe depression) to +3 (severe mania). It gives examples of how people with bipolar disorder feel and think (and what they say) when they're in these various states. Not every example or descriptive label in the table need apply to you for you to be able to use the corresponding scale number. Rather, try to figure out which category of depression or elevation best describes how you feel on a given day.

Mood Descriptors

(0) *"WNL" (within normal limits).* This is your baseline: Your mood is not elevated or depressed, your energy level is normal for you, sleep is normal, and you're able to carry out your daily work and other tasks with little or no difficulty. You have no other obvious symptoms of your mood disorder.

Elevated Mood

(+1) *Mildly elevated.* You are feeling giddy, cheerful, or energized, or somewhat more irritable or anxious or nervous than usual, but you are not really impaired; you have more energy and more ideas, and you feel more self-confident but have been able to work effectively and relate normally to others. "I'm more restless/animated/talkative today than usual," "I'm making more phone calls," "I'm getting by with a little less sleep" (for example, 1 or 2 hours less than usual), "I'm more easily distracted today," "I'm snapping at people more," "I'm more frustrated by little things," "I'm somewhat revved up or wired," "My mind is clicking along a little faster," "I'm feeling sexier," "I'm more optimistic," "I'm hypomanic."

(+2) *Moderately elevated.* "High" or moderately manic; your mood is euphoric or very irritable and anxious, and people have told you it seems inappropriate; you feel like breaking things; you feel heavily goal driven and hypersexual and your thoughts are going very fast; you have significant difficulty focusing on your work; you are having run-ins with people (they seem to be moving and talking too slowly); people are complaining that you seem angry or grouchy or are moving way too fast; you have yelled at others inappropriately. You are sleeping as little as 4 hours per night and not feeling tired. "I'm feeling very impatient today," "I think I can get by with a lot less sleep," "I'm very preoccupied with sex," "My mind is working faster than ever," "I have so much to say and I hate being interrupted," "I'm feeling irritated, angry at everything."

(+3) *Severely elevated/manic.* Euphoric or aggressive; you are laughing constantly or your irritability is out of control; you have had loud verbal or physical fights with people; you feel like you are exceptionally talented or have special powers (for example, the ability to read people's minds, to change the weather); you are constantly moving about and cannot sit still; you cannot work or get along with others; you have gotten in trouble in public, have been stopped by the police, or have been taken to the hospital; you are sleeping little or not at all.

(cont.)

Mood Descriptors (*cont.*)

Depressed Mood

(–1) *Mildly depressed.* You are feeling slightly slowed down or sad; you have trouble keeping certain negative thoughts out of your head; you feel more self-critical; you want to sleep more or are having slight trouble falling or staying asleep, and you feel somewhat more fatigued than usual; you wonder if life is worth living; things don't seem as interesting as they usually do; you can still work effectively and are relating normally to others, even though you may feel less effective; your depression is not obvious to others.

(–2) *Moderately depressed.* You are feeling very sad, down in the dumps, hopeless, moderately slowed down, or uninterested in things for most of the day; you are sleeping more or having a lot of trouble falling asleep or staying asleep (for example, waking up regularly in the middle of the night); fewer and fewer things are of interest to you; you are ruminating a lot about current or past failings; you are feeling grouchy and irritable; you have significant difficulty getting your work done (missing days at work or school or being less productive); your concentration is impaired; others comment that you seem morose or slowed down or that you're speaking slowly; you have considered suicide and have thought of various methods.

(–3) *Severely depressed.* You feel deeply sad or numb; you have lost interest in almost everything; you are experiencing severe suicidal feelings: you wish to die or have made an attempt on your life; you feel extremely hopeless; you believe you have sinned terribly and should be punished; you can't work, concentrate, interact with others, or complete self-care tasks (for example, bathing, washing clothes); you stay in bed most of the day and/or cannot sleep and have severe problems with lack of energy.

Sources: Sachs and Lafer (1998); Williams (1988); Young et al. (1978).

Effective solution: If you are not sure your mood chart rating is reasonable, ask someone who knows you well (perhaps a family member or your partner) if he or she would agree with your rating on any given day.

Mood charting requires a bit of practice. You may be a person who is naturally able to judge for yourself whether you are feeling manic or depressed, and you may be easily able to describe the experience to others. Alternatively, the descriptive label *manic* or *depressed* may not fully capture the way you feel. If this is the case, take time to learn the mood chart and numerical scales and try to see if you can equate the terms used in the chart with your particular way of describing mood states. For example, *depressed* can mean the same thing as "crashed"; *elevated* can mean the same thing as "wired."

Practice by seeing if you can apply a mood descriptor to your mood today and yesterday, using the scale of −3 to +3. If you feel that your mood varies considerably during the day, make a "best" and a "worst" rating (for example, you may be at a −2 in the morning and a −1 or 0 by evening). If your mood has been both elevated and depressed on the same day, make two ratings, indicating the highest and lowest points.

In choosing your level, try to think about the least and most depressed or manic you've ever been in your life and determine where these states fit on the scale. For some people, the worst period ever might have been a −1; for others it might have been a −3. If your mood has never gone above or below a 2, use these as benchmarks for judging your mood today and throughout the week.

Compare your depression level today against that of a typical day (your baseline, or how you feel most of the time, which would rate a 0). Then compare your mood to other days when you felt blue or out of sorts but not impaired (−1), days when you have felt impaired but could still function with significant difficulty (−2), and, if applicable, days when you felt so down that you could not work at all or interact with others (−3). These comparisons should help you determine today's rating. Likewise, try to think of the most manic or hypomanic you've ever felt. If you were ever severely manic and in the hospital, your rating at that time would have been a +3.

If you have ever been elevated to the extent that you were having trouble functioning at work, your rating would be a +2. If you have been "wired" and "upbeat," but this state did not cause run-ins with others or make it difficult to sleep, a +1 (hypomanic) probably applies. In other words, think in terms of your own personal benchmarks.

Step 2: Recording Your Anxiety and Irritability

You'll notice that the mood chart also asks you to rate your anxiety and irritability levels on a 0–3 scale. There are two reasons to do this. First, anxiety and irritability can be the first signs of a new manic, mixed, or even depressive episode. Second, some medications may produce these symptoms as side effects (for example, the SSRI antidepressants). So, it's a good idea to track these symptoms, even if you're not sure how they are related to the cycling of your bipolar disorder.

Examples of "1" levels of irritability include feeling somewhat snappish or grumpy, but not to the extent that you can't function alongside people. A "2" would mean moderate irritability that causes problems for you at work or at home. A "3" would mean that you were severely irritable and angry to the extent that you were having real trouble functioning. People at a "3" are having physical altercations with others, are destroying property, or have been threatened with arrest. Likewise, a "1" anxiety rating would mean feeling mildly jittery, apprehensive, and perhaps scared but able to get along with minimal extra effort. A "2" would mean moderate anxiety that makes it difficult to work, read, socialize, or perform daily chores; however, you can still function with extra effort. A "3" would mean overt panic and severe, incapacitating anxiety.

Step 3: Recording Your Hours of Sleep

Along with your mood rating, make a daily rating of how many hours of sleep you had the previous night. If you're rating your mood for, say, Thursday, record the hours you slept from Wednesday night to Thursday morning. If your sleep is intermittent, try to estimate the actual number of hours you were asleep. Your recall of your prior night's sleep may be most accurate when you first wake up in the morning.

If you take naps regularly, separately recording nighttime and daytime sleep will allow you to investigate whether napping in the afternoon makes it harder to sleep that night or makes your mood worse by the end of the day.

After a week or more of doing this charting, you may begin to see how your sleep and mood are related. Many people are surprised at the result. Amy, for example, had always assumed that lack of sleep caused her to get more depressed, yet she found from her mood charting that sleep loss was more consistently associated with her hypomanic periods (note the shift on day 10 of her chart).

Step 4: Taking Daily Notes on Life Events and Social Stressors

If you feel that your mood has been influenced by one or more events or interactions with others, record these on your chart under "Daily Notes." Some of these may be significant (for example, breaking up with your partner, quitting your job), and others may seem minor (having a change in work hours; racing to the airport to catch a plane; getting stuck in a traffic jam). Record all events that you feel may be important, even if they seem as if they would be inconsequential for many people. For example, Amy found that even relatively routine quarrels with her father were associated with a mild drop in her mood (to a –1). The purpose here is to observe the connection between specific events and specific mood changes. When reviewing the day and filling out your chart, consider questions such as the following:

■ "What happened right before I last felt irritable or hypomanic?"

■ "What happened right after my irritable mood set in?"

■ "What happened right before my mood spiraled downward?"

When you're recording stressors, recall one issue raised in Chapter 5: it can be difficult to tell whether stress was the cause or the effect of your mood. Over time, mood charting may help you determine the timing of events in relation to changes in your mood. For example, did you race to the airport and then feel an increase in your energy level and mood, or were you feeling speedy before you raced to the airport? Did you get into an argument with your father and then feel down about yourself, or were you feeling down and irritable before you got into the argument? Don't worry for now if you're not sure which caused which. Instead, just try to identify the factors that coincide: stressful events, mood states, and sleep patterns.

The "Daily Notes" section is also a good place to record your alcohol or drug use. If you drank or smoked marijuana on a specific day, record that information as an event even if your intake seemed trivial (for example, "drank one beer" or "had a margarita"). Then you can observe for yourself whether, and to what degree, alcohol or marijuana use affects your mood the next day. You may also learn whether you are using substances, in part, to alleviate a negative mood state from the previous days or week.

Step 5: Recording Your Treatments

Record all of the medications and dosages you are supposed to take at the top of the left columns of the chart, including medications that are not specifically for your bipolar disorder (for example, blood pressure pills). In the boxes corresponding to the day of the month you're rating, record the number you actually took. This will help you, your physician, and other members of your treatment team know if inconsistencies in your use of medications are affecting your day-to-day mood. Amy missed her evening dosages on the night she went to the concert and the next evening as well, which probably contributed to her mood instability. As discussed in Chapter 7, most people miss a medication dosage once in a while, but it's important to keep track of these seemingly minor inconsistencies. Likewise, place a check mark next to any days when you attended a psychotherapy session. As with medication, some people are quite regular and others are quite irregular in their therapy attendance.

You may be taking some of your medications "as needed." For example, some people take a medication like clonazepam (Klonopin) only when they can't get to sleep. Indicate "as needed" on the top left column of your mood chart next to medications that fit this description. Some people find that their mood is lower on the day after they have taken an as-needed medication. Others find that certain as-needed medications (for example, the allergy medication pseudoephedrine) make them feel temporarily energized, wired, or hypomanic or interfere with their sleep.

Your physician will be able to use your medication records in a number of ways. Let's imagine that he or she has prescribed divalproex and an SSRI antidepressant. Let's also imagine that your chart indicates improvements in your mood a week or two after you started the SSRI, but then you began to report "roller-coastering" or rapid cycling of your emotions and energy levels. If all of this is documented on your chart, your physician may decide to discontinue the antidepressant or adjust your dosage as a way of stabilizing your mood.

Step 6: Recording Your Weight and Menses

Two other pieces of information will help round out your mood chart. First, record your weight at least once during the month. It's best to weigh yourself on the same day each month so that you can see whether your medication, stress, or mood cycling is connected with changes in your weight. If you are gaining weight on an atypical antipsychotic (for example, quetiapine [Seroquel]), your physician may choose to switch you to a different medication within the same class (for example, risperidone [Risperdal]) or adjust your dosage. If you are a woman, circle the days on which you had your period. You and your doctor may wish to examine whether your mood cycles begin before, during, or after the onset of your menses (also see Chapter 12).

Evaluating Your Mood Chart

Share your completed mood chart with your therapist or physician during each visit. Together, you can evaluate the influence of certain stressors on your mood, the influence of sleep disturbances, and the effects of various medications and your consistency with them. Even if you're not meeting regularly with your doctor or therapist, make a point of examining the chart at the end of each week to see if any patterns jump out at you. Keeping the chart over a year or more will enable you to develop longer-range hypotheses about which biological or social factors are provoking shifts in your mood (for example, periods of greater alcohol or marijuana use, the onset of winter or spring, the Christmas holidays, periods of increased work or school stress).

Problems with Mood Charting

Mood charting can feel reductionistic: it does not do justice to the many varied experiences you have on a daily basis. It is also very present-focused. Some people feel that their mood shifts are related to factors that can't be recorded easily on the chart (for example, traumatic events in the recent past or in childhood). Even with these limitations, however, mood charting is a very efficient way of summarizing a great deal of information very succinctly for yourself and your doctor. If you are using mood charting as a supplement to your personal psychotherapy, think of it as a point of departure for exploring larger issues that affect your mood. For example, events such as minor disagreements with a partner can have profound effects on your mood if they trigger fears of separation or loss. You may wish to explore these larger issues with your therapist.

Mood charting can also be difficult to remember to do every day. Try to pick one time each day to complete your chart and stick to this time on a day-to-day basis. Some people fill it out right before getting ready for bed; others tie mood charting to a specific daily activity (for example: just after finishing dinner, after walking the dog, before watching the evening news). Avoid choosing the worst moment of the day to fill out the chart if that moment does not represent how you've felt for the whole day. So if you usually feel quite unhappy when you first wake up but feel better within half an hour or so, pick another, more representative time of day. Avoid trying to fill out a month's worth of mood charts just before your doctor appointments, as people sometimes do. The more accurate the information you convey to your doctor, the better the treatment decisions you and your doctor can make.

> **Effective solution:** Try these tips to get the most out of your mood charts:
>
> ■ Fill out the chart at the same time every day to make it a habit.
> ■ Don't pick the worst moment of your day.
> ■ Don't try to fill out days' worth of charts right before your doctor appointments.

Maintaining Wellness Tip No. 2: Maintaining Regular Daily and Nightly Routines

> *"I really feel that I benefited from psychoanalysis. I was in it four times a week. But I don't think it was all that learning about my childhood. There was something very therapeutic about getting on the subway and having a place to go to in the morning, seeing the same therapist every day, seeing the same attendant in the parking lot, getting back in my car at the same time ... I found all of that structure very comforting."*
>
> —A 40-year-old woman with bipolar II disorder

In Chapter 5, I discussed the beneficial effects on your mood of external "time keepers" and the potentially negative effects of events or social demands that disrupt your daily routines and sleep–wake cycles. *Actively maintaining daily and nightly routines is one of the most important behavioral changes you can undertake— aside from regularly taking your medications—to help keep you in the driver's seat in managing your disorder.* In this section, I discuss the *social rhythm stability* approach to maintaining wellness.

Keeping a Social Rhythm Chart

The Social Rhythm Metric (SRM) is a more time-consuming device than the mood chart, but it is also potentially more informative (Monk et al., 1990). In this chart, you keep track of when you eat, sleep, exercise, and socialize, and make ratings of your daily mood. With time, you can work on stabilizing your daily routines as a means of stabilizing your mood. This involves planning your regular activities for predictable times of the day or night.

The SRM was developed as a central part of Ellen Frank and David Kupfer's work on interpersonal and social rhythm therapy (IPSRT). As discussed in Chapter 6, Frank and her colleagues have shown that the combination of IPSRT and pharmacotherapy is effective in improving the course of bipolar disorder (Frank et al., 2005). I was trained in Frank's social rhythm therapy approach some years ago and have become convinced of the value of daily rhythm tracking and stabilization for persons with bipolar disorder.

The purpose of social rhythm tracking is to allow you to discover the relationship between changes in your daily routines, levels of interpersonal stimulation, sleep–wake cycles, and mood. Over several weeks or months, you will begin to see certain patterns emerge (as Amy did). For example, you may find that changes in your activity levels or sleep patterns presage the development of new episodes. In the beginning phases of mania you may observe a gradual decrease in the time you spend sleeping and an increase in the time you spend exercising. Likewise, you may find that as you recover from a manic or depressive episode, your activity and sleep patterns naturally go back to the way they were before you became ill. In other words, your sleep and activity patterns can be a sign of whether your mood problems are getting better or worse.

As with the mood chart, it's best to fill out the SRM every day and review it each week by yourself and with your therapist or psychiatrist. Keeping the social rhythm chart on a regular, ongoing basis will enable you to spot shifts in your daily routines and sleep–wake cycles that may be of subtle importance in determining your mood.

The chart on page 169 was completed by Leslie, a 40-year-old woman with bipolar II disorder. First notice the upper left-hand corner, where she has made a daily mood rating on a scale of −5 to +5. In this respect it is like the mood chart. But notice that there are 17 activities listed on the left side; most people will do some portion of these every day. Indicate in the boxes what time you did the following activities: woke up, had your first cup of coffee, went to work, went to school or did some other daily activity, ate lunch, exercised, came home, ate dinner, and went to bed. These daily routines, in part, drive your sleep–wake habits (Frank, 2005). For example, if you have a shifting work schedule that demands that you work from 8 A.M. to 4 P.M. one day and then 4 P.M. to 12 A.M. the next, your bedtime and wake time will be correspondingly altered from day to day, and your mood may change

THE SOCIAL RHYTHM METRIC (SRM)
MacArthur Foundation Mental Health Research Network I

Please fill this out at the end of the day.

Day of Week: _Sun_   Date: _5-28_

ACTIVITY	Check If DID NOT DO	CLOCK TIME	A.M.	P.M.	Check If ALONE	Spouse/ Partner	Children	Other Family Members	Other Person(s)
MOOD RATING (Choose one): _-2_ — Scale: -5 -4 -3 (-2) -1 0 1 2 3 4 5, Very Depressed / Normal / Very Elated		**TIME**		**Check**		**PEOPLE** 1 = Just Present, 2 = Actively Involved, 3 = Others Very Stimulating			
SAMPLE ACTIVITY (for reference only)		6:20	√			2			1
OUT OF BED		9:30	√		√				
FIRST CONTACT (IN PERSON OR BY PHONE) WITH ANOTHER PERSON		10:00	√						2
HAVE MORNING BEVERAGE		9:30	√						1
HAVE BREAKFAST		10:00	√						2
GO OUTSIDE FOR THE FIRST TIME		10:45	√						3
START WORK, SCHOOL, HOUSEWORK, VOLUNTEER ACTIVITIES, CHILD OR FAMILY CARE	√								
HAVE LUNCH		12:00							3
TAKE AN AFTERNOON NAP	√								
HAVE DINNER		7:30		√	√				
PHYSICAL EXERCISE		5:30		√	√				
HAVE AN EVENING SNACK/DRINK		9:00		√	√				
WATCH AN EVENING TV NEWS PROGRAM		10:00		√	√				
WATCH ANOTHER TV PROGRAM	√								
ACTIVITY A _Phone conversation_		9:30		√					3
ACTIVITY B									
RETURN HOME (LAST TIME)		7:00		√					2
GO TO BED		10:00			√				

A social rhythm chart.

Reprinted by permission from Monk et al. (1991). Copyright by Elsevier Science.

(up or down) in the days that follow. In contrast, if you eat, exercise, work, and interact with others at fairly regular times of the day or evening, you will come to expect sleep at a certain time.

The SRM also asks you to record *who did each of these activities with you and how stimulating they were.* The degree to which your interchanges with others are provocative, conflict ridden, or otherwise stimulating, versus low key or laid back, can be important determining factors in the degree of stability you experience in your emotional states and possibly even your sleep. Say you ate dinner with your spouse or partner but had an argument, and then the two of you went to opposite ends of the house (rated a "3" on stimulation); you would probably have more trouble falling asleep that night. Compare that night to another night when you and your spouse had a relaxing dinner together (which might be rated a "1"—"others just present").

High levels of stimulation from other people can feel quite positive but still affect your mood or sleep–wake cycle negatively. Deborah, age 26, found that her evening waitressing job, which she enjoyed a great deal, contained highly stimulating bursts of activity (usually 3-hour blocks in which she was in great demand by the patrons). She consistently had more trouble falling asleep after getting home than she did on nights when she wasn't working. She had an easier time when she was assigned the early evening shift.

Katherine, age 42, enjoyed the intensive contact with people she had through her job in the clothing section of a department store. However, the social stimulation rose to almost intolerable levels during the weekends prior to the Christmas holidays, and she found herself becoming increasingly irritable. She learned not to schedule any social activities on the weekend evenings following these workdays as a way of modulating her exposure to stress and stimulation.

Leslie's Example: Evaluating a Social Rhythm Chart

Although only 1 day is shown in Leslie's example on page 169, we can develop some hypotheses about factors that affected her mood states. For her, a mixed mood state is a day of depression, along with agitation, nervousness, and irritability. Note that even though the sample day occurred during the spring, when daylight hours were longer, she had a relatively short day (woke up at 9:30 A.M. and went to bed at 10 P.M.). She was sleeping too much. She also had several high-stimulation interactions during the day (including an argument over the telephone with her ex-husband about their child and a confrontation with a roommate whom she felt was being inconsiderate). She had at least one alcoholic drink when alone. In addition to her biological predispositions, these factors may have partially determined her agitated, depressed mood.

It is possible that these events and activities resulted from her mood state (for example, she might have been anxious and irritable and therefore more prone to confrontations). To help determine which caused which, Leslie collected social rhythm and mood information on herself over a period of several months. She began to see how provocative interactions with certain people, sleep patterns, and alcohol combined to change her mood, as well as how her mood states affected the timing and frequency of these events and habits. She became increasingly certain that alcohol before bedtime and sleeping more than 9 hours combined to make her nervous and irritable and more prone to run-ins with people.

"How Can I Regulate My Daily Routines?"

The next step is to devise strategies that help you regulate your daily routines. Keeping regular routines sounds straightforward, but if you've ever tried to do it, you know that significant challenges are likely to arise. You can do this alone, but your spouse or even your therapist can help you develop target times for various activities such as sleep and exercise.

The first, most important ingredient is to go to bed at the same time every night and wake up at the same time every morning. Try to maintain this pattern on weekends, even when you'd rather sleep late. Of course, there will be times when getting to bed at your target hour or waking up at a specific time is impossible, such as when you travel, have social plans on a weekend, have a sick child, or need to get up extra early to pick up someone at the train station. Some of these events will be controllable by you (for example, whether to go to the early or late showing of a certain movie) and some will not (for example, the timing of an airline flight). If your schedule is shifted by an hour or two on a given night, try to reinstate your original sleep–wake target times as soon as possible.

Try to maintain your sleep patterns even if events conspire to make you change them. For example, if you have lost your job, try to get up at the same time you would have gotten up when you were going in to work. If your new job requires different hours (say, getting to work by 8 A.M. instead of 9 A.M.), adjust your bedtime to an hour earlier. It's best to ease into your new schedule gradually rather than suddenly.

> **Effective prevention:**
> Maintaining a regular routine revolves around keeping a consistent sleep schedule: go to bed and get up at the same time every day as much as you possibly can.

You can also work with your therapist to *anticipate events that will change your daily routines* and plan ways to regulate yourself once these events occur. For example, if you know that you may be changing jobs soon or traveling more in the near future, you can anticipate that your sleep will be disrupted. Make plans, in advance, to go to bed and wake up at consistent times even after these disruptive events have occurred.

Second, if you have been having trouble sleeping (see the section on sleep, page 174), try to avoid *sleep bingeing,* in which you catch up from all the lost sleep during the week by sleeping more on weekends. You'll probably find that sleep bingeing makes your depression and anxiety worse). It also makes it harder to sleep the next night.

Third, try to see if you can maintain the same hours each day at work or school. For example, try to take classes during the same interval each day. Try to avoid having all of your classes on one or two days and none on the other three. To parallel your regular job hours, try to exercise at the same time (for example, just after work) rather than late in the evening on one night and then early in the morning the next day. Try to have a regular period to unwind before going to bed. Avoid having your most stimulating interactions with partners, friends, or coworkers right before you try to go to sleep.

Practical Challenges to Maintaining Regular Routines

There are practical problems to be solved, of course. The courses you want to take may be offered at all different times of the day or night. You may have a job that requires a lot of travel, necessitates long shifts on weekends, requires work at home in the evening on some nights but not others, or involves changing shifts. An example is a contract nursing job, in which people are often called for a full 8-hour shift only an hour before the shift is to start. Restaurant jobs often have shifting schedules as well. In Chapter 13, you'll find some suggestions for negotiating work hours with your employer in light of the limitations your disorder can impose.

Here are examples of how some of my patients have kept regular social rhythms even when facing the demands of school or job. Walter had an open discussion with his employer about his mood disorder. His employer agreed to keep him on the 8–5 daily shift at his computer programming job, rather than the constantly variable shifts that were typical. Juanita, who traveled frequently, always tried to get the same number of hours of sleep each night, even when she was in a new time zone. Maintaining her sleep habits required a degree of assertiveness, given that she was often encouraged by her traveling coworkers to stay out late.

Candace (discussed further on pages 181–182) found that her weekends involved long periods with little contact with others, and her depressions usually became worse then. Scheduling low-key activities with friends or acquaintances during weekend days gave her a greater feeling of consistency in routines from the week to the weekend and helped improve her mood. Likewise, Wesley, who became depressed after breaking up with his girlfriend, found that scheduling activities with other people each morning or, at minimum, taking trips to a coffee shop by himself helped get him out of bed by a certain time.

The SRM can help you design a daily schedule of sleeping, eating, exercising, and socializing that is comfortable and feasible, given the demands of your current social, family, and work life. Try to set goals for when you plan to go to bed and when you want to wake up and try not to deviate from these plans by more than 30 minutes to an hour, even when there are rewarding activities (for example, parties, late-night movies) that you feel would improve your mood. Other members of your family, if living with you (your spouse or partner, for example), may be able to help you design this program and stick to it.

Resistance to Tracking and Keeping Regulated Routines

Some people complain that social rhythm tracking is tedious and reminds them of doing homework assignments for school. Like most treatment and self-management techniques, the SRM is not without its costs in terms of time and effort. But as you get used to it, you will find that you can do it at the end of the day in about 5 minutes. With time, you may find that certain items on the chart are more important to record than others. For example, your bedtime, wake time, job hours, and exercise times may be critical in determining your mood stability, but your mealtimes or TV habits may be less central.

In my experience and that of other clinicians, the bigger issue that people with bipolar disorder face is the trade-off involved in regulating their daily routines: it means giving up a degree of spontaneity. People sometimes wonder, "Why can't I have the same kind of 'devil may care' attitude that others have? If everyone else is staying up until 2 A.M. to party, why can't I?"

These reactions are understandable. For Amy, keeping a regulated routine made her feel that she was different from everyone else. On the other hand, she came to realize that the unpredictability and social stimulation she craved was like a drug. She usually had a "mood hangover" the next day.

There is comfort in knowing that you are doing something proactive to manage your disorder. You will almost certainly see benefits in terms of your mood stability and productivity when you structure your days and nights. With time, a regulated routine will give you a sense of security and control over your fate.

Even apart from the issue of mood stabilization, some of my clients find that social rhythm tracking helps them manage their disorder and lifestyle in ways they hadn't expected. For example, Carmen, age 29, found that SRM tracking helped her develop more consistent medication-taking habits, which until that point had been haphazard and unpredictable. After filling out his chart for several weeks, Arthur, 35, observed that "I have a habit of jamming in too many things to avoid depression, but then I get like a car that's run out of gas. I want contact with people, but I can get to the point where I'm doing too much. I need some more consistency, and I need not to be constantly overstimulated and running away from myself."

It is not only people with mood disorders who have to stay on regular, regimented schedules. Parents usually need to follow very predictable routines to manage the daily activities of their children. Athletes need to stick to well-regulated training schedules. People who become expert performers, such as accomplished professional musicians, have often developed highly regimented routines to help them accomplish their craft (see, for example, Krampe & Ericsson, 1996).

Nonetheless, if you're finding a regimented routine too stifling, discuss this with your doctor. There may be compromises that can be made. Perhaps you can identify the point at which fluctuating routines negatively affect your mood. For example, a 30-minute departure from your bedtime may make no difference, but 90 minutes might make a big difference. Try to see if you can identify the range of fluctuation in routines within which you can function and still feel stable.

"OK, Now That I'm Going to Bed on Time, How Do I Fall Asleep?"

"I toss and turn, look at the clock, sneer and snort through my nose, walk around the house ... do my yoga, do my meditation, turn on Poker After Dark *... but I still can't sleep. It irks me to no end that my wife can just lie down and she's out. I almost want to wake her up to make her suffer like I am, but I don't ... It goes like this every night, and then, of course, I'm a wreck at work the next day."*

—A 51-year-old man with rapid cycling bipolar disorder

For some people with bipolar disorder, getting to bed at the right time isn't the main problem. The problem is falling asleep and staying asleep. There is nothing more frustrating than lying awake and trying to fall asleep. Sleep disturbance is a key symptom of bipolar disorder and sometimes can be a side effect of antidepressant or psychostimulant medications. It can also be due to substances like caffeine, excessive sugar, tobacco, or alcohol, especially if these are ingested close to your bedtime.

Your doctor may decide to give you medications for sleep, such as clonazepam or zolpidem (Ambien), or even major tranquilizers like quetiapine. Although these medications often work well, not everyone likes to take them because you can become addicted or tolerant (that is, you may need a bigger dosage over time to achieve the same effect, or you may become unable to sleep without them). But you and your physician may decide that a sleeping medication is the best alternative to keep sleep disturbance from contributing to your worsening mood state.

Fortunately, there is a literature on behavioral interventions for sleep problems. Michael Otto and his colleagues at the Harvard Medical School

> **Effective solution:** To cope with sleep disturbance:
>
> ■ Keep stress out of the bedroom.
> ■ Give yourself time to unwind before sleep.
> ■ Never "compete" to get to sleep.
> ■ Use muscle relaxation techniques.
> ■ Adjust your sleep cycle before travel.

and Massachusetts General Hospital (2008) have developed recommendations for ways to improve sleep if you're suffering from bipolar disorder (see sidebar on this page). Some of these sleep techniques would be applicable to people without bipolar disorder as well.

Examples of "stress in the bedroom" include having arguments with your spouse, preparing work assignments for the next day while in bed, examining your next day's work schedule, checking the stock market pages, checking your e-mail or text messages one last time, eating a large meal, and making last-minute phone calls. These activities should be avoided right before bedtime. More generally, try to keep the last hour just before sleep free of stressful activities so that you can unwind and relax. If possible, try to arrange your bedroom so that noise is blocked out (for example, the telephone is turned off, no radios are playing) or wear earplugs. Paradoxically, activities that people often take for granted as necessary for falling asleep may actually contribute to sleep disturbance. For example, many people watch the evening news in bed before turning out the lights, but the news overstimulates them and cranks them up. Likewise, many people feel they can't fall asleep without reading a book, yet sometimes reading, even if it's only a novel, can get the brain running in all sorts of different directions. If you've been reading a good murder mystery, it may be hard to put down and stop thinking about! Likewise, most people believe that regular exercise contributes to good sleep because it tires you out and relaxes your muscles. But it can also keep you awake if you exercise right before bedtime—try to give yourself as much as 3 hours between finishing your exercises and going to bed.

If you want to investigate which activities are contributing to your sleep problems, try nights with and without these activities and record the changes on your mood chart or SRM (for example, write "no TV" on Thursday night and "yes TV" on Friday night and record your sleep for each). Try to see if you can detect whether doing or not doing certain activities affects your sleep and mood.

Some people feel that falling asleep is like an athletic competition, like running a race in a certain time. Being unable to sleep makes them feel inadequate or incompetent, and performance anxiety begins to accompany their attempts to sleep. Try not to think of your ongoing sleep disturbance as something you're doing to yourself, but rather as a biological sign of your disorder. Rather than wrestling with yourself about being unable to sleep, experience the physical sensations of being in bed, including how your body feels, how you experience the covers over you, or how the pillow feels against your head. If you have access to a relaxation tape or meditation exercises, you may wish to use these to help you experience the physical sensations that lead to sleep (Otto et al., 2008).

Many people have trouble sleeping when they travel. If you fly from the West Coast of the United States to the East Coast, you may arrive when everyone else is going to sleep, but for you it is three hours earlier. Transatlantic travel (for example, flying from Chicago to Paris) is particularly difficult for people with bipolar disorder because there is such a dramatic shift in circadian rhythms. But travel is often unavoidable.

One way to combat this travel disruption is to gradually adjust your internal time clock to the new place you're going, before you actually leave. So, over the course of the week before you travel to a later time zone, go to bed an hour earlier than usual, then an hour and a half, and then 2 hours earlier, and so forth. By the time you arrive, it may be easier to adjust to the hours of the new time zone. This procedure usually works best if you'll be in the new time zone for more than a few days.

There are other strategies you can use to improve your sleep, some of which go beyond the scope of this book. If you've been having difficulties, consider reading self-help books specifically oriented toward sleep issues, such as Paul Glovinsky and Art Spielman's (2006) *The Insomnia Answer: A Personalized Program for Identifying and Overcoming the Three Types of Insomnia,* Colin Espie's (2006) *Overcoming Insomnia and Sleep Problems,* or Lawrence Epstein and Stephen Mardon's (2006) *The Harvard Medical School Guide to a Good Night's Sleep.*

Maintaining Wellness Tip No. 3: Avoiding Alcohol and Recreational Drugs

Ruth, a 32-year-old woman who had just been diagnosed with bipolar I disorder, had a severe problem with drinking that usually began when she was relatively free of bipolar symptoms. Typically, romantic relationships with men or conflict-ridden business entanglements were the background of these episodes. Her drinking binges were so severe that she often had to be hospitalized and detoxified. She eventually was court ordered to undergo an Antabuse program, in which she was required to come in twice a week to take a medication that made her vomit if she drank.

Her own view was that her bipolar disorder was making her drink. Many observers, including her doctors and family members, felt that it was the other way around: that her drinking came first and led to her mood cycling. She constantly complained of the pain of the mood swings and their associated anxiety, but her symptoms co-occurred so consistently with drinking that it was difficult to tell which were due to the bipolar disorder and which to the alcohol. In fact, her family wasn't even convinced she had bipolar disorder and thought it was one of many excuses she had given over the years.

During one interval, Ruth became convinced that she should give up alcohol and stayed abstinent for almost 6 months. Her mood swings were much improved during this interval: she still had a mild depression but no mania or mixed symptoms. She was able to obtain a regular waitressing job and began functioning better than she had in a long time.

During this period of recovery, however, Ruth came to the conclusion that she had no real problem with drinking. She began to reinterpret her past almost exclusively in terms of her new bipolar diagnosis, denying any causal influence of alcohol. For example, she labeled her past alcohol binges as "rapid cycling" and "self-medicating." She reasoned that she wouldn't again lose control of her drinking since her mood disorder had become stable.

About 5 months into her period of abstinence, she traveled to Palm Springs for a weekend with her new boyfriend. Quite deliberately, she discontinued her Antabuse program 5 days before the trip. Within 1 week she was back in the hospital in need of detoxification. Her depression was much more severe upon her hospital discharge, and she was court ordered, once again, into the Antabuse program.

Alcohol and Drugs: What Are the Risks?

Most psychiatrists and psychologists agree that if you have bipolar disorder, you should avoid alcohol and recreational drugs altogether. As discussed in Chapter 5, alcohol and drugs interfere with the effects of your medications and worsen the course of your illness. If you use alcohol and drugs, you are likely to become inconsistent with your medication regimen and will have more trouble becoming stable as a result (Strakowski et al., 1998). Worst of all, alcohol and drug use puts you at a much greater risk for committing suicide (Fawcett et al., 2000; see also Chapter 11).

Some doctors will tell you that you can drink alcohol in very small quantities (for example, a single glass of wine with dinner). There may be people with bipolar disorder who can do this and stay stable, but, to be honest, I know very few. I tend to take the more extreme view that *not drinking at all and not using any drugs (including marijuana) is one of the best ways to maintain wellness.* I have no moral qualms about people drinking or using marijuana; my concerns stem entirely from watching too many people with bipolar disorder destroy themselves with substances. People with bipolar disorder are more strongly affected—in terms of their mood stability and behavior—by small amounts of alcohol or substances than their age-mates. This is especially the case if they indulge in alcohol or drugs when their mood states are already starting to fluctuate.

Many people with bipolar disorder, like Ruth, have a codiagnosis of alcohol or drug abuse or dependence (the *dual diagnosis* situation). People with dual diagnoses must learn to become abstinent, because the two disorders can worsen each other, much as they did for Ruth. If you have previously had problems with alcohol or drugs, consider joining a 12-step program such as Alcoholics Anonymous (as Ruth eventually did) or Narcotics Anonymous. These groups can serve as powerful resources in helping people maintain abstinence. If you don't like groups, 12-step and other programs for addictive behavior (for example, motivational enhancement therapy; Miller & Rollnick, 2002) can often be obtained on an individual basis.

Spencer, age 45, struggled with his desire to drink for many years. However, through couple educational therapy sessions about his disorder and through mood charting, he learned to recognize his signs of mood cycling: subtle increases in irritability and anger, lethargy, and insomnia. During these cycling intervals, he learned to drink nonalcoholic beer when he was with his wife and friends who were drinking. He eventually gave up drinking. He summarized his experience this way:

"I used to be a two-drink-a-night person, every night, for many years. I finally came to the conclusion that I just couldn't do it. It wasn't some moral thing; it was actually just a simple decision that drinking created a state in me that was miserable. For two days after drinking even just small amounts I would feel irritated with everybody, emotionally exhausted, and want to sleep all day. The price I was paying was too high. But before I could quit, I had to have hard evidence that alcohol was worsening my life, that it was something I didn't need to do to myself. I finally saw alcohol as a big contributor to my anger and my problems with people. Without alcohol, I can decide if I want to work on my anger; it's within my power to do so. With alcohol, the anger just takes me over."

Beliefs about Drinking, Drug Abuse, and Bipolar Disorder

People often have mistaken beliefs about alcohol, drug substances, and bipolar disorder. Some of these are listed in the box on page 179.

I've heard people with bipolar disorder claim that marijuana or cocaine is just as effective as a mood stabilizer such as lithium or divalproex in controlling their mood states. They argue that alcohol calms them down, reduces their anxiety, or improves their depression; they argue that marijuana boosts their mood when they are depressed. One patient said, "For me, alcohol is like the ropes that keep the hot air balloon from going up ... and on the other side is like a disguise covering over the depression."

Some people do drink or use drugs to make themselves feel better, but whether these substances are really doing the trick—as opposed to making their moods worse—is another question. We know that alcohol worsens depression (as in the examples given above). People who have both bipolar disorder and alcohol problems also have more rapid cycling, mixed symptoms, and anxiety or panic than those who do not drink. Alcohol can also interfere with sleep, which can worsen mania.

People often assume, as Ruth did, that their depression came first and that they use alcohol or drugs for the purpose of self-medicating this depression. For many people with bipolar disorder, however, the alcohol abuse precedes the depression rather than the reverse (Strakowski et al., 2000). For some, a vicious cycle takes over: They drink heavily and get depressed and anxious, then stop drinking and experience a recurrence of depression or panic symptoms that is attributable to the alcohol withdrawal. Then they try to self-medicate these mood symptoms with more alcohol. This pattern makes the course of both disorders much worse.

Marijuana, although not as toxic as alcohol for persons with bipolar disorder, can also be detrimental to your mood stability. In Strakowski and colleagues' study (2000), marijuana use was associated with manic symptoms, whereas alcohol use

---

Mistaken Beliefs about Bipolar Disorder and Alcohol or Drug Abuse

▪ Alcohol or drugs can be used as mood stabilizers.

▪ Hard drugs like amphetamine, LSD, or cocaine can be used as antidepressants.

▪ Substances cannot worsen your disorder if your mood has been stable.

---

was associated with depressive symptoms. One patient put it this way: "Marijuana makes me think and think and think, and then it keeps me from sleeping. It's like a catalyst for something in me." Marijuana can also interfere with your attention and concentration as well as your ability to remember to take your medications. Some people find it makes them lethargic and unmotivated. In other words, there is no evidence that the medical uses of marijuana should extend to bipolar disorder!

Rationalizing their heavy drug use, some people claim that LSD (acid), amphetamine (speed), cocaine (crack), and Ecstasy are really antidepressants. They argue that these drugs can help their depression more than a standard antidepressant such as Prozac. Some even know about studies showing that LSD stimulates the action of certain serotonin receptors or that amphetamine prolongs dopamine activity, as some antidepressants do. But they are misinterpreting the clinical implications of these studies. Even though many street drugs do affect the same neurotransmitter systems as antidepressants, street drugs do not produce true mood stability. Instead, they tend to produce short-term bursts of neuronal activity accompanied by elation or irritability (much like mania or hypomania), rather than truly alleviating depression.

Some people with bipolar disorder use substances to intensify the elated and grandiose aspects of their hypomanic or manic states. They feel driven toward further stimulation and novelty. Cocaine and amphetamine are especially likely to be used in this way. The result is often a severe increase in manic or mixed symptoms or the initiation of rapid cycling states, sometimes leading to hospitalization.

You may believe that taking alcohol or drugs is fine as long as you have been feeling well for a period of time. This was Ruth's logic, and she tested it frequently by going "off the wagon" whenever she had a period of mood stability. For her, ordinary life seemed very drab. The up-and-down periods that alcohol brought were preferable to feeling that life had become ordinary and boring. Many people whose bipolar disorder is stable report that alcohol and drugs provide a relief from their feelings of emptiness. It is true that substances often activate the reward circuitry of the brain. But the relief is temporary at best, and the same substances can trigger negative mood states that are far more unpleasant than boredom.

The exercise on page 180 may help you identify what makes you want to drink or use drugs (McCrady, 2007). Try to identify:

A Maintaining Wellness Exercise: Identifying Triggers for Alcohol and Drug Abuse, Your Responses to Those Triggers, and the Consequences

List the type of alcohol or the drug you use most frequently (*examples:* beer, wine, marijuana, Vicodin, cocaine).

_____

_____

List the *situations* in which you are most likely to get drunk or high (*examples:* being alone; being out with friends; parties; Friday afternoon after work; with specific people).

_____

_____

List the *feelings* you ordinarily have right before you drink/get high (*examples:* depressed, anxious, irritable, excited).

_____

_____

Describe your *expectations* about what this drink/drug will do for you (*examples:* it will make me relax and ease up with people; help me deal with difficult situations; decrease my depression; help me sleep; make me think more clearly).

_____

_____

Describe the *actual consequences* of your drinking/drug use the last few times. Try to distinguish (1) what happens immediately after you drink/get high (*examples:* relaxed me, got me into an argument, alleviated my depression, made me feel more social) versus (2) the delayed effects (made me feel more depressed the next day, had hangover, got to work late).

Immediate effects:

_____

_____

Delayed effects:

_____

_____

_____

- triggers for use (for example, being with people whom you want to impress)
- the feelings you want to alleviate (for many people with bipolar disorder, depression or anxiety)
- your expectations
- the immediate consequences of using the drug/alcohol (for example, feeling relaxed, feeling more confident, forgetting your medications)
- the extended or delayed consequences of use (for example, sleep disturbance, missing work the next day, feeling irritable, drowsy, or anxious several days later)

Amy learned to avoid certain situations and people who, she believed, made her drink more. Earl, who smoked marijuana heavily, learned to plan to do things during times of the day when he was most likely to get high (typically late afternoons after he finished his classes). Bethany learned to challenge her belief that alcohol alleviated her depressions. When she systematically evaluated the results of her drinking, she concluded that she felt better at first but more irritable and depressed later. She began to think of alcohol as a cause rather than an effect of her mood problems.

> **Effective solution:** Think of drinking or drug use as one event in a sequence of events rather than as a singular, isolated act. Then you'll be in a position to think about changing this sequence.

Maintaining Wellness Tip No. 4: Relying on Social Supports

Candace, a 49-year-old woman with bipolar II disorder, suffered from an ongoing depression that was not alleviated by antidepressants or mood stabilizers. After becoming frustrated with the myriad medications she had tried, she consulted a psychotherapist, who observed that she was quite socially isolated: she had broken up with her boyfriend 2 months earlier, she had few new friends or even acquaintances, and she had become disconnected from her parents and her two sisters. Her therapist encouraged her to try some new social activities, which she strongly resisted doing. Her weekends were largely spent alone in her apartment, where "my thoughts eat me alive."

Candace had few hobbies in her current life but had played soccer in college. With some reluctance, she joined a group who played soccer on weekends. She felt awkward at first. "They're not my kind of people," she observed. At the beginning she had to force herself to go. Little by little, however, she found that her weekends became more structured because of the soccer practices. Although she never admitted to enjoying the company of members of the team, she did notice that her mood brightened when she participated in an activity with them.

At first she thought this was due to physical exercise, but she found that her mood also brightened when she went to potluck dinners or movies at the team members' houses. She eventually disclosed her illness to a few of her teammates, who "weren't fazed like I thought they'd be." With time, the group became like a second family to her, and she began dating one of the men. After playing with the team for 6 months, she acknowledged in one of her therapy sessions that her chronic depression, while still present, was not as bad as it had been before she had made these connections.

Social support—feeling emotional connections with people with whom one regularly interacts—is an important protective factor against depression. Having a group of people you know well, whom you trust with knowing about your bipolar disorder and whom you see with some regularity, will help you do better in terms of the cycling of your disorder.

New research: Sheri Johnson and colleagues at the University of Miami (1999) found that after an episode of depression, people with bipolar disorder who had good social support systems recovered more quickly and had less severe depression symptoms over a 6-month period than those with small or nonexistent support systems.

You may be a person who seeks out others naturally, or you may prefer spending time by yourself. Either way, when you're depressed, it is hard to interact with anybody. Unless you have a social support system in place when you're well, you may find it hard to reach out for the very help you need when depression strikes. Likewise, maintaining regular contact with your social support group when you're well will do much to prevent future depression. When you encounter the inevitable conflicts that come up with family members or coworkers, your friends and supportive relatives can be like a landing pad for comfort and steadiness. They provide a counterpart to, and minimize the impact of, stressful conflicts.

I don't want to oversimplify things by implying that just having people around you is all that counts. As I discussed in Chapter 5, high levels of conflict with certain members of your core circle, particularly family members but also with close friends, can be associated with a more difficult course of your illness. It is empathic, give-and-take relationships with members of your core circle, and just plain low-key social time, that will best protect you from depression. Needless to say, that won't always be possible. Chapter 13, on family and work relationships, will acquaint you with skills to help you maximize the positive influences of your social support system.

Your Core Circle

As you'll see in the next chapters, your social supports can be critical in keeping your illness from cycling out of control. But first, let's identify who these people are.

Complete the exercise on page 184, "Identifying Your Core Circle." You may be surprised at your list! For some people, the core circle consists of members of a church or synagogue, or a group devoted to a particular hobby (as was the case for Candace), or people at school. Other people regularly rely on and socialize with just a few friends or family members. It isn't simply the number of people in your life that protects you from a drop in your mood but the quality of these relationships and the regularity of the contact.

Maintaining Friendships While Avoiding Alcohol or Drugs

What if your social circle is one that relies heavily on alcohol or drugs? Dispensing with alcohol, marijuana, or hard drug use can indeed have negative social implications. For example, some people find it hard to go out with their friends without drinking (this was the case for Amy). Some say that their friends devalue their efforts to stay sober. If these problems apply to you, consider discussing your dilemma with one or more trusted friends. Do they understand about your disorder and the likely impact of alcohol or drug use?

If you're not comfortable disclosing the disorder to any of your friends, consider giving other justifications for why you don't want to drink. Many people today respect any measure taken to improve physical and mental health and fitness, so saying you're trying to lose weight, or that drinking at night discourages you from getting up and working out when you want to, or that when you drink you don't have the mental sharpness you need at work the next day, might keep them from pushing you further.

Many of my clients report that giving up alcohol or drugs does make socializing with certain people more awkward. Very few, however, experience outright rejection if their friends understand their motivations: They are abstaining out of a desire to take care of their health—rather than to judge or place themselves above others.

■

Think about managing your disorder in stages. Some techniques are best applied when you're well (this chapter) and others during various phases of your illness (Chapters 9–11). In previous chapters I emphasized the importance of maintaining consistency with your medication regimen and your psychotherapy sessions. The strategies covered in this chapter for maintaining wellness—mood charting, keeping regular sleep–wake routines, avoiding alcohol and drugs, and relying on social supports—can enhance the effects of your psychiatric treatments in keeping your mood stable. In the next three chapters you'll see how the lifestyle management techniques discussed here can be adjusted when you feel your moods start to spiral upward or downward.

Identifying Your Core Circle

List all the people you consider *friends*—those you feel you can confide in (talk to, get emotional support from) and whom you see or have phone contact with at least once a week. List their phone numbers in the second column.

_____   _____

_____   _____

_____   _____

_____   _____

_____   _____

List which *family members* you see regularly and feel comfortable confiding in. List their phone numbers in the second column.

Lynette Larett   (801)618-8018
(Sister)

_____   _____

_____   _____

_____   _____

If you were ever in trouble (for example, having a medical emergency) and needed somebody to help you, whom would you be most likely to contact and in what order (list them in order of preference, from first to fourth)? List their phone numbers in the second column.

Kristina Marie (365)445-2078
Boyce Supervisor
from Key

_____   _____

_____   _____

Are there any *groups* of people who could help you feel less lonely or assist you if you were having any kind of emergency (*examples:* church or synagogue groups, support groups like Alcoholics Anonymous, groups dedicated to certain activities—art, cooking, foreign languages, or sports)?

Kristina Marie
Boyce (365)445-2078
Supervisor at
Key Residential

_____   _____

_____   _____

9

Heading Off the Escalation of Mania

Robert, 45, managed a successful landscape architecture firm. He'd had three manic episodes in the 4 years since he had been dating his current girlfriend, Jessie, with whom he was now living. Two of his episodes involved hospitalizations. He maintained close contact with his two kids from a previous marriage, 18-year-old Angie and 22-year-old Brian. Jessie had no children.

His most recent manic episode, which had led to a hospitalization, involved an identifiable set of warning signs. The first sign he reported was becoming disinterested in his job and irritable with his coworkers, about whom he had become mistrustful. This was a difficult time to become disinterested; his business was flourishing due to a new housing development project he had been involved in planning. During the earliest stages of his manic episode, he described being aware that something was wrong: his thoughts began to race and he was full of great ideas. He had still been able to sleep most of the night, however, and saw no need to call his psychiatrist.

According to Jessie, Robert became "overly expressive" and "took on this physical dominance stance" during the 1-week interval prior to his hospitalization. For example, he attended Angie's basketball game and "was the loudest one in the bleachers. At some point the coach asked him to leave." On another evening Jessie and Robert had gone to a fast-food restaurant in which he had "barked" his order at the waitress. He later apologized to the waitress. Jessie and Robert discussed his escalating behavior and Robert admitted that he was being "hyper" but also felt good: "I'm seeing things more clearly than ever before."

They finally agreed to call his doctor, whom he hadn't seen face to face in almost a year. Robert's doctor talked with him by phone but didn't really ask questions about his mood state, focusing instead on his feelings about his work situation. She concluded that "you need some rest. You sound exhausted." No changes were recommended in his medication regimen, which consisted of relatively low dosages of divalproex (Depakote) and verapamil (Isoptin, a calcium channel blocker).

Things took a turn for the worse when Robert, irritated that his son, Brian, had not returned his calls, went down to the record store where Brian worked. He and Brian had a verbal showdown next to the cash register, involving much profanity. Brian's boss angrily told Robert and Brian to "take it somewhere else." Brian was quite upset and told Robert never to come see him at work again.

In the next few days, Robert's behavior escalated dramatically. His movements became rapid and frenetic. He became angry, paranoid, and fixated on grandiose notions about a music career, even though he had been playing the guitar only occasionally, as a hobby. He bought an expensive Fender Stratocaster guitar but then impulsively traded it at a guitar show for an instrument worth much less money. He and Jessie began to have bitter arguments in which, according to Robert, "she took on this angry, resentful, removed tone but also got controlling and know-it-all." He impulsively moved out of their apartment and went to live at his office. He called her, in tears, one night to say he had begun to panic because he thought he was dying or that he might kill himself. Jessie called the police, who found him in his office staring fixedly at the ceiling. They escorted him to a local state hospital. He stayed there for 2 weeks before being discharged on a new regimen of divalproex (at a higher dosage) and the antipsychotic risperidone (Risperdal).

A manic episode can wreak havoc with a person's life. It can drain finances, ruin marriages and long-term relationships, destroy a person's physical health, produce legal problems, and lead to loss of employment. It can even lead to loss of life. The fallout can be long-lasting: William Coryell and his colleagues at the University of Iowa Medical Center (1993) found that the social and job-related effects of a manic episode are observable for up to 5 years after the episode has resolved itself.

If you think back to your last manic (or hypomanic) episode, you will probably recall that it was quite exhilarating at the time. There may be a part of you that wants to re-create the manic phases for the euphoric, energized, confident feelings that accompany them (see also Chapter 7). When your mood was escalating, your thought processes probably seemed very purposeful and brilliant to you, even if others found them bizarre. You probably enjoyed the feeling of being highly energized and goal driven. Perhaps you even knew you were getting manic but didn't want to shut off the intoxicating feelings. This was the case for Robert, as it is for many people with bipolar disorder with whom I've worked.

In retrospect, you probably feel that, if it had been possible to prevent or at least minimize the damage associated with your manic episodes, you would have done so. After his hospitalization, Robert expressed a great deal of remorse at the toll his manic episodes were taking: Jessie was threatening to leave him, and his son Brian was not talking to him. His relationships with his employees were damaged as well.

If you have not had full manic or mixed episodes but only hypomanic ones (that is, you have bipolar II disorder), little damage may have been done during your activated states. Nonetheless, you may have found that hypomanic episodes—much like their more severe counterparts—bring on major depressions in their aftermath. The adage that "what goes up must come down" applies only too well to bipolar disorder.

Because of their biological bases, you can't fully prevent manic or hypomanic episodes from occurring altogether. *But you may be able to control how severe they get and limit the damage they cause. You can learn to "head them off at the pass" by recognizing when they are starting to occur, and then putting into motion plans for preventing yourself from spiraling upward even further.* In Robert's case, there was a brief window of opportunity in which his early warning signs were apparent and more could have been done to prevent his escalation into a full-blown episode. You'll learn more about how Robert and Jessie learned to anticipate and derail his worst manic symptoms later in this chapter.

If you can successfully implement a plan to prevent or decrease the severity of your manic episodes, then your family, job, and social functioning will almost certainly improve. Some aspects of this plan will involve things you do on your own. Some will involve the actions of your family members and significant others. Still other aspects will involve your doctor and therapist (if you have one). *When mania is escalating, you will need the help of others because it will be hard to rein in yourself.* It's best to make relapse prevention plans when you're well, because when you are escalating you will have a difficult time recognizing the potential dangers associated with your behavior and what to do to curtail the upward cycle.

I think of a developing manic episode as like a train leaving a station. When the train is starting to move out of the station and someone wants to get off, the conductor still has time to stop the train before it reaches full speed. But if he waits too long, the train will be on its own trajectory and passengers will be stuck on the train until it stops or crashes on its own. Manic episodes can feel like this train. The key is to be able to tell when the train has started to move and to try to get off it before it's barreling down the tracks.

The Relapse Prevention Drill

How important is it to know when you are getting manic? One study indicated that there were two predictors of rehospitalization in bipolar disorder: not taking medications and failing to recognize the early signs of relapse (Joyce, 1985). On a more hopeful note, people with bipolar disorder who receive educational interventions with their relatives, such as learning to identify early warning signs of mania and then seeking mental health services, are less likely to have full recurrences of mania over 2 years or more than those who do not receive this kind of education (Miklowitz et al., 2003; Rea et al., 2003) (see the box below). As Robert said, once he and Jessie had begun to implement a successful relapse prevention plan, "I used to think I was in the driver's seat when I was manic, but that was just the illness talking. Now I think I'm in the driver's seat when I can stop myself from getting manic."

In this chapter, you'll learn a three-step strategy for getting off the train before mania takes you for a harrowing ride. The method, called a "relapse prevention drill," was developed by Alan Marlatt (Marlatt & Donovan, 2007) for the treatment of alcoholism relapses. The relapse drill was used successfully in our studies of family-focused treatment for people with bipolar disorder (see Chapter 6).

A relapse drill is like the fire drills you took part in back in school. Like fire drills, relapse drills are formulated when everything is safe and going well so that you know exactly what to do should a disaster occur. The relapse drill involves a series of steps you take to try to prevent the damage that could be done by an anticipated event:

■ Identify your prodromal symptoms.

■ List preventative measures.

■ Create a written plan or contract detailing the prevention procedures.

In the first step, *identifying your prodromal symptoms,* you make a list (usually with the help of others) of early warning signs that signal the beginning of a manic period. Identifying warning signs may also involve identifying the circumstances that elicit these symptoms (for example, drinking heavily, missing medication dosages, missing your therapy or physician appointments, encountering stressful work situations).

New research: Margaret Rea and our group at UCLA (Rea et al., 2003) studied two types of therapy for people with bipolar I disorder who had just had an episode of mania. One was the 21-session family-focused therapy I've described elsewhere; the other was a 21-session individual therapy. People who got family-focused therapy as well as medications had fewer hospitalizations and longer well periods between recurrences than those who got individual therapy and medications, even though the individual therapy had much of the same content as the family sessions (for example, learning to recognize the onset of new episodes). Involving family members did much to derail new manic episodes because family members were often the first to recognize when people were becoming ill. It is much harder to do that on your own.

In the second step, *listing preventative measures,* you brainstorm with your relatives about what actions to take if one or more prodromal signs appear (for example, call your psychiatrist, go in for an emergency medical appointment, arrange for others to take care of your children). These actions involve you, your doctor, and members of your core circle (see also the examples in the sections that follow).

In the third phase you, your significant others, and your doctors put the first and second steps together and *develop a written plan, which is a kind of contract, for what to do when you feel a manic episode coming on.* It's important that all key players have ready access to the contract so that they can help you put it into action when you are beginning to escalate—since that is when you're least likely to seek help.

This chapter focuses only on the prevention of manic episodes. This material is also relevant to preventing hypomanic episodes, which, while doing less damage, often have a similar set of warning signs and can be derailed with some of the same preventative strategies. The next two chapters discuss ways to prevent or minimize the downward spiral of depression. But before I get into the actual mechanics of developing a contract, let me say something about a sensitive issue that may have already occurred to you: the discomfort of relying on others when you are becoming ill.

A Little Help from Your Friends

"I start yelling and then I'm suddenly happy again, my sleep gets all disturbed, my thoughts go so fast I can't grasp them. I get high-spirited and strong-willed. But the weirdest thing to me is that I don't even know I'm ill, and why would I take my medications if I'm not ill? My husband always knows first, my sister next, and then my best friends. I'm always the last one to know when I'm getting manic."

—A 33-year-old woman with bipolar I disorder

The loss of insight into yourself is a neurological sign of mania—people don't see anything abnormal about their behavior when at the height of an episode, and sometimes even when they're cycling upward or coming out of an episode (Ghaemi et al., 2000). It's much like when someone has a stroke but is unaware of the memory deficits that follow, or when someone is hypnotized or in a dream state and doesn't realize he or she is acting differently. Because of this lack of insight, close relatives (your parents or siblings), a spouse or romantic partner, and friends are often the first to recognize your developing mania, seeing things in your behavior that you cannot (see the quotations from relatives on pages 191–192). For that reason, it's essential to involve them in the three steps of the relapse drill process. Refer back to the exercise in Chapter 8 in which you were asked to list those family members and friends whom you feel you could trust in an emergency.

Close relatives should be involved in the care of any person with a chronic ill-ness, whether it is a psychiatric disorder or a traditional medical disorder like heart disease or diabetes. We know from research in health psychology that people who have the best health care practices tend to engage family members in changing their unwanted habits. For example, their family members encourage them to eat healthy foods, avoid smoking, or get exercise. However, involving others is a double-edged sword: accepting the help or oversight of another person will probably cause you a certain amount of psychological distress (Lewis & Rook, 1999).

What is this distress about? Most people resent the idea of having others— particularly their close relatives—in a position of authority when they start to become ill. In the extreme, it can feel like agreeing to have someone else take away your independence. These are understandable reactions shared by people with many other medical illnesses. For example, people with insulin-dependent diabetes dislike the idea that someone else might have to inject them if they go into shock. People with high blood pressure or cardiovascular diseases dislike the idea that a spouse might control their food or salt intake.

People with bipolar disorder seem especially prone to feeling this way. I have heard the statement "I hate the idea of giving up control to anyone" from many clients, whether the control is being given up to a lover, a spouse, a doctor, or (espe-cially) a parent. I think there are several reasons why the issue of control is so salient to people with bipolar disorder. First, when you experience the internal feelings of chaos that mood fluctuations cause, it can become especially important to feel like you're at least in control of your outside world. Second, the feelings of confidence and power associated with the early and later stages of mania make you especially prone to rejecting the advice, opinions, or direct help of others. Third, many people with bipolar disorder have had bad experiences in the past when others—however well intentioned—tried to exert control over them during emergencies.

If your reaction to involving others is negative, think about why you feel this way. What bothers you most about leaning on others? Is the issue really about con-trol or personal autonomy? Is it about competition? Do you fear that there will be "strings attached" to the help? Alternatively, do you feel that you already ask too much of that person? In addressing the issue of whom to choose to help in emergen-cies, my clients have said: "The only person who would probably do this for me is exactly the person I don't want to have any more control over my life—my mother"; "My relationship with my wife is such that there's always a price to pay. If I lean on her, she'll slam me in some other way"; and "My brother and I have always been competitive. If he were to step in when I got manic, it would be kind of like saying, 'You won.'" It's important to try to understand what issues are at stake for you when you seek help from family members.

With these issues in mind, there are various ways that you can make the involve-ment of others feel more acceptable. *First, remember that you're asking them to step in when you get sick, not when you are healthy and competently running your day-to-day life.* You may fear that if you let others control one difficult interval in your life, giving up control in other areas will soon follow. You may fear that your wife, husband, or family member will always be hovering over you and making sure you eat, sleep, work, and socialize according to his or her rules. But the truth is that you are giving up control over only a fragment of your life, and for only the brief period during which you are escalating into mania. In fact, you may want to make this point clear to them: that you are asking for help *only* when you become ill, not when you're well.

Second, try to involve people with whom you do not have a long history of control battles. If you have a history of severe conflicts with your mother or father over independence, involve your siblings or close friends instead. There may be members of your core circle whom you see frequently who would know if something was going wrong, and whom you would trust with a degree of decision-making capacity during a time of crisis.

A practical problem that can come up when relying on social supports is that no one in your core circle may see you often enough to know, within a brief time, whether you are showing the early warning signs of mania. If your relatives live far away or speak to you only by phone, they may not observe the subtle changes that constitute your manic escalation, or they may not have the practical resources (for example, access to your physician) to be able to help. Clients have handled this by relying more heavily on local friends or roommates to perform the same functions or by giving long-distance relatives the phone numbers of their therapist or physician, with instructions to call if the relative has concerns.

If you do not have local connections with significant others, then it becomes all the more important to observe your own mood and behavior and seek help from your doctor when you need it. Some people use the fluctuations on their mood charts (Chapter 8) to determine when to increase contact with their therapist or physician. You may observe very minor increases in your mood as the episode is building, even over intervals as short as a few days. Although subjective, these observations can still inform your treatments and are far preferable to ignoring your illness and letting it take its own course.

Step 1: Identifying the Early Warning Signs of Mania

"He gets disconnected and withdrawn, kind of overwhelming, irritable ... in your face, loud, insensitive. He almost sounds like someone else in his body. But at this point I know what it looks like."
—The wife of a 50-year-old patient with bipolar I disorder

"I start thinking that I made mistakes at my job [as a refrigerator repairman] ... I start wondering if I wired things incorrectly and then thinking that the refrig-

erator in someone's house will blow up and burn them ... I start wondering whether I've just thought things or said them out loud. It makes me pull away from everybody. I get tight-lipped."
   —A 60-year-old man with bipolar I disorder with psychotic features

"She's usually shy, but when she's getting high she gets in people's faces; she gets imposing, overly emotional and effusive, like telling her whole life story to a bank teller ... I can see other people backing off and sort of looking at me, but she doesn't know that's how she's coming across."
   —The husband of a 37-year-old woman with bipolar I disorder

Defining Your Prodromal Phase

Recall that in Chapter 2, I described the manic syndrome as involving changes in mood, energy or activity levels, thinking and perception, sleep, and impulse control. Think about the beginning phases of mania as involving any or all of these. The *prodromal phase,* usually defined as the period from the first onset of symptoms to the point at which symptoms reach the height of their severity, can last a day or two to even a week or several weeks. During this prodromal phase, your symptoms will probably be mild and not necessarily troublesome—and therefore difficult to detect. They are usually muted versions of the symptoms of a full manic episode. I encourage my clients to err on the side of caution: the appearance of even one mild prodromal symptom is often a signal to seek help.

> **Effective prevention:** It is during the prodromal phase that the train has only just begun to leave the station and you have the most control over your fate. That's why it's important to prepare yourself to recognize even the mildest symptoms of mania.

In a study of the prodromal phases of manic episodes, Emily Altman and our group at UCLA (1992) observed people with bipolar disorder over a 9-month period following a hospitalization and rated their symptoms every month. Some had manic episodes during the observation period. The patients who developed mania showed very mild increases in "unusual thought content" in the month before their full episodes. These unusual thoughts were reflected in statements the patients made during clinical interviews regarding their beliefs in the influences of spirits, psychic powers, or the occult; their overly optimistic schemes for making money quickly; their feeling that others were staring or laughing at them; or the belief that their mind was sharper than everyone else's (in other words, mild psychotic symptoms). These changes in thinking were mild, and in some cases even the person expressing them could admit the ideas sounded odd or unrealistic. So, *observable changes in the content of your thinking and speech may be a clue that you are beginning to escalate.*

A survey by Grace Wong and Dominic Lam (1999) at the Institute of Psychiatry in London asked people with bipolar disorder to describe their early warning signals prior to previous manic episodes. The most frequent signals reported were reduced sleep and an increase in activity, both reported by over 40% of the respondents. Less frequently, people reported feeling euphoric or irritable, having racing thoughts, or being energetic and productive (goal driven) in the interval just before their episode.

It appears that many people with bipolar disorder can describe how they behave when they're getting manic, at least when they're asked after the fact. The harder question is, how do you know ahead of time what symptoms you should be looking for? *One way to increase the probability that you or others will recognize a developing episode is to make a list, when you're well, of early warning signs recalled from your last few episodes.* In other words, take advantage of the greater insight you have into your illness when you are well. This kind of objectivity will be harder to summon when you are heading into an episode, but having the list available may help you view your escalating mood, thoughts, and behaviors in a different light. Soon I'll talk about what you can actually do when these prodromal signs appear.

The following exercise will help get you started recording your prodromal symptoms. Your early warning signs, of course, may be different from the ones listed in the exercise. Nancy experienced the onset of her hypomanic episodes as an increase in anxiety and worry. Pete reported that, despite feeling speedy and internally stimulated, he withdrew more when he was escalating because he knew that he would alienate other people once he became manic. Heather became obsessed with a certain movie star and began "seeing things out of the corner of my eye."

It is important to distinguish the early warning signs of mania from those of depression, which usually involve feeling slowed down, fatigued, self-critical, hopeless, or uninterested in things (see the next chapter). Holly reported periods of increased irritability and anxiety prior to manic episodes but misidentified these as signs of depression. Prior to learning more about her disorder, she used to self-medicate her irritability with over-the-counter remedies such as fish oil or SAM-e. During one period of escalation she even convinced an internist to prescribe an anti-depressant, which made her manic symptoms much worse. With time, she observed that irritability and anxiety usually portended mania rather than depression, and she learned to rely on more traditional prevention methods, such as increasing the dosage of her mood stabilizer.

If you've had only one or two episodes, you may have difficulty listing your prodromal symptoms. Your family or friends may be able to help you here, as may your doctor. Chapter 2 describes how different mania can look to people who have the disorder than it looks to their family members or doctors. You may not agree with your relatives that a certain behavior (for example, your aggressiveness) or thinking pattern (for example, distractibility) characterizes you when you're getting manic, but it's better to list these behaviors or thinking patterns if they might in some way help your relatives recognize your episodes early. Likewise, record your own views

Listing Your Prodromal Signs of Mania or Hypomania

With the help of your close friends or relatives, list a couple of adjectives describing what your *mood* is like when your manic or hypomanic episodes first begin (*examples:* up, happy, more aware, willful, more reactive, cranky, irritable, euphoric, anxious, wired, cheery, like a yo-yo, pumped up).

_____

_____

Describe changes in your *activity* and *energy* levels as your manic episode is developing ("goal-directed behavior"). Include changes in how you relate to others (*examples:* call lots of people, make lots of new friends, take on more projects or start multitasking, talk more and faster, get in people's faces, tell people off, feel "horny" or very sexually driven).

_____

_____

_____

Describe changes in your *thinking* and *perception* (*examples:* thoughts race or at least go faster, sounds get louder, colors get brighter, I think I can do anything, I think others are looking at me or laughing at me, I get more interested in religion or the occult, I feel really smart and confident, I start thinking about many new ideas involving money, other people seem boring and closed-minded, I get extrasensory perception, I have psychic abilities, I think about hurting or killing myself, I ruminate about things, I get easily distracted).

_____

_____

_____

Describe changes in your *sleep* patterns (*examples:* sleeping 2 hours less than usual but not feeling tired the next day, waking up a lot during the night, staying up late and relying on catnaps during the day, not needing sleep).

_____

_____

Describe anything you've done in the last week that you wouldn't ordinarily do (*examples*: spent a lot of money or invested money on impulse, got one or more speeding tickets or drove recklessly, had more sexual encounters with partner or other partners, gambled money).

_____

_____

Describe the *context* (any changes, events, or circumstances) associated with these symptoms (*examples:* an increase in your work stress, stopping or becoming inconsistent with your medications, missing your doctor's appointments, starting to drink or use drugs, starting a new project, changes in your work hours, travel across time zones, more family or relationship conflicts, starting a new relationship or ending another one, changes in your financial circumstances).

_____

_____

_____

of your early warning signs or eliciting circumstances even if these views don't coincide with what your relatives think.

Robert, the man discussed at the beginning of the chapter, reported feeling very sexual and having racing thoughts before he had changes in his mood. His girlfriend, Jessie, saw it differently: she thought he became irritable first, then loud and physically intrusive. Another person with bipolar disorder, Tom, said that his manias almost always involved religious preoccupations and paranoia. His parents described him as "getting a certain look in his eyes" and "muttering stuff underneath his breath." The physician who treated Alan, the 60-year-old refrigerator repairman who believed that others could hear what he was thinking, felt that Alan's "bouncy, upbeat quality" was his first prodromal sign. Characterizations like these are helpful in rounding out what your prodromal phases look like from your own vantage point and the vantage point of others.

If you have bipolar II disorder, you may wonder whether your hypomanias really have a definable beginning and end. Hypomanic episodes can be very subtle, and, because they do not significantly interfere with your day-to-day functioning, they can be hard to distinguish from your usual state. However, even hypomania involves observable physical, cognitive, and emotional changes relative to your ordinary state. Typical prodromal symptoms of hypomania are sleep loss (sometimes a change of only an hour or two), increases in energy levels, increases in the speed of your thoughts or speech, a feeling of creativity or being able to "think outside the box," and irritability or impatience. Perhaps you can recall when these changes last occurred and you knew something was different.

Identifying the Context in Which Your Early Warning Signs Occur

You may have an easier time describing your prodromal signs if you also record information about the context in which they occur. For example, Robert felt that his irritability during his last manic episode was closely tied to increases in his work demands and annoyances expressed by coworkers, who had begun pressuring him about the company's financial outlook. For Ruth (see Chapter 8), manic cycles were nearly always precipitated by alcohol usage, sometimes even in small quantities. In the exercise above, there is a space to record any eliciting circumstances (usual or unusual) that you or any of your relatives think may be associated with your early warning signs.

Identifying circumstances associated with your prior manic episodes can help you minimize the impact of the next one. If you know that a particular circumstance (for example, an increased workload due to the Christmas holidays) was associated with your last episode (even if you don't think it caused your illness), you may want to become more vigilant about your feeling states or behavior during the next interval in which a similar source of stress occurs (for example, the next time you know your work demands will increase). This kind of vigilance can help you determine when you should ask for medical or other kinds of help, time off, or other accommodations (also see Chapter 13).

Teresa worked as an accountant. She came to realize that tax season, with its much longer work hours, was a trigger for her manic episodes. Prior to tax season, she obtained a prescription from her doctor for a tranquilizing medication (in her case, quetiapine [Seroquel]) to be started if she was unable to sleep, experienced racing thoughts, or felt overly goal driven. She was also able to arrange a few days off in the middle of tax season when she felt her mood escalating. As a result, she could get through tax season without a full episode, although she remained aware of an underlying energized state that was only partially masked by the medication.

Step 2, Part A: Preventative Steps You Can Take Yourself or with Others' Help

The focus of this section is on preventative steps you and your significant others can take at the appearance of one or more early warning signs. I've separated this section from the next (Part B), which concerns negotiating help from your doctor and the mental health system. Later, we'll put Steps 1 and 2 together into a written contract (Step 3).

Not all of the following preventative steps will apply to you. For example, you may be a person who has trouble with money but not with sexual indiscretions. You may have a history of making impulsive life decisions but have never driven recklessly. Your individual pattern of prodromal symptoms may dictate which of the following preventative measures are most urgent and which can wait. So, for example, if your prodromal symptoms are irritability and a decreased need for sleep, you may want to see your physician immediately, but asking someone else to hold on to your credit cards may not be as essential (unless irritability and sleep disturbances have, in the past, heralded a drive toward haphazard investments).

Managing Money

"One time I took a cab way downtown, tipped the driver 50%, and then bought two very expensive dresses at a department store that I thought was having a big sale. It turned out they weren't. I bought the dresses anyway, without knowing anything about the materials I was buying or whether the prices were good, without taking anyone with me, which I would have done normally. I spent over a thousand dollars, which we didn't have. I eventually took one of them back, but [when I was manic] I destroyed the other one by leaving an iron on top of it."

—A 55-year-old woman with bipolar I disorder describing a manic episode

Bipolar disorder makes managing money much harder than it would ordinarily be. When people are becoming manic, and especially when they are fully manic, they often go on spending sprees and invest wildly. In many ways this is one of the more humorous symptoms of bipolar disorder. In *An Unquiet Mind*, Jamison offers good examples of the thinking behind spending sprees. But as she recounts, spending sprees and foolish business investments can damage your life and contribute to your feelings of hopelessness after the manic episode has cleared.

Mania tends to generate "hyperpositive thinking," in which you overestimate your abilities to achieve (for example, make a lot of money) and underestimate the risks (for example, going into debt) of your behavior (Mansell & Pedley, 2008). When you have hyperpositive thoughts, it can be hard to step back and evaluate them objectively. In fact, some people equate *imagining* being able to do something with actually being able to do it. If you can imagine making a lot of money very quickly, how much harder could it be to actually do it? You and your significant others can become attuned to noticing when your thinking takes on an overly optimistic or hyperpositive turn. Do you suddenly believe you have found quick answers to financial problems that have been plaguing you for years? Are you becoming more and more enthralled with "get rich quick" or "pyramid" schemes? Do you find yourself unusually preoccupied with money or merchandise, driven to purchase expensive things (see the example of Robert and his electric guitars)? Do you think that you must have those things, sooner rather than later, or else you will be "ripped off"? Have you come to believe that your finances are virtually unlimited? Do you feel impatient or frustrated with your spouse when he or she tells you that you can't afford something?

You may not be able to prevent these thoughts from occurring, but here are some concrete steps you can take when they first appear:

- Have someone else hold on to your credit cards.
- Avoid trips to the bank unless you are going to take a trusted person with you.
- Stay away from your favorite stores.
- Avoid watching television stations whose primary purpose is to sell you goods.
- Don't give your credit card numbers or bank account information to telemarketers or investment counselors who call you with their special deals (an advisable practice even when you're feeling well, of course!).
- Avoid investing in the stock market altogether or making sudden changes in, or withdrawals from, your retirement accounts.
- Stay away from online stock trading.

In other words, decreasing your access to the *means* of implementing your plans makes it less likely you will actually carry them out.

Another practical maneuver is to arrange, when you're well, to make it logistically difficult for you to get a hold of large sums of money in a short period of time. There are several ways to do this, including keeping your money in small amounts spread across several accounts in different banks, or keeping the majority of your money in a joint account that requires a cosigner for a withdrawal. Karla, a 35-year-old woman with bipolar I disorder, made the following agreement with her boyfriend, Taki: Karla obtained three bank debit cards from their three shared accounts. Each of her cards was labeled with an expense category (for example, "clothing") and had a posted spending limit. The two agreed to determine which purchases she had already made and how close she was to the spending limit in each category on a weekly basis.

Effective prevention: Consider the 48-hour rule: Wait 24 hours after two good nights of sleep before making a purchase that exceeds a certain limit (Newman et al., 2001). During these 48 hours, discuss the intended purchase with as many as three trusted people (a family member, a friend, and a doctor or therapist). During the waiting period, ask yourself:

- "If someone else wanted to do what I am intending to do, what advice would I give that person?"
- "What is the worst thing that could happen if I wasn't able to follow through with my plans?"
- "What is the worst thing that could happen if I did carry them out?"

The passage of time, your own critique of the situation, and the input of others may help you evaluate the likely success of your financial decisions.

If you work closely with an investment counselor, it may be possible to entrust him or her with information about your illness so that he or she can stop you from investing too wildly or irrationally. Consider asking him or her to set an upper limit on how much money you can exchange within a single transaction.

Of course, maintaining these kinds of controls over your finances implies that your thinking is still fairly rational and that you can make good decisions. Rational thought is often possible during the early prodromal phases of mania (another reason to catch your episodes at the beginning). But as you may know, once your symptoms have accelerated, it becomes difficult to make logical decisions of any type and you may become highly resentful of anyone else's intervention. If you get your significant others involved *early* in the escalation process, and trust them enough to take your credit cards, provide final signatures on investments, or offer input into your spending decisions, you may be able to avoid a major financial collapse. Remember that most major financial decisions require a second opinion even in the best of circumstances.

Giving Up the Car Keys

Are your manic episodes usually characterized by reckless driving? This is the case for some people and not for others. One male client put it succinctly: "My highs almost always go along with some problem involving my car." If you do have a poor driving record, your early warning signs may signal the need to stop driving for now. Mania—much like drinking alcohol—makes your driving unsafe for yourself and others. You are at especially high risk for an auto accident if you are in a manic state and are also drinking and driving, as some people do. This is yet another arena in which it helps to have others' input. Your significant others can collaborate in helping you make good judgments about whether you can drive safely. While you will resent that your spouse or siblings have access to the car and you don't, remember that it is only for the limited time until your manic or hypomanic symptoms have cleared. Your doctor's input will also be valuable if he or she knows your driving history.

Avoiding Major Life Decisions

When you have one or more early warning signs, avoid making decisions that could affect your or others' futures, particularly if these decisions involve meetings with people who have a degree of "fate control." Now is not the time to ask your boss for a raise or a change in job duties—you are likely to come across to him or her as demanding and entitled (see also Chapter 13 on strategies for coping in the work setting). If you are an employer, delay your decision to assemble your employees to inform them of major structural changes in the company. Likewise, avoid making decisions about your family life that could lead to long-term consequences, such as getting married, divorced, deciding to have children, buying a new house, moving to another city, changing careers, or deciding to home school your kids.

It's hard to make these agreements with yourself, and even harder to implement them when you feel so good, so optimistic, and so elated. The decisions you feel pressed to make when you are getting manic seem like great ideas at the time, even though to others—or even to yourself when you're well—the ideas seem unrealistic and extremely risky. Try to think of the pressure to make these decisions, along with your feeling of greater mental clarity, as a part of your illness (especially if you also notice other symptoms, such as distractibility, racing thoughts, or an increase in your sex drive). People with bipolar disorder almost invariably make their best life decisions when they're in the remitted, euthymic state, and they usually end up regretting those decisions they made while manic.

Avoiding Risky Sexual Situations

"*I was getting real manic and got tired of being around Carol and the kids, so I went out to a bar. I ran into this old girlfriend and got drunk with her. We wound up in bed that night. I can't believe I did that—I'm not that kind of person! It seemed like such a great thing at the time. Of course, I felt terrible about it later and it really hurt my relationship with Carol. Even though she knows about mania and its biology and all that, she blames me for getting myself in that situation in the first place. She thought it was what I really wanted to do and the mania just gave me the excuse to do it."*

—A 46-year-old man with bipolar I disorder, recently separated from his wife

Like many rewarding endeavors, sex has a particular pull when you're getting manic. This can be true even if you're a person who is sexually conservative in your stable times. People get themselves into very risky sexual situations when they are escalating, and sometimes the emotional results—which can include feelings of shame, humiliation, and anger—worsen their cycling mood state. And, as you know, impulsive encounters carry a high risk of contracting sexually transmitted diseases.

As discussed in Chapter 2, mania is more a goal-driven state than a happy one. When you feel strongly pulled toward rewards, it's hard to step back and ask whether you're making healthy decisions for yourself or whether you really want those things. Some people benefit from knowing that they're prone to sexual "acting out" when they're in the prodromal and active phases of mania. Knowing this about yourself is the first step toward controlling it.

The best way to avoid dangerous sexual situations is to spend as much time as possible with people you know and trust, who can talk you out of impulsive sexual encounters. That is, when you go out at night, go with a friend who knows about your illness and who can "run interference" when you start to show poor judgment. Make special efforts to stay away from alcohol and street drugs: there is nothing worse than "self-medicating" an escalating mood with caffeine, drugs, or alcohol, which will almost certainly contribute to your mood escalation and lower your threshold for acting on a sexual impulse. Encourage your friends to take you home if they think you're making foolish decisions. Ultimately the decision to have or not have sex with someone is yours alone, but limit setting from others (even if quite irritating to you at the time) can help keep you from getting into encounters that you'll regret later.

Effective solution: The fact that becoming manic can increase your sex drive doesn't mean you have to avoid sexual activity. In fact, sex can be a good outlet for your energy if it is with the right person at the right time. The key is not to allow your mania to drive you toward irresponsible or risky sex.

Some people report that their primary romantic relationships improve when they get manic or hypomanic because they become more sexually engaged with their partners. Others report that an increase in their sexual encounters with their partner contributes to their upward escalation into mania. But, for

most people, being manic doesn't mean having to avoid sex with their regular partner.

A Reminder to Use Your "Maintaining Wellness" Strategies

When you are in the early stages of mania, it is essential to implement the strategies for maintaining wellness outlined in Chapter 8. I won't reiterate them all here;
suffice it to say that now is an especially important time to maintain a regular daily
routine. Try as hard as you can to get a full night's sleep (your doctor may be able to
recommend sleeping medications) and to keep your hours consistent from the week
to the weekend. Avoid stressful interactions with other people, particularly family
members, to the extent possible. Stick closely to your medication regimen. Continue
to chart your mood on a daily basis to identify changes in your mood status as early
as possible.

Step 2, Part B: Preventative Maneuvers Involving Your Doctor

Collaborating with your psychiatrist to prevent or diminish the impact of your
manic episodes is more complicated than it sounds. Most psychiatrists will tell you
that you should call them for an emergency medical appointment when you think
your illness is getting worse. This sounds like a "no-brainer." But the reality is that
you may not believe you are really ill or that your illness is bad enough to warrant
a phone call. Alternatively, you may not feel comfortable calling your doctor, especially if he or she is new to you or if you have had bad experiences with calling him
or her in the past.

Even if you see the need for emergency care, you may have doubts about how
much your doctor will really help you. You may fear that he or she will recommend
medication changes that have worse side effects than the ones you already experience. You may fear that he or she will immediately hospitalize you, which would
cause you social embarrassment at work or at home. Of course, you are more likely
to avoid hospitalization if you call your physician early than if you wait until the
point of no return. But calling during an emergency requires a certain amount of
trust that the physician will approach you compassionately and take steps that will
alleviate, not worsen, your symptoms. This section deals with strategies for collaborating with your physician during emergencies.

"When Should I Call, and What Should I Say?"

A good rule of thumb is to call as soon as you feel like your mood or energy
level has changed upward or downward, or if you believe (or if a significant other
believes) that you've developed one or more prodromal symptoms. *In other words,*

err on the side of getting help when you or others think you might need it, rather than assuming you don't and being wrong.

Make sure your doctor's phone numbers (or the numbers of the clinic where he or she works) are easily accessible, including his or her emergency contact information. There are places on your mania prevention contract (at the end of this chapter) to record this information. Most physicians have a "backup" doctor available for patients' emergencies during vacations or on weekends. Usually the phone numbers of this backup physician are included in the message on your doctor's or the clinic's emergency phone line. When you do reach your physician or his or her backup, be ready to recount any prodromal symptoms you think you have developed.

Below is a telephone interchange between a person with bipolar I disorder, Chad, and his psychiatrist, Dr. Eastwood.

Chad: Yeah, I think I'm going off again.

Dr. Eastwood: What's going on?

Chad: I'm taking my medication, but I'm having all sorts of thoughts and stuff.

Dr. Eastwood: Thoughts about what?

Chad: Like about the past. About my dad and his death and stuff.

Dr. Eastwood: How's your mood, Chad? Any changes?

Chad: Yeah, just more pissed off, getting grouchy, yelling at the kids. I just don't know if I wanna do the whole family thing anymore.

Dr. Eastwood: How's your sleep been the last few nights?

Chad: OK, but not great; can't stay asleep very long. I've been pacing at night and stuff. Thoughts going a mile a minute. Bed's not comfortable.

Dr. Eastwood: Sounds like a lot's going on right now. Anything else I need to know? Are you thinking about hurting yourself? Do you feel like you need to be in the hospital?

Chad: No, not there yet. Just upset and stuff. Mad, can't sleep.

Dr. Eastwood: How have things gone with your medications?

Chad: I missed my lithium this morning, took it this evening.

In this interchange, Dr. Eastwood has done a quick assessment and concluded that Chad may be in the prodromal phase of a manic or a mixed episode. At this stage, Chad's escalation can be treated on an outpatient basis, which Dr. Eastwood did by setting up an emergency medical appointment, increasing the dosage of Chad's lithium, and adding a small dose of an antipsychotic medication. A blood test revealed that Chad's lithium level was low, even though Chad said that he had been taking the medication relatively regularly. These changes to his medication regimen did the trick without a host of new side effects. Within a week, Chad's mania had stopped escalating and his depression subsided, and he began to return to his baseline state.

Chad did a good job of describing his prodromal symptoms. Dr. Eastwood guided him toward describing these symptoms and his medication usage. She was fairly task oriented and kept Chad from going off the track. Notice that Dr. Eastwood did not pursue any psychotherapeutic issues over the phone, such as Chad's feelings about his father or his current family. Expect that when you call your physician under emergency circumstances, in most cases he or she will not conduct a psychotherapy session with you. This may be frustrating because you may feel that certain personal issues are important in explaining your symptoms. Many people believe, as Chad did, that their manic symptoms are triggered by feelings of loss. But the emergency phone call to your physician is mainly for the purpose of evaluating whether a change in medication is necessary or, in more extreme circumstances, whether you need to be hospitalized. In a session with your therapist, once your symptoms have settled down, he or she may be able to help you make sense of how current or past stressors or losses are contributing to your escalating mood.

"What If I'm Uncomfortable with My Physician?"

Robert, described at the beginning of this chapter, did not particularly like his physician and saw her infrequently. Perhaps as a result, this doctor was not as helpful as she could have been in preventing his manic episode. Had he been in contact with a doctor with whom he had a good relationship, a face-to-face session might have been arranged quickly, with more positive results.

Not everyone feels comfortable calling his or her doctor during an emergency, and during a manic escalation your discomfort may be exaggerated (most emotions become more dramatic during mania). One of my clients, Holly, had long-standing frustrations with her doctor. She called Dr. Nelson on a number of occasions when she felt she was cycling rapidly. Typically, Dr. Nelson did not call her back. She considered switching physicians but wasn't convinced she had given Dr. Nelson a fair try.

I encouraged Holly to talk over this dilemma with Dr. Nelson, a man whom I had experienced as very approachable. But Holly felt uncomfortable broaching the topic, fearing that he was going to "fire me as a patient." I finally interceded and called Dr. Nelson when Holly developed mixed affective symptoms and suicidal thoughts. Dr. Nelson told me that he had tried to talk to Holly on a number of occasions but that *she* hadn't returned *his* calls. He also found that when he gave Holly advice on how to control her symptoms, she would become angry and uncooperative. So there were frustrations on both sides.

Eventually, we scheduled a meeting involving Holly, Dr. Nelson, and me. We hammered out a series of agreements regarding what steps would be taken if she developed mixed or manic symptoms in the future. Dr. Nelson gave an additional phone number to Holly, and explained, again, his emergency and backup/vacation policies. There is still tension in their relationship about handling emergencies but to a lesser degree. Ultimately, Holly's treatment was made more successful by the direct contact between her psychiatrist and psychotherapist (see also Chapter 6).

Your best option is to talk over your concerns with your physician until you feel reasonably comfortable about contacting him or her in an emergency. Explain your fears about new medications, side effects, or the need for hospitalization (discussed more on pages 206–207). If your "bottom line" is that you would never call this person when you're feeling bad, find another physician.

"Should Somebody Else Call for Me?"

When you feel exhilarated, excited, and goal driven, you may see no reason to destroy this by taking what the physician has to offer—which is usually more medication. For this reason, it may make sense for someone close to you to make the call to your psychiatrist or GP. Give members of your core circle some leeway in deciding when to make this call, recognizing that you may not agree that your physician's help is needed. It is my strong impression—both in my clinical practice and in our research studies—that people who have allowed members of their core circle to call their doctors in emergencies have had better outcomes (Miklowitz et al., 2000). For example, Paul, the husband of Lorraine, a 64-year-old woman with bipolar I disorder, routinely called his wife's doctor whenever she became giddy, delusional, or agitated. Lorraine's doctor was usually able to deal with the escalation over the phone by making adjustments to her prescriptions instead of hospitalizing her.

Contact between your relatives and your doctor may require mutual understanding about treatment policies. Your doctor should make clear to you and your relatives the circumstances under which they should call (for example, when you are clearly escalating, when you are refusing all your treatments). Your relatives may have a set of unrealistic expectations, such as the following: your doctor will call them as soon as you've missed an appointment or as soon as you've reported *any* symptoms; your doctor will discuss any planned medication adjustments with them before making them; they can call whenever there has been a family argument or

> **Effective prevention:** Consult your physician as to whether a friend or close relative can accompany you to your medical visits. If you have become confused or distractible due to your symptoms, your significant other may be better able to recall the physician's recommendations when you need to implement them later.

whenever they want to know something about bipolar disorder. These are assumptions your physician may not share. Remember to sign a release-of-information form for your doctor, allowing your chosen relative to exchange information with him or her.

"What Will My Doctor Do?"

During an emergency session, your physician will probably take the steps outlined in the sidebar. He or she will start by assessing your symptoms and reevaluating your medication regimen. Your doctor may decide to make changes to your regimen over the phone if an appointment can't be arranged. A major intent of catching and treating your symptoms early is to help you avoid hospitalization, but if this is not possible, your doctor can help you arrange one.

He or she will usually begin by asking you the kinds of questions Dr. Eastwood asked Chad. Physicians vary on which symptoms they emphasize (some focus on mood and others on activity levels or sleep), but generally, the more you can speak to your doctor in the language of prodromal symptoms (for example, racing thoughts, goal-driven behavior, decreased need for sleep), the more he or she will know what to recommend. Your physician will probably want to know if you have missed any dosages of your medication, and you should be as honest as possible about this. It's not at all uncommon for people to miss dosages (especially if they are expected to take a lot of pills) when they are becoming manic or hypomanic.

If you are on lithium, divalproex, or (less frequently) carbamazepine (Tegretol), your doctor may ask you to get your blood level tested. He or she will most likely be interested in your "trough" level, which is usually collected 10–14 hours after your last dose (people who get their blood level checked just a few hours after taking their last dose may appear to be getting enough medication when, in fact, they are not). For example, if you have been taking lithium and your trough level is 0.6 milliequivalents per liter or less (see Chapter 6), the doctor may conclude that you've missed dosages or that your dosage is too low to be therapeutic. Then he or she may recommend that you increase your lithium dosage as a way of preventing further

Steps Your Physician Will Take to Prevent the Escalation of Mania

- Perform an assessment of the severity of your symptoms.
- Evaluate blood levels of certain of your medications (lithium, divalproex).
- Make changes to your regimen, including adding or subtracting certain medications or increasing the dosage of current medications.
- Arrange a hospitalization if necessary.

escalation. Because it may take a few days before your blood level is processed, your doctor may decide not to wait for that information before changing your dosage, especially if he or she has been collecting blood level information from you all along. If possible, your doctor may increase the frequency of your treatment sessions during the interval in which your symptoms are worsening.

If your physician increases the dosage of your primary mood stabilizer, you and your significant others will want to become familiar with the signs of neurotoxicity (see also Chapter 6), which are the medical complications associated with getting too much of a medication. For lithium, these symptoms include drowsiness, severe nausea, abdominal discomfort, severe diarrhea, blurry vision, slurred speech, muscle twitching, or being confused as to where or who you are. For divalproex, they include severe dizziness, drowsiness, irregular breathing, severe trembling, or coma. For carbamazepine, they include double vision, unsteadiness when walking, or feeling dizzy. If you show any of these symptoms, your doctor should be notified immediately—by you or a member of your core circle—so that he or she can adjust, or even take you off, these medications.

Your doctor may add some of the medications discussed in Chapter 6, including atypical antipsychotics with mood-stabilizing properties such as quetiapine or risperidone, or benzodiazepines such as clonazepam (Klonopin) or lorazepam (Ativan). These medications may help bring you down from an activated, agitated state, improve your sleep, and treat delusional thinking (for example, paranoia). If you are on only one mood stabilizer, your doctor may add a second one (for example, adding divalproex to lithium). These decisions are often based on physician choice rather than research data. For example, we do not know whether simply increasing the dosage of lithium or divalproex is more or less effective in preventing relapses of mania than taking the two mood stabilizers together.

Don't be surprised if your physician believes that the best treatment for your escalating mania is to stop taking one of your current medications rather than to start you on a new one. If you are getting manic and are believed to have rapid cycling (four or more episodes per year), the most effective intervention may be to discontinue your antidepressant if you are on one. Your physician is unlikely to start you on an antidepressant when you are escalating (see Chapter 6). Your physician may also recommend that you discontinue your antipsychotic medications or your periodic use of caffeine or bronchodilators such as Proventil.

"When Is Hospitalization Required?"

Many people with bipolar disorder never need to be hospitalized. In addition, alternatives to inpatient hospitalization—such as partial hospital or day hospital programs—have emerged in recent years as short-term strategies for emergencies. These programs provide close monitoring of your symptoms and treatment response without the need to enter an inpatient facility. But if your manic symptoms escalate to a certain point of disruptiveness, or if you are actively suicidal or dangerous to others, there is a good chance that your doctor will recommend that you be hospitalized for a period of time. You are more likely to be hospitalized if you are manic (or mixed) than if you are hypomanic or depressed.

It is very common for people in manic episodes to believe that they don't need to be hospitalized. Often they insist on leaving very soon after they are admitted, thinking they are closer to recovery than their doctors or others think. Perhaps you have had some of these experiences. But if your doctor believes that you are at imminent risk of hurting yourself or someone else, or are otherwise unable to take care of yourself, it is his or her professional, ethical, and legal responsibility to seek permission from a judge to continue inpatient treatment, under a court order if necessary. You won't feel good about this course of action, but it may be necessary to preserve safety for yourself and others.

If your doctor does recommend hospitalization, it is usually easiest if he or she calls the hospital to arrange for an inpatient bed. In some cases, you or your family members may have to make the arrangements (for example, if your doctor hasn't seen you in some time or doesn't have hospital admitting privileges). As a relapse prevention maneuver, keep the phone number of the recommended hospital's emergency room and your insurance cards in easily accessible places (see the Contract for Preventing Mania exercise on pages 210–211).

Nowadays, many people have managed care health insurance plans that stipulate which hospitals can or cannot admit them, and for how long. Before signing up for a new insurance policy, it is important to find out if the psychiatrist whom you see is "in network" and if the hospitals at which he or she has admission privileges are providers within the plan. Otherwise, your health insurance policy could require you to be admitted to a different hospital from the one your doctor might recommend.

"What Will Happen to Me in the Hospital?"

If you do have an inpatient hospitalization, you will probably meet on a daily basis with an inpatient psychiatrist (who may or may not be your regular doctor). You should expect some individual or group counseling sessions concerning life issues, relapse prevention, and posthospital adjustment. In the best-case scenario, family or spousal visits are encouraged and become an integral part of the treatment plan.

Hospitalization can be a scary proposition. Many people fear that psychiatric hospitals are like snake pits—a place where things are dirty, people are violent, the nurses are cruel, shock treatment is mandatory, and little help is delivered. Although this is largely a distortion based on the past, hospitals do vary considerably in quality, just as do the doctors and nurses who work within them. Many hospitals are excellent and provide state-of-the-art mental health care. Others are underfunded, employ out-of-date models of intervention, and are not oriented toward treatment as much as the protection of others. If you have been in a hospital more than once, you probably have had diverse experiences, depending on which hospital you went to and the condition in which you were admitted.

Consider the following if you need to be hospitalized. First, many people confuse being hospitalized with being institutionalized. The latter usually means that a person is kept in a hospital for months or years at a time, under court order. Nowadays, psychiatric hospitalizations are very short, averaging about a week long.

Second, the treatment you receive in the hospital is usually geared toward controlling your acute symptoms (including suicidal thoughts or intentions) and keeping them from worsening to reduce the immediate risk to you and those around you. Hospitalization also allows you to "dry out" if you have been drinking or using drugs during your manic escalation. Your inpatient stay will enable you to start a new regimen of medications or newly adjusted dosages, "wash out" your existing medications, or try other treatments (for example, electroconvulsive therapy or, in some hospitals, rapid transcranial magnetic stimulation [rTMS] if you are acutely manic, mixed, or depressed and not responding to mood stabilizers, antipsychotics, or other agents). However, your stay will probably not be long enough to know if your new regimen is effective in the long term.

Third, hospitalization is not a personal failure. You have a biological vulnerability to manic or depressive episodes that is not fully under your control, and it is not your fault if you need hospitalization. Being hospitalized does not mean that others have to run your life from now on. Instead, it signifies the temporary giving up of control for a short period of time. You will have your life back soon enough, especially if you are successful in collaborating with your doctor to develop an effective posthospital plan.

Finally, hospitalization can provide you with a much-needed rest or break from the stressors of your day-to-day life. Although you'd no doubt rather spend a week in the Bahamas, a short or even a longer hospital stay can give you time to think through what is and isn't working about your treatment plan. It can also give you distance from your relatives, which you (and they) may need from time to time. Robert's hospitalization helped him rethink his feelings about Jessie and

Effective treatment: If your doctor, therapist, and family members believe hospitalization will help you, you may find it less frightening and more acceptable if you remember the following:

- Being hospitalized is not the same as being institutionalized; it lasts a very short time.
- Hospitalization can be the best way to get acute symptoms under control.
- Agreeing to be hospitalized does not signal the end of your control over your own life.
- Hospitalization can provide a needed break from daily stresses and family conflicts and give you a chance to gain a new perspective.

his children, and upon being discharged, he felt more resolved to make things work. It will be hard to take this view when you are first admitted to a hospital, but later you may have quite a different view of the experience.

Step 3: Developing a Mania Prevention Contract

Now let's put together everything discussed so far in this chapter into a written contract for relapse prevention. The following exercise asks you to summarize what you have concluded about your prodromal phase, the steps you and your significant others can take to prevent relapse, and emergency procedures involving your doctors. Consult with your family members, spouse, doctor, and other trusted persons to make sure that everyone understands what he or she is being asked to do.

When filling out this contract, try to include as many options as possible. Some of the options will probably seem more comfortable to you than others, but it's better to write them all down even if you don't end up using them. Encourage your significant others to be open about what they do and don't feel comfortable doing when you're cycling into mania. Write into the contract only those responsibilities you and they are willing to accept. Alternatively, list all of your possible options and rank them from top to bottom in order of preference. Ask everyone to sign the contract.

Troubleshooting Your Contract

Things improved for Robert after his hospital discharge. He found a new psychiatrist, Dr. Barnard, who met with him several times after his discharge to help him optimize his medication regimen. Robert and Jessie also met with a psychologist, who helped them develop a relapse prevention contract. Together they developed a list of his prodromal symptoms, which included mild irritability, mistrustfulness, standing too close to people and talking too loud, a sudden disinterest in his job, an increase in his sex drive, and a subjective feeling of mental clarity. They made a distinction between these early warning signs and signs of his full-blown manias, such as feeling elated or expansive, socially inappropriate outbursts of anger, spending excessively and impulsively, grandiose beliefs about his musical talents, severe loss of sleep, and a firm denial that anything was wrong. They also agreed on the environmental circumstances associated with his escalations: an excessive workload, family arguments, and financial problems.

Robert and Jessie negotiated a series of prevention steps. One of these involved giving Jessie the freedom to call his psychiatrist if Robert appeared to be escalating. They also agreed that when his symptoms were still mild, Jessie would help get him away from his immediate stressors (for example, encourage him to take a few days off work with her). They agreed, as a couple, to try to maintain regu-

Contract for Preventing Mania

Your physician's name: _____ Phone number, office: _____

Phone number, emergency: _911_,_____

Your therapist's name: Britnani_____ Phone number, office: _____

Phone number, emergency: _____

Name of local hospital: U of U_____ Emergency room number: _____

Your insurance carrier: Medicare+Medicade Policy number: _____

Group number (if applicable): _____

1. List your typical early warning (prodromal) signs of a manic episode (from the exercise on page 194 above).

   _____

   _____

   _____

2. List the circumstances in which these prodromal symptoms are most likely to occur.

   _____

   _____

   _____

3. Ask one or more members of your core circle to add any other early warning signs they've observed, and, if relevant, the circumstances in which these signs first appeared.

   _____

   _____

   _____

4. List what behaviors you can perform when these symptoms start to appear (*examples:* calling your doctor; getting your blood level tested; sticking closely to your medication regimen; trying to get regular sleep; getting back on a structured daily and nightly routine; avoiding alcohol, drugs, or caffeine; giving up your credit cards and car keys; avoiding major financial or other life decisions; avoiding risky sexual situations).

   _____

   _____

   _____

   _____

(*cont.*)

5. List what behaviors your relatives, significant others, or friends can perform (*examples:* call your physician, talk to you in a supportive way, tell you what you are doing that worries them, tell you how much they care about you, keep you from overscheduling yourself, call the hospital emergency room, remind you to take your medications, accompany you to doctor's appointments, take care of your children, accompany you when you go out at night, help manage your money, help you stay on a regular sleep–wake cycle, help you stay away from alcohol or drugs).

_____

_____

_____

_____

6. List what you would like your psychiatrist to do (*examples:* meet with you on an emergency basis, take your blood level, revise your medication regimen as appropriate, call the hospital and arrange for admittance, if necessary).

_____

_____

_____

_____

Signatures   Date

_____   _____

_____   _____

_____   _____

_____   _____

lar sleep–wake routines, especially when one or more of his prodromal signs were observable. Finally, Robert consented to have Jessie accompany him to the hospital emergency room, if it became necessary.

Robert did not stay episode free, however. His next manic episode began about 2 months later, but this time he and Jessie caught it earlier. Once again, he refused to make an appointment with his doctor. He admitted that he was probably escalating but didn't want to take any more medication. He and Jessie began to argue. As Robert later described it, Jessie became "rigid ... finger-pointing, serious, not loving." Jessie got increasingly more desperate when she found that Dr. Barnard was out of town. She called Dr. Barnard's backup, who prescribed an increase in the dosage of Robert's antipsychotic medicine, risperidone. Robert agreed to the medication adjustment, which kept him from going back into the hospital. Nonetheless, more damage was done to their relationship, and Jessie considered leaving. Robert also had more conflicts with his coworkers and other family members during this interval.

A meeting with his psychologist, arranged about a week after Robert changed his medication, focused on troubleshooting the relapse prevention plan. Robert, who was still hypomanic, complained that the plan hadn't worked because of Jessie's emotional stance. He said that he needed her to be "kinder and gentler" in her approach. The psychologist asked him to be more specific, and he said, "I want her to tell me she loves me, and in a more tender way tell me that she thinks I need help and why, even if I'm not receptive." He added that he wished she wouldn't take his irritability so personally and instead see it as part of his disorder. Jessie, in turn, expressed frustration that he hadn't gone to his medication appointments when Dr. Barnard had been in town. "I want him to go for me or for our relationship, if he won't do it for himself, knowing that I'm speaking out of caring for him." She wasn't sure if she could take a gentler emotional stance when dealing with his escalating mood. "It's hard to smile at a bus that's about to run you over," she said.

The psychologist encouraged Robert and Jessie to practice communicating in the way the other wished: Jessie trying to be more tender in her approach and Robert ceding a degree of control to her. They also discussed the potential involvement of other family members, such as Robert's son, at times of emergencies. Robert decided, however, that he wanted to shield Brian as much as possible from his illness and didn't want his son interacting with his doctors. Jessie agreed.

When she returned from her trip, Dr. Barnard met with Robert and Jessie and told them of a medication plan to undertake if Robert had one or more prodromal signs and could not immediately get in to see her: increase his dosage of risperidone and add a benzodiazepine (Klonopin) for sleep. She wrote a prescription with a plan for increasing the dosage, with the understanding that Robert would come in to see her as soon as possible after initiating the new dosing schedule. These modifications were written into their modified contract (for example, "Robert to increase risperidone dosage; Robert to call his doctor or be willing to let Jessie make the call if he will not; Jessie to try to recognize Robert's irritability as part of the manic syndrome"). Robert and Jessie agreed to reexamine the contract every three months and revise it as necessary.

Robert has continued to have mood cycles, but his episodes increasingly resemble hypomanias rather than manias. He feels he has a good relationship with Dr. Barnard and his psychologist, and he and Jessie are still together and working on their problems. He has explained his bipolar disorder to his son, who, with time, is becoming more understanding.

Think of your mania prevention contract as a work in progress. The prevention steps can be defined, agreed upon, and practiced when you're healthy, but no one can be certain how well they will work until you put them into action. Knowing your prodromal signs, being responsive to the feedback of others, and knowing when to ask for help are all central to making the contract effective in real life.

> **Effective solution:** If you have a manic episode despite having a prevention contract in place, take time afterward to review what went wrong and how the contract should be revised.

If you do have a manic episode despite your prevention contract, sit down with your doctor, family, or therapist after the dust has settled and try to decide what did and did not work. Were you unable to reach your physician or a backup physician? If so, ask your doctor to recommend medication adjustments that you can make on your own the next time you start to escalate. Ask him or her to write down your emergency medicine plan in prescription form, with the understanding that you will follow the plan when your early warning signs appear (for example, "increase my Zyprexa dose when I feel agitated and unable to sleep") and arrange an in-person meeting as soon as possible thereafter.

Were there other problems that prevented the contract from working? For example, were you hostile to significant others, who then threw up their hands and refused to help any further? Were your relatives unnecessarily controlling? Alternatively, did you ask for help but no one was available? If so, perhaps you can think of other relatives or friends to whom you are less likely to react negatively when you are escalating or who might be available with little notice.

Was the contract ineffective because you found the recommendations made by significant others unacceptable? If so, how could the contract be modified to make these recommendations more palatable? For example, Gabriel refused to see a certain doctor whom his parents insisted he see. He was, however, willing to see a doctor he had found by himself. Being able to see his preferred doctor was added as a modification to his mania prevention contract. You will find that the contract has a much greater chance of succeeding if you have had input into each step, have listed choices of strategies rather than only one single strategy, and can troubleshoot and revise the contract as you go along.

■

Because of the influences of your individual neurophysiology, you should not expect to be able to fully prevent manic episodes. *But you have a window of opportunity in the early stages of manic escalation in which you may be able to decrease the severity of your oncoming episode.* Being able to identify your episodes early and receive emergency treatment will give you a greater feeling of autonomy in the long run, even if it means having to give up control to others in the short run. A written contract, especially if it is developed and filled out when you are feeling well, will enhance the likelihood that your and others' prevention efforts will be successful.

Depressive episodes have a different quality. They do not come on suddenly and often last longer than manic episodes. But as is true for mania, identifying and combating the early warning signs of depression will help you feel more in control of your disorder. In Chapter 10, you'll see how you can use the support of your core circle, along with certain personal strategies such as behavioral activation and cognitive restructuring, to try to keep your depressions from becoming more serious or debilitating.

10

Halting the Spiral of Depression

One day you realize that your entire life is just awful, not worth living, a horror and a black blot on the white terrain of human existence. One morning you wake up afraid you are going to live. ... That's the thing I want to make clear about depression: It's got nothing at all to do with life. In the course of life, there is sadness and pain and sorrow, all of which, in their right time and season, are normal—unpleasant, but normal. Depression is in an altogether different zone because it involves a complete absence: absence of affect, absence of feeling, absence of response, absence of interest. The pain you feel in the course of a major clinical depression is an attempt on nature's part (nature, after all, abhors a vacuum) to fill up the empty space.

—Elizabeth Wurtzel, *Prozac Nation* (1994, p. 22)

In bipolar disorder, depression can occur in "pure" form—in which you feel extremely sad, slowed down, lethargic, fatigued, or numb—or as part of a mixed episode, which means you feel both the symptoms of depression and those of mania. Many writers have described the despair of depression, both the bipolar and unipolar (major depressive) forms (for example, Jamison, 1995, 2000; Solomon, 2002; Styron, 1992; Thompson, 1996). What is important for you, however, is that you learn to recognize the early warning signs that *your* depression is recurring. The central goal of this chapter is to give you psychological self-management techniques that you can use to greatest benefit during the early phases of depression, before it becomes incapacitating. When self-management techniques effectively improve your mood during these early stages, you may be able to avoid the medical interventions that are usually required when depression reaches its most severe point.

Medical interventions usually include antidepressant agents, higher dosages of mood stabilizers, ECT, and hospitalization. For reasons that are discussed in Chapter 6, it's best to avoid some of these alternatives if you possibly can (for example, antidepressants, which can inadvertently lead to rapid cycling). Nonetheless, it's essential to consult your physician about these medical alternatives if self-management or your personal psychotherapy is not keeping your depression from getting worse.

In the next chapter, I talk about suicidal episodes and how to combat them. Suicidal thoughts and impulses are a very common component of the bipolar syndrome. They are nothing to be ashamed of—virtually everyone with this disorder has thought about suicide at some point. Fortunately, there are ways to protect yourself from sinking further when you begin to feel suicidal.

Mostly, this chapter is about hope. Depression is a painful aspect of the human condition, and people with bipolar disorder experience it more intensely than virtually anyone else. To make matters worse, the pain may not be obvious to those around you, and they may want you to just snap out of it. You can't do that, but there are some things you *can* do—often with the support of others—to help combat it.

Bipolar Depression: An Illness, Not a Character Flaw

Alexis, a 37-year-old woman with bipolar II disorder, had been dealing with an ongoing depressive state for years—a state that occasionally became worse and incapacitated her. She had tried to alleviate her depression through various antidepressants, medicinal herbs, cognitive therapy, group treatment, and, at times, "exercising to a fault ... driving myself constantly until my body gave out." Her depressions were usually accompanied by self-accusations about being weak, not having the courage to face up to her problems, and not being able to accomplish her goals. She had heard that depression had a strong biological basis, especially in bipolar disorder, but had never really connected this fact to her situation.

A breakthrough occurred in her therapy when her clinician said to her, "If you had diabetes, would you be blaming yourself for not being able to control your blood sugar levels?" She began to entertain the idea that she needed to "make an end run around my depression" rather than trying to get rid of it and feeling like a failure for not being able to do so. When she started thinking of her depression as a physical illness that was caused by factors not entirely within her control—and something she needed to learn to live with—her mood began to improve, albeit gradually. She learned that accepting the reality of her depression was not the same as giving in to it or becoming immersed in it.

She eventually recognized that, when depressed, she needed to slow down, take care of herself (sleep regularly and balance her pleasurable versus work activities), "give myself a break," and not try too hard to drive her depression away with frenetic activity. She has never been entirely free of depression, but now she has a different perspective: "I can now ignore those old tapes in my mind telling me I'm a bad person. I now see that this is the depression talking."

If you had a bad case of the flu, what would you do? Most of us would take time to convalesce and not expect too much of ourselves while recovering. Likewise, if you were suffering from chronic pain, such as severe back problems, you would probably give yourself a break in terms of your physical expectations of yourself by declining to lift heavy objects, not sitting in the same position for hours, and carefully selecting a "back-friendly" form of exercise. In all likelihood you would pay close attention to those things that helped alleviate your pain and avoid those that made it worse.

Why don't we do the same for ourselves when we're in emotional pain? One of the keys to coming out of depression is to *show kindness to yourself.* Try to think of bipolar depression in the same way you would think of a flu, chronic pain, or perhaps a long-term medical illness such as diabetes. No one would think of blaming a diabetic for not being able to control the way his or her body processed sugar. No one would blame a person with epilepsy for having seizures. Likewise, you should not blame yourself for having depression. As discussed in Chapter 5, bipolar depression is strongly influenced by biochemical, genetic, and neurological factors. It is *not* the product of a character flaw, personality defect, or lack of moral fiber.

Even the well-known explanatory concept of depression as the result of low self-esteem is suspect with regard to bipolar depression. Many people think that if you're depressed, you must not think much of yourself. This low estimation might characterize the way you feel when you're depressed, but you may feel quite differently about yourself when you're well. In other words, low self-esteem is not a trait. Rather, it may just be a symptom of your depression. In fact, one of the leaders in our field, Martin Seligman, of the University of Pennsylvania, has compared self-esteem to a fuel gauge: It is a measure of how we're doing at any one time—how much fuel is in the tank—but it can change depending on what we are able to accomplish (Seligman et al., 1996).

Depression is not due to an unwillingness to accept responsibility, fears of coping with reality, laziness, cowardice, or weakness. It is an illness. To be sure, there are things you can do to make yourself feel better or at least stop your depression from worsening. But the fact that you have depression in the first place, or that you're having a difficult time making it go away, probably says more about your biology than it does about your effort, willpower, or self-esteem. Knowing this basic fact about depression will not make it disappear, but may make it easier to cope with.

Different Styles of Coping with Depression

As you read this chapter and the next, you'll see that I recommend a diverse set of techniques for coping with depression. These involve changes in your behavior and thinking as well as in your relationships with others. You'll see that some of the techniques involve distraction. Distracting yourself in a positive manner means seeking out and engaging in activities that keep you busy, give you pleasure, and help keep your mind off your pain and anguish. Examples include spending time with others with whom you feel close, exercising, listening to music, reading, and relaxing.

Some of the coping strategies involve emotion-focusing. That is, you learn to recognize that you're depressed and experiencing pain and you teach yourself to look at it, label it, and accept it without becoming overwhelmed by it, as Alexis learned to do ("mindfulness"). Emotion-focused coping can also involve talking about your feelings with people who are supportive and empathic.

A third strategy, cognitive coping, involves learning to combat and challenge negative thinking patterns about specific situations or events (for example, self-blaming thoughts) and considering alternative ways to view these situations or events. As you'll see, these strategies are not mutually exclusive. In fact, the people who do best with bipolar depressions seem able to sample from all three, using different strategies at different times.

Are You Depressed Right Now?

Depression is not just sadness. As you know if you've had a serious depression, it can be a blunted, empty, inhibited state marked by loss of interest in most things, an inability to experience pleasure, and withdrawal from everybody and everything (see the quote by Elizabeth Wurtzel that opened this chapter). Some people don't even feel sad when they're depressed. Instead, they just feel numb. If you've had mixed episodes, you're probably familiar with the feeling of being fatigued and drained but also charged up, irritable, and anxious ("tired but wired"). In the same way that mania is not always a happy state, depression is not always a sad state. But unlike mania, depression is almost never enjoyable or intoxicating.

Try filling out the Quick Inventory of Depressive Symptoms Self-Rating Scale (Rush et al., 2003) that follows. This scale is intended to measure the severity of your depression as you've experienced it in the past week. Fill out the scale according to how you've felt most of the time and tally your total score, which can range from 0 (not at all depressed) to over 21 (very depressed). The four answers to each item are coded from 0 to 3; you get the total test score by summing the following:

- The highest number from questions 1–4
- The number from question 5
- The highest number from questions 6–9
- The total of each question from questions 10–14
- The highest number from questions 15–16

Quick Inventory of Depressive Symptoms

Please check the one response to each item that best describes how you have felt for the past 7 days.

1. Falling Asleep:
   - ❑ I never take longer than 30 minutes to fall asleep.
   - ❑ I take at least 30 minutes to fall asleep, less than half the time.
   - ❑ I take at least 30 minutes to fall asleep, more than half the time.
   - ☑ I take at least 60 minutes to fall asleep, more than half the time.

2. Sleep during the night:
   - ❑ I do not wake up at night.
   - ❑ I have a restless, light sleep with a few brief awakenings each night.
   - ☑ I wake up at least once a night, but I go back to sleep easily.
   - ❑ I awaken more than once a night and stay awake for 20 minutes or more, more than half the time.

3. Waking up too early:
   - ❑ Most of the time, I awaken no more than 30 minutes before I need to get up.
   - ❑ More than half the time, I awaken more than 30 minutes before I need to get up.
   - ❑ I almost always awaken at least one hour or so before I need to, but I go back to sleep eventually.
   - ☑ I awaken at least one hour before I need to, and can't go back to sleep.

4. Sleeping too much:
   - ☑ I sleep no longer than 7–8 hours/night, without napping during the day.
   - ❑ I sleep no longer than 10 hours in a 24-hour period including naps.
   - ❑ I sleep no longer than 12 hours in a 24-hour period including naps.
   - ❑ I sleep longer than 12 hours in a 24-hour period including naps.

5. Feeling sad:
   - ❑ I do not feel sad.
   - ❑ I feel sad less than half the time.
   - ❑ I feel sad more than half the time.
   - ☑ I feel sad nearly all the time.

6. Decreased appetite:
   - ❑ My usual appetite has not decreased.
   - ❑ I eat somewhat less often or lesser amounts of food than usual.
   - ☑ I eat much less than usual and only with personal effort.
   - ❑ I rarely eat within a 24-hour period, and only with extreme personal effort or when others persuade me to eat.

7. Increased appetite:
   - ❑ My usual appetite has not increased.
   - ❑ I feel a need to eat more frequently than usual.
   - ❑ I regularly eat more often and/or greater amounts of food than usual.
   - ❑ I feel driven to overeat both at mealtime and between meals.

(cont.)

219

8. Decreased weight (within the last 2 weeks):
   ☐ My weight has not decreased.
   ☐ I feel as if I've had a slight weight loss.
   ☑ I have lost 2 pounds or more.
   ☑ I have lost 5 pounds or more.

9. Increased weight (within the last 2 weeks):
   ☐ My weight has not increased.
   ☐ I feel as if I've had a slight weight gain.
   ☑ I have gained 2 pounds or more.
   ☐ I have gained 5 pounds or more.

10. Concentration/decision making:
    ☐ There is no change in my usual capacity to concentrate or make decisions.
    ☐ I occasionally feel indecisive or find that my attention wanders.
    ☑ Most of the time, I struggle to focus my attention or to make decisions.
    ☐ I cannot concentrate well enough to read or cannot make even minor decisions.

11. View of myself:
    ☐ I see myself as equally worthwhile and deserving as other people.
    ☑ I am more self-blaming than usual.
    ☐ I largely believe that I cause problems for others.
    ☐ I think almost constantly about major and minor defects in myself.

12. Thoughts of death or suicide:
    ☐ I do not think of suicide or death.
    ☑ I feel that life is empty or wonder if it's worth living.
    ☐ I think of suicide or death several times a week for several minutes.
    ☐ I think or suicide or death several times a day in some detail, or have actually tried to take my life.

13. General interest:
    ☐ There is no change from usual in how interested I am in other people or activities.
    ☐ I notice that I am less interested in people or activities.
    ☐ I find I have interest in only one or two of my formerly pursued activities.
    ☐ I have virtually no interest in formerly pursued activities

14. Energy level:
    ☐ There is no change in my usual level of energy.
    ☑ I get tired more easily than usual.
    ☐ I have to make a big effort to start or finish my usual daily activities (for example, shopping, homework, cooking or going to work).
    ☐ I really cannot carry out most of my usual daily activities because I just don't have the energy.

(*cont.*)

15. Feeling slowed down:
    - ☑ I think, speak, and move at my usual rate of speed.
    - ☑ I find that my thinking is slowed down or my voice sounds dull or flat.
    - ❑ It takes me several seconds to respond to most questions and I'm sure my thinking is slowed.
    - ❑ I am often unable to respond to questions without extreme effort.

16. Feeling restless:
    - ❑ I do not feel restless.
    - ❑ I'm often fidgety, wringing my hands, or need to shift how I am sitting.
    - ❑ I have impulses to move about and am quite restless.
    - ❑ At times, I am unable to stay seated and need to pace around.

Generally, people who have scores between 0 and 5 are not likely to be depressed. Those in the 6–10 range are mildly depressed; 11–15, moderate; 16–20, severe; and 21 or over, very severely depressed. If you are in the severe or very severe range, you will almost certainly need attention from your doctor or therapist; some people in this range require hospitalization. Scores lower than 20 often warrant treatment as well, both medical and psychological. Also, your score may change from one week to the next. This is the nature of depression, particularly of the bipolar type.

If you scored in the mild-to-moderate range, the self-management techniques described in this chapter and the next will be particularly relevant to you right now. But they may also be helpful if you are not feeling depressed (i.e., below 6) but want to develop skills for preventing or alleviating episodes of depression in the future.

How Does Your Depression Wax and Wane?

Depression comes and goes in different ways for different people. It is helpful to know that for some people depressive onsets are dramatic, whereas for others the onsets are subtle. If your onsets are subtle, it may not always be clear to you (or your significant others) whether your depression is a new episode or the continuation of an existing one. With experience, you may learn to distinguish minor differences over time in the severity of your depressed mood or your energy and activity levels.

In the first type, which I call the *classic recurrent* type, a full-bore depression or mixed disorder develops either following a period of time in which you've been functioning at your baseline (or what, for you, is your typical mood state) or just after a manic episode, with little or no break in between. The onset of this depressive episode is usually not as sudden as the onset of a new episode of mania or hypomania. Instead, it usually involves a gradual winding down of your mood state over a period of days, weeks, or even months, until you reach a state of full clinical depression or mixed disorder. For some people the onset can be tied to specific life events (see Chapter 5).

In the other type, called *double depression,* you have an ongoing state of sadness (dysthymia) that may have been present for years and is quite unpleasant but still allows you to function. Then a major depressive episode develops on top of this state of dysthymia. This new episode of bipolar depression is kind of a "slow burn": it develops gradually and perniciously, almost imperceptibly from day to day. When this severe depression remits, you may return to a milder state of depression or dysthymia rather than to a depression-free state. This cycle can be quite frustrating and demoralizing.

Notice that in describing these course patterns, I don't refer to depression as a change from normal mood. In my experience, people with bipolar disorder do not ever feel like they get to a state of normal mood. In fact, they feel that their moods are always fluctuating. Many say that they are always somewhat depressed. Of course, it's not entirely clear what normal mood means for the typical person— some people seem to feel fine most of the time, whereas others are always somewhat anxious, angry, bored, disappointed, or sad.

Whether you have classic recurrent or double depression, it is important to learn to recognize your prodromal signs of a new episode. As discussed in Chapter 9, prodromal signs are those early indicators that your mood state is changing. If you live in an ongoing state of dysthymia, the prodromal signs of a new depressive episode will be more subtle than those experienced by people with classic recurrent depressions and will mainly reflect changes in the *degree* to which you experience depressive symptoms (for example, the seriousness of your suicidal thoughts). Nonetheless, knowing how to intervene when these signs appear can be central to your mood stability and well-being. You may be able to implement the self-care strategies in this chapter to keep the depression from becoming as bad as it otherwise might become or to make your "rebound" dysthymia more tolerable. It is important to keep these targets in mind—*the fact that your depression doesn't disappear entirely is not a sign that you have failed in your attempts to cope with it* (see the earlier example of Alexis).

How Do You Know If You're Getting More Depressed?: The Mood Spiral

One symptom of depression seems to feed on others: negative moods like sadness and anxiety, along with the physical symptoms of depression like lethargy or insomnia, produce negative thinking (for example, negative "self-statements," the harshly critical, accusatory voice in your head), and vice versa. The combination of negative mood, negative thought patterns, and physical changes can make you feel less motivated to try hard, which can make you withdraw and, in turn, worsen your negative thinking and mood. This undesirable pattern is called the mood spiral. Consider the following experiences of two people with bipolar depressions.

Denise, a 27-year-old with bipolar II disorder, was typically mildly depressed and pessimistic in her day-to-day life, despite being loyal to her regimen of lamotrigine (Lamictal) and paroxetine (Paxil). Her more serious depressions had a gradual but predictable course. Her first sign of a depressive recurrence was ruminating about things that were realistic but blown out of proportion. For example, prior to her most recent episode, she felt slighted by a colleague at work and angry at herself for not having responded adequately to the slight. She expanded the significance of this minor event into thinking that no one at work liked her and that her coworkers thought she was crazy. She then became very self-critical, claiming it was her lack of interpersonal skills that led others to dislike her. Her depressed mood worsened, and she had more and more difficulty going to work. Her performance started to deteriorate, and she developed insomnia. Sick days followed. Eventually she took a leave from her job and became inactive and withdrawn in her home. At this point she became tearful and suicidal.

Denise eventually came out of her depression through a combination of medication changes (for example, an increased dosage of her mood stabilizer), regular psychotherapy, and behavioral activation exercises assigned to her by her therapist. These exercises usually included spending time with friends and neighbors, various forms of light physical exercise, and activities that involved her young niece.

Carlos, age 35, had bipolar I disorder with classic recurrent depressions. He'd had numerous episodes and learned to recognize the symptoms that signaled the onset of a depressive episode with mixed features. His prodromal signs took the form of mild fatigue, sleepiness, and poor concentration. These signs were usually intermixed with feelings of anxiety, dread, and a restless "jumping out of my skin" feeling.

Fortunately, when he had been well, Carlos and his therapist had put into place a prevention plan for staving off his worst symptoms. His plan included getting on a regular bedtime/wake-up routine, eating more protein and fewer carbohydrates, avoiding alcohol and street drugs, scheduling at least one contact each day with a person who could give him positive input, and taking breaks from work when he needed to. He also kept a "thought record" (see page 235) in which he recorded examples of self-blaming statements or overgeneralizations about his situation (for example, "My life has never had any joy or fulfillment"). He also learned to counter these thoughts with more adaptive ones ("I'm going through a tough time ... I've dealt with this before and come out of it ... Depression is going to color the way I feel about things").

The exercise on the facing page will help you list the prodromal signs of your depression (your mood spiral). The list is not exhaustive, and spaces are left for symptoms that are not included here. In completing the exercise, try to think back to the last time you became depressed. If you are currently depressed, you may be able to recall the earliest phases of your depression. What were its first signs? If you were already depressed when the new episode developed, how did you know it was getting worse? As you did when listing your prodromal signs of mania (Chapter 9), include the input of your spouse or another family member or friend who observed you during the early phases of depression.

Notice how the prodromal signs of depression differ from the signs of mania discussed in Chapter 9. The depressive warning signals usually involve feeling slowed down, negative, unmotivated, uninterested, mentally sluggish, and hopeless. The mania signals involve feeling sped up, goal driven, energized, mentally swift, and, often, overly optimistic or grandiose. Some people experience the buildup of mania and the descent into depression simultaneously, culminating in a mixed episode.

Keep your list of depression warning signs in a place where you can find it later. If you feel your mood or energy level start to shift, refer back to the list to see if you are experiencing a new onset of depression. You can then move on to introducing self-care strategies when one or more of these signs appears. As you did with your mania list, share this list with your close relatives (your spouse, trusted friends, parents) so that they can learn to recognize when you're getting depressed and are in a position to offer help (for example, listen supportively, look after your kids, provide a distraction, help you to stay active).

Self-Care Strategy No. 1: The Behavioral Activation Method

"When I get depressed, it's hard for me to even be out in public. I withdraw, I get tired, I think in very black-and-white terms, I discount anything good that happens. But I've learned not to give up. I know that 12 in the afternoon is my worst time, so I force myself to go to the gym then. I just pray no one will talk to me. On other days I'll just have coffee with a friend. It's tough, I dread it, I feel like I'm so down and I can't do this, I just can't. But, without a doubt, it helps me."

—A 41-year-old woman with bipolar II disorder

Behavioral activation is one of the most important components of cognitive-behavioral therapy (CBT) (Martell et al., 2010). There are two assumptions behind behavioral activation. First, depression results in a loss of pleasurable activities or *positive reinforcements.* That is, being depressed makes you less likely to do the sorts of things that will help you get something positive from your environment. Second, the lack of these reinforcements worsens your depression and makes you

Listing Your Prodromal Signs of Depression

List a couple of adjectives describing what your *mood* is like when your depressive episodes first begin (*examples:* sad, anxious, fearful, irritable, grouchy, downhearted, blue, "blah," flat, numb, bored).

grouchy

Describe changes in your *activity* and *energy* levels as your depressive episodes develop (*examples:* feeling slowed down, withdrawing from people, moving more slowly, talking more slowly, doing fewer things, having little or no sex drive, feeling fatigued, feeling "tired but wired").

No comment

Describe changes in your *thinking* and *perception* (*examples:* thoughts go more slowly; can't get interested in things; colors seem drab; people look like they're moving too fast; feel self-doubting, self-critical, or self-blaming; feel guilty; regret past deeds; feel hopeless; concentrate poorly; feel dumb; can't make decisions; think about hurting or killing myself; ruminate and worry about things).

feel numb,

Describe changes in your *sleep* patterns (*examples:* wanting to sleep more, waking up in the middle of the night or not being able to fall asleep easily, waking up an hour or two earlier than usual).

Don't get enough sleep most of the time.

Describe anything else that seems different when you're getting depressed.

when a pet has to get put down for their sufferings. Or when a person dies.

want to withdraw even more. It is certainly true that being depressed makes it very difficult to get yourself to do anything. But it's equally true that, in combination with your biological predispositions, not engaging with your environment keeps you depressed and eventually makes you feel worse.

Depression has a way of spoiling your experience of things you used to love to do. They just don't seem fun anymore. Sometimes the events that make you depressed (for example, the ending of a relationship) result in limiting your contact with people whose company you used to enjoy and decreasing your access to activities that used to give you pleasure. All of this will make you feel like withdrawing. But when you're depressed, the worst thing you can do is stay in bed, sit at home, and avoid people. It's certainly understandable that you'll want to do these things, and you may have to from time to time. But if this state of inactivity dominates your life, your depression will only get more severe. "The more we do, the less depressed we feel; and the less depressed we feel, the more we will feel encouraged to do things" (Lewinsohn et al., 1992, p. 74).

The goal behind behavioral activation is to try to increase your contact with your physical and social environment, to the point where you start feeling better about yourself. Of course, you need a regular slate of routines and pleasurable activities even when you're well (Chapter 8), but it's especially important to introduce activating exercises when you recognize a worsening state of depression. In this section, I'll give you a brief set of instructions for implementing the behavioral activation method.

Make a List of Pleasurable Activities

Start by examining the previous week or, if you prefer, take notes on yourself for the forthcoming week. Your mood chart should help you track information about your daily habits. Ask yourself the following:

- "Are my days characterized by a lack of structure?"
- "Are there long periods of time when I have nothing to do?"
- "Are there particular points during the day when I feel down?"
- "Are the mornings long expanses, with nothing to look forward to?"
- "Do I dread the weekend because there is nothing to do?"
- "Is the beginning of the workday inviting just because it gets me out of the house?"

Alternatively:

- "Have my days been dominated by too many activities, most of which are required by my work or family life but which I don't find rewarding?"

- [If you're not working:] "Has there been a good balance between pleasant activities and 'must do' activities?"
- "Am I engaged in enough positive, rewarding activities to keep my mood from spiraling downward?"

Next, try to list as many pleasurable or engaging activities as you can. It can be hard to think of pleasurable things to do when you're depressed, but filling out the form below will get you started. At the bottom you'll find a list of examples of activities many people find pleasurable when they're feeling down. List all of the activities that could be pleasurable for you, even if they don't seem feasible (for example, you

Listing Pleasurable Activities

List as many activities as you can think of that you would find rewarding and pleasurable. Include activities that keep you engaged with other people, activities that increase your sense of competence, and activities that might allow you to experience emotions other than depression.

more roadtrips
more time with
my family more
often.
more yard or
Estate Sales
with my mom
and Mark

(*Examples:* taking a walk, going to a church or synagogue group, playing a musical instrument, walking the dog, watching a TV program, going to the library, talking on the phone to a friend, talking to a therapist, playing a sport, watching a comedy movie, having sex, riding a bicycle, visiting the Humane Society, listening to music, practicing a hobby, sitting in a café, cooking, driving, sewing, dancing, working at a homeless shelter, writing in a journal, taking photographs, taking a class, painting or drawing, soaking in the bathtub, eating at a restaurant, listening to a relaxation tape, shopping, hiking, gardening, praying, meditating, going for a swim, eating lunch outside, attending a lecture, washing your face or hair, lying out in the sun, playing with a pet)

Source: Lewinsohn et al. (1992).

may really enjoy fishing, but there is nowhere to fish nearby). Some people find self-awareness exercises, such as mindful breathing, to be relaxing and "centering" (see below, "A 3-Minute Mindfulness Breathing Exercise"). You may want to try these as well.

Just because you list a number of activities doesn't mean you should try to do all of them. In fact, the objective here is first to make a list of pleasurable events and then to introduce one each day, or perhaps more than one if you feel up to it. Make a particular effort to list activities that have the potential to (1) keep you engaged with other people and make you feel valued or respected (for example, hiking with a friend), (2) give you a sense of competence and purpose (for example, taking a piano lesson or a foreign-language class), and (3) make you likely to experience emotions other than depression (for example, watching a humorous movie, being out in nature, riding a bicycle). Keep in mind that what is pleasurable to other people may not be pleasurable to you, and vice versa (see the extended list provided by Lewinsohn et al., 1992). Try to list only activities that you want to do and know you would enjoy.

A 3-Minute Mindfulness Breathing Exercise

Behavioral activation strategies can be supplemented by exercises that get you in touch with your body, your breathing, and your surroundings within the present moment, or what we call "mindful awareness." Try the following the next time you feel mildly anxious or down:

■ Find a comfortable chair to sit in: sit with your back upright and your hands on your thighs, not touching the back of the chair. You can also lie on your back.

■ Close your eyes or stare at an object in the room. Spend 60 seconds being aware of the noises in your room—the sound of the air conditioner or heating, sounds from the street, music, people's voices. Ask yourself, "What am I experiencing in my thoughts, my emotions, and my body?" Acknowledge to yourself each sensation, thought, or feeling, whether pleasant or unpleasant.

■ Now, for the next 60 seconds, focus on your breathing. Keep focusing on your in-breath and out-breath, like you were riding a wave. It's inevitable that your mind will wander. If your attention shifts to thinking of other things, notice what took you away but gently escort yourself back to your breathing.

■ Now, for the next 60 seconds, shift your attention to your entire body—your belly, feet, legs, thighs, buttocks, stomach, chest, neck, and facial expression. Notice your posture and the sensation in different parts of your body as you breathe in and out. If your mind wanders, gently escort your awareness back to your body and breathing.

■ Slowly open your eyes and come back in contact with the room.

Adapted by permission from Segal et al. (2002). Copyright by The Guilford Press.

Note to the reader: If you'd like to learn more about using mindfulness meditation as a coping strategy, we recommend Williams and colleagues' (2007) *The Mindful Way Through Depression.* This book will take you through numerous meditation practices, of which this one is just an example.

Scheduling Pleasurable Activities

Next, choose one or two activities from this list to do each day of the next week (see the "Scheduling Pleasurable Activities" exercise below). Pick the day you will do each activity and set a target time in the "Day of the Week" column. If you feel that one activity per day is too much, choose one to do every other day or even one every 3 days, and build up from there.

Effective prevention: Engaging with your social and physical environment—behavioral activation—can help halt the downward spiral of depression.

If you're feeling very depressed or low in energy, pick easy activities such as putting on a favorite piece of clothing, taking a bath, or spending 5 minutes outside in the sun. It will feel therapeutic to be able to do something small for yourself each day, or every few days, when it feels impossible to do more.

Scheduling Pleasurable Activities

Day of the week and target time	Pleasurable activities	Actual time of day each activity was done	Mood before and after each activity (−3/+3)	
Monday	1. _____	1. _____	_____	_____
	2. _____	2. _____	_____	_____
Tuesday	1. _____	1. _____	_____	_____
	2. _____	2. _____	_____	_____
Wednesday	1. _____	1. _____	_____	_____
	2. _____	2. _____	_____	_____
Thursday	1. _Lynette+I_	1. _9:30AM_ Looking at plants	_____	_4+_
	2. _____	2. _____	_____	_____
Friday	1. _____	1. _____	_____	_____
	2. _____	2. _____	_____	_____
Saturday	1. _____	1. _____	_____	_____
	2. _____	2. _____	_____	_____
Sunday	1. _____	1. _____	_____	_____
	2. _____	2. _____	_____	_____

Some activities and events require coordination of your and other people's schedules, extensive travel, money, and reservations made well in advance (for example, concert tickets, ski lessons). You may find it easier to choose activities that do not require such planning. Perhaps activities that require planning can be introduced later.

Try to pick activities that will not disrupt your work routine or your sleep–wake cycle. For example, if you like to exercise, avoid doing it in the evening, especially right before you go to bed. If you enjoy conversations with a specific person but feel wired or energized by these talks, avoid them after a certain time of night. Try not to be too ambitious (at least, at first) in scheduling activities early in the morning.

Next, record the actual time of day that you completed each activity. Record your mood on the –3 (severely depressed) to +3 (severely manic) scale that you used for your mood chart in Chapter 8. Rate your mood before you begin the activity and again as soon as you are finished. For example, if your activity was gardening, record how you felt just prior to going out to the garden and then give yourself another rating for the hour or so after finishing. Make copies of this form before filling it out so that you can use it in subsequent weeks.

Notice that I've asked you to keep track of your high as well as your low moods. As you know from previous chapters, certain activities can contribute to manic symptoms. For example, exercise generally improves a person's moods, but some people exercise to excess and become hypomanic. It's important to keep data on yourself so that you can determine whether certain activities improve your mood or "overcorrect."

Troubleshooting Your Plan

After scheduling pleasurable events for a week or more, evaluate whether the plan is working. Are your mood ratings more positive on the days in which you did one or more pleasurable activities? To determine this, complete the "Impact of Your Behavior Activation Plan" exercise (below), in which you rate each day in the last week on the –3 to +3 scale and make a check mark next to the days you completed at least one of your planned activities. If your mood varied considerably during any given day, use the rating that you think best characterizes the whole day, rather than how you felt at a particularly tough moment. Then calculate an average mood rating for the days that you did, and did not, complete your activities. You should be able to tell from this overview whether your activity plan has had a beneficial impact on your mood in the last week.

If your plan is not working yet, consider the possibility that you are choosing events that are too hard, that require too much planning, or that you don't really enjoy. For example, if you have included taking a foreign-language class but don't really like the process of learning a language, you may not want to include this activity. Also, consider the balance between activities you must do and those you

Impact of Your Behavior Activation Plan

Day of the week	Mood that day (−3 to +3)	Check (✓) if you followed your activity plan
Monday	_____	_____
Tuesday	_____	_____
Wednesday	_____	_____
Thursday	_____	_____
Friday	_____	_____
Saturday	_____	_____
Sunday	_____	_____

Average mood rating for the days you followed your plan _____

Average mood rating for the days you did not follow your plan _____

really want to do. If your depression is related to the absence of pleasurable events as well as the avoidance of unpleasant activities that have to be done (for example, sweeping the garage, preparing your taxes), introduce a combination of pleasurable and required activities into your schedule. Start slowly: Don't try to schedule a "must-do" activity every day. Work your way up to a reasonable balance, such as two pleasurable activities and one required activity per day.

If things have gone well for you so far, and you've noticed that your mood has improved (or, at minimum, your prodromal depressive symptoms haven't worsened), start introducing more pleasurable activities into various parts of your day. You may find, for example, that you feel better if you have something pleasurable to do during the lunch hour (for example, sitting at an outdoor picnic table) as well as something to look forward to when you get home from work, school, or other activities. If you are not working or going to school, it's especially important to have rewarding activities at the beginning and end of the day so that some structure is introduced into your routines.

Effective solution: If it just seems too difficult to get involved in a pleasurable social activity, avoid pushing yourself too hard and start with a couple of nonsocial activities you find easy to do.

The behavioral activation method may seem somewhat superficial or too obvious. You may feel, "Of *course* I should be doing those things—the problem is that I *can't!*" When your depression is gradually worsening, it becomes especially important to reengage with your environment and do the things that give you a different experience of your emotions. The key is not to push yourself too hard with these activities. Don't try to do too many all at once. At first, pick a few you can do easily (for example, taking a short walk, listening to music, taking a bath, bird-watching, playing cards). Then work on building up to a reasonable number each day, until you find yourself looking forward to the next day because of the pleasant activities you've scheduled. Troubleshoot the plan at the end of each week to determine why it didn't work. On your first few tries, you probably won't be able to complete certain aspects of the plan. Try not to get discouraged; it may take a few weeks to formulate a plan that really works for you.

Even if it sounds simple, you may be surprised at how well your plan helps to prevent your depression from spiraling. In all likelihood, you'll get a feeling of mastery from making your plan work, which will make you want to extend it further.

Self-Care Strategy No. 2: The Cognitive Restructuring Method

You are probably aware that mood states are affected by the things you tell yourself—by what we call *cognitions* or *self-statements*. Many studies have shown that negative thinking is associated with depressed and anxious moods. People with depression often have negative *core beliefs* about themselves (for example, "I'm not a likable person"), about people in general (for example, "people are generally motivated by selfish concerns"), and about their future ("I'm never going to accomplish my goals/be loved/be healthy"). The assumption of CBT (Beck et al., 1987) is that certain events provoke distorted *automatic negative thoughts* that reflect core beliefs about one's unworthiness or unlovability. These automatic thoughts and core beliefs are important in causing and maintaining depressed mood and behaviors (for example, withdrawing from others). In cognitive restructuring, you hold your assumptions up to the light to see if they are logical and accurate or if there are other ways to make sense of your experiences. You may recall my discussion of CBT in Chapter 6; it is one of the most effective treatments for depressive and anxiety disorders.

The relationship between thoughts and mood states is probably not one-way: depressed moods also generate distorted thoughts and increase a person's access to negative memories or images (Gotlib & Krasnoperova, 1998). J. Mark Williams and his group at Oxford University (2008) have proposed that negative mood states, even when minor, increase access to negative networks of information that then worsen our mood, culminating in more serious episodes of depression. In turn, learning to modify negative thoughts and replace them with more adaptive or balanced cognitions—or, at minimum, learning to observe your thoughts and gain some distance from them—can go a long way toward alleviating your negative mood states.

Cognitive restructuring involves a sequence of techniques. First, you identify the automatic thoughts or self-statements associated with certain disturbing situations or life events and link these thoughts with your mood states. You will probably find that certain thoughts or images are more powerful than others in provoking your emotional reactions (*hot cognitions*). Second, you evaluate the evidence for and against these automatic thoughts. Next, based on this for/against evaluation, you learn to replace your original thoughts with self-statements that provide a more balanced interpretation of your experiences. Last, you observe the effects of these new self-statements on your mood.

This method is *not* a matter of blithely replacing bad thoughts with good ones, which many people find superficial and unrealistic. *Instead, it involves thinking up alternative or more balanced ways of understanding the things that have happened to you and looking at your situation from a number of different vantage points.* A simple example: some people automatically blame themselves when someone else treats them badly, without considering the possibility that this other person is having a bad day or often behaves in a similar manner with other people.

In this section, I describe the method of cognitive restructuring and outline exercises to help you learn it. Like the pleasurable activity scheduling, cognitive restructuring will probably have its greatest power once you have noticed the appearance of one or more depressive prodromal symptoms, before your depression gets really severe. If you want to explore this method further, I suggest consulting the book *Mind Over Mood* by Dennis Greenberger and Christine Padesky (1995).

Step 1: Identifying Negative Thoughts

Jake, age 49, struggled with severe bipolar depressive episodes that alternated with mixed episodes. When he was feeling well, he was a popular coach of a children's soccer team. But when he felt he'd had a bad day of coaching (for example, his concentration had been poor or the kids had not responded to his suggestions), his mood would sink. He became aware of a self-statement that went like this: "I'm just no good with kids. I have major character flaws that they can see in me." Sometimes, just the word *character* would pop into his mind, and he would feel his mood drop. *Character* became a hot cognition closely tied to his mood state of depression.

There had been a few minor run-ins with parents that he had exaggerated in his mind, such as when a father of one of the team players had snapped at Jake for not allowing his son more time on the field. Mostly, Jake was quite good with children, and the kids and parents on his team frequently expressed their appreciation of him. Nonetheless, his thinking and resulting mood contributed to his growing desire to quit coaching altogether. When asked to recount why he thought he had a bad character, he tended to focus on one or more mistakes he had made and magnify or overgeneralize these mistakes ("I was impatient with one of my kids. I was too hard on him. I can't work well with people because I can't be patient with myself").

The first step in cognitive restructuring is to become aware of the thoughts, images, or memories that crop up when you have experiences that negatively affect your mood. Be particularly attuned to experiences involving your work, family, or close relationships. Take a look at the thought record exercise on page 235, which we'll be completing throughout this section. Pick out three negative experiences you've had in the past week and record them in the table (column 1). Rate the intensity of your mood (column 2) in reaction to these events on a scale of 0% (not depressed) to 100% (very depressed). (Alternatively, use the −3 to +3 scale introduced in Chapter 8 if you're more comfortable with that rating format.) List other moods you may also be feeling (for example, anxiety) and rate their intensity. Try to distinguish how you felt during or immediately after the event, not how you felt that entire day.

Now see if you can recall any negative self-statements that came into your head right before you started feeling bad, or notice and record any that come into your mind now as you review the events. Write these in the "Automatic Thoughts" column. To help you "snag" these statements or automatic thoughts, try to be attuned to questions like these (Greenberger & Padesky, 1995):

■ "Why did this event happen?"
■ "What was going through my mind just before I started to feel this way?"
■ "What does this event say about me or what others think of me?"
■ "What does this mean will happen in my future?"
■ "What is the worst possible reason this could have happened?"

Don't be surprised if you're not immediately aware of any thoughts or images. You may find that you can't quite remember how you felt or what you thought after a particular event. If you are having trouble remembering, practice by focusing on recent events that caused you to have strong emotional reactions (for example, rejections from a romantic partner, run-ins with people, problems with your boss at work). These events are probably most closely associated with certain identifiable hot thoughts. Try talking or writing about this experience to see if you can identify *thoughts* as opposed to feelings.

You may find it helpful to carry a note pad or handheld digital recorder to record your thoughts when you experience emotion-provoking events. This kind of online recording will increase your chances of tracking thoughts accurately, rather than trying to reconstruct them after the fact. With time, as you become more familiar with this thought-tracking method, you will no longer need recording devices.

Some people are more visual, and their hot thoughts come in the form of disturbing images (for example, a picture of themselves as a child being picked on by other kids on the playground). For others, specific words are hot thoughts. For Jake, it was the word *character*. For Suzanna, it was the word *crazy*. If single words or images

Thought Record

1. Situation	2. Moods	3. Automatic thoughts (images)	4. Evidence that supports the hot thought	5. Evidence that does not support the hot thought	6. Alternative/balanced thoughts	7. Rate moods now
Whom were you with? What were you doing? When was it? Where were you?	Describe each mood in one word. Rate intensity of mood (0–100%).	Answer some or all of the following questions: • What was going through my mind just before I started to feel this way? • What does this say about me? • What does this mean about me? my life? my future? • What am I afraid might happen? • What is the worst thing that could happen if this is true? • What does this mean about how the other person(s) feel(s)/think(s) about me? • What does this mean about the other person(s) or people in general? • What images or memories do I have in this situation?	Circle hot thought in previous column for which you are looking for evidence. Write factual evidence to support this conclusion. (Try to avoid mind-reading and reinterpretation of facts.)	Ask yourself questions to help discover evidence that does not support your hot thought (e.g., "When I am not feeling down, do I think about this type of situation any differently?")	Ask yourself questions to generate alternative or balanced thoughts (e.g., "Is there an alternative way of thinking about or understanding this situation? If someone else was in this situation, how would I suggest that they understand it?" Write alternative or more balanced thoughts. Rate how much you believe in each one (0–100%).	Copy the the feelings from Column 2. Rerate the intensity of each feeling from 0 to 100%.

are associated with your mood changes, record them in the "Automatic Thoughts" column, and see if you can expand them into a full sentence (for example, "as long as I act this way, people will always think of me as being crazy").

Let's imagine you had an unpleasant conversation with your father last week and that you have been ruminating about it, on and off, since then. Record the event as "Conversation with Dad that didn't go well" in the "Situation" column. Let's also assume your resulting depressed mood was 70% (quite depressed) out of a possible 100% (extremely depressed). For the "Automatic Thoughts" column, you would record the self-statements or images that came up during the conversation or immediately after it. Examples might include "I never will be able to live up to his expectations" or "I let him down again," both of which might fuel your low mood.

Step 2: Challenging Negative Thoughts

Now let's work on modifying your automatic thoughts. Your thoughts can be considered hypotheses, rather than hard facts, about certain events. Complete the next two columns, "Evidence That Supports" and "Evidence That Does Not Support" your hot thoughts. Be a scientist observing your own thought process (Greenberger & Padesky, 1995): Is there any evidence for or against your conclusion that you let your dad down or can't live up to his expectations? Did your father say anything that indicated differently? Have you had any experiences with your dad recently that would show that these conclusions are not always true? Are you discounting any-

thing positive that he said? Could your sad mood have made you view the conversation differently from what it really was? Would you have viewed it differently in a different mood state? Was the outcome of the conversation really within your control?

The next step is to complete the column titled "Alternative/Balanced Thoughts." This is the chance to consider alternative

> **Effective treatment:** Think of your thoughts as hypotheses that can be proven or disproved once you collect real-world information about them. Try to design small experiments to see if you can evaluate them.

viewpoints that are more balanced (as opposed to distorted), even if you don't believe them fully. Try writing down all of the other causes, explanations, or conclusions you could have drawn from this event, and rate each of them on a 0–100% scale as to how credible you find them (100% means you believe this alternative explanation fully, 0% means not at all). Examples might include: "I think Dad was just in a bad mood that day and I got defensive" (40%); "We got on the touchy subject of money, which always makes us both uncomfortable" (70%); and "Dad expressed disappointment in me, but some important things came to light that we needed to talk about" (50%). Once you have generated and reflected on these alternative thoughts, make new ratings of your moods (depression, anxiety, or any other emotions you listed in column 2) using the same 0–100% (or −3–+3) scale.

In developing alternative thoughts, consider the following strategies. Write a sentence that summarizes all of the "for" and "against" evidence for your cognition about this event. Consider what advice you would give another person who was in the same situation, had the same thoughts and moods, and had given you the same for/against evidence. Consider the best, worst, and most likely (realistic) outcomes if your hot cognition turns out to be true. For example, if the hot cognition "I let Dad down again" turns out to be true, a worst-case outcome might be that he reminds you of your failings the next time you talk to him and you end up feeling even worse; a best-case outcome might be that he apologizes and admits he was wrong, and you feel great; a realistic outcome might be that you feel tension the next time you talk to him but that you effectively steer the conversation toward more comfortable topics.

> **Effective treatment:** To come up with alternatives to negative thoughts:
>
> ■ Write lists of evidence for and against the negative thought.
> ■ Think of how you'd advise someone who had the same negative thought.
> ■ Consider the best, worst, and most likely outcomes of your negative thought if it came true.

Jake, the soccer coach, learned to evaluate the evidence for and against his automatic, self-blaming thought that "I'm no good with kids." There was plenty of evidence to the contrary, given the many positive comments he received on an ongoing basis from his wife, the players, and their parents. He was able to generate more balanced thoughts: "Sometimes the kids get uncooperative when I'm not feeling my best"; "Coaching can be a difficult task no matter how good you are"; "Today the kids were getting overstimulated and weren't in the mood to learn"; "I'm never going to be able to please all the parents." His mood tended to improve upon introducing and repeatedly restating to himself these countervailing thoughts.

Another person with bipolar disorder, Katrina, age 41, had emigrated to the United States from Hungary. A year after arriving she obtained a job at an inner-city school teaching teenagers who were developmentally disabled. During a particularly difficult day, three of the boys in the class cursed at her and told her she was the worst teacher they'd ever had. By day's end, she felt quite depressed and anxious and didn't want to go back to work. She took two days off, citing "mental exhaustion." She recounted thoughts in reaction to this event, such as "Maybe I shouldn't be a teacher ... I don't know if I have the strength and willpower ... I'm not effective; I can't deal with it by myself ... I don't belong; I can't make it." She identified "I'm not effective" as the most powerful, emotion-provoking hot thought.

In examining the evidence for and against this thought, Katrina cited the fact that she'd had to call in the school counselor to help mediate the conflict, that the kids liked her only when she was being friendly and casual but not when she was actually teaching, and that she seemed more powerfully affected by this incident than the other teachers thought she should be. She was also able to generate evidence against her hot cognition, including the fact that she had received positive evaluations of her teaching from the school administration and that her earlier teaching experiences in Hungary had been quite positive. She admitted that "the kids are troubled and angry at everybody" and "I've seen them curse out other teachers." She also recalled that the incident began after one of the boys had verbally taunted another boy in the class.

She eventually settled on more balanced views that did not rule out her own role in causing the incident but that included the contrary evidence: "I'm a good teacher, but I have a difficult set of students that anyone would have a problem with ... I sometimes struggle with my own boundaries and how to set limits with people ... I'm new at this, and it's hard not to get my buttons pushed ... I'm still making a difference in their lives, and they're teaching me a lot about myself even though they hurt my feelings sometimes." Her mood in reaction to the confrontation improved significantly upon reviewing these balanced thoughts. Over time, as her depression lifted, she focused on the larger question of whether she wanted to teach, which had become confused in her mind with whether she was good at it.

What's Different about Thinking Patterns in Bipolar Depression?

So far, the cognitive restructuring method I've described could apply to almost any form of depression or anxiety. The method applies well to bipolar disorder, but bipolar depressions tend to be much more severe than those experienced by people going through life transitions. So, in constructing your alternative or balanced thoughts, consider the role of your disorder—particularly, its biological and genetic underpinnings—in modulating your view of the causes of negative events. Do inherited vulnerabilities of brain circuitry explain your behavior in certain situations better than character flaws? Could your emotional reactions in the heat of the moment have been due to overactivation of the amygdala rather than your inability to deal with people?

Jake, for example, recognized that soccer coaching did not go as well when he experienced the physical signs of depression or anxiety (for example, poor concentration, headaches, low energy). On days in which his coaching and athletic performance were impaired, he introduced balanced thoughts, such as "I can tell that my mood and energy are off kilter today; this is one of those days I can't expect as much from myself ... This is not about my flawed character; it's about my biology ... My depression is causing me to view things more pessimistically than I have to—it doesn't follow that I'm not a good person because I can't control my moods." Although he was never happy with himself when coaching didn't go well, these thoughts gave him a sense of self-acceptance when his moods interfered with his high performance standards.

Katrina worried that "I'm too emotionally unstable to be a consistent figure in their [her students'] eyes." Indeed, negative interactions with her students probably had a more powerful effect on her mood states than might be the case for a person without bipolar disorder, but through no choice of her own. She learned to internally rehearse the self-statements "I'm going to have more severe ups and downs than the ordinary teacher," "Not all of my emotional reactions will be under my control, but that doesn't mean I can't teach," and "I'm good at what I do, and there is a great deal of meaning in it." She also recognized the need to give herself more time to relax and decompress after work than might be required by some of her coworkers.

Consider another example. Say you've had a string of negative interactions with your employer over the last week but generally have had good relations with him or her. Is it possible that your irritability with your boss derives from depressive or mixed symptoms rather than your "short fuse," "angry nature," "problems getting along with people," or "problems with authority figures"? I am not saying, "Blame everything on your bipolar disorder." I'm recommending that you take a more balanced perspective on the factors influencing events in your life, *including* your disorder.

To sum up, cognitive restructuring has the potential to help you alleviate your depressed mood by identifying and revising the automatic thoughts that trigger low mood states. The role your bipolar disorder may play in stimulating your emotional reactions to persons, situations, and challenging events should not be underestimated. In combination with behavioral activation methods, cognitive restructuring has the potential to help alleviate your depression or, at minimum, keep it in check.

This chapter has introduced you to important self-management tools for coping with your depression. Implementing these tools—identifying your early warning signs, scheduling pleasurable and/or activating events, and reconsidering the way you think about, and respond to, the events in your life—can go a long way toward controlling the negative spiral of depression.

Don't be too concerned if you don't take to these methods right away. They require guided practice and skill before they feel natural. If you have access to a cognitive-behavioral therapist, consider doing these exercises with his or her guidance at first.

The next chapter addresses an issue that many—in fact, most—people with bipolar disorder confront at one time or another: suicidal thoughts or actions. This topic is, for many, an uncomfortable one. But as with many other attributes of bipolar disorder, you will put yourself in the driver's seat once you are able to understand suicidal impulses as symptoms of your illness that require management. You will see the special role of psychotherapy, medication, social supports, and self-management tools in alleviating feelings of hopelessness and suicidal despair.

11

Overcoming Suicidal Thoughts and Feelings

"I had been getting more and more depressed and had thought about killing myself, but somewhere in there I decided to finally do it. One night I came home from work to my apartment and went through a whole ritual. I had decided I was going to do it by overdosing on my lithium, since that's the drug I had the most of. I took it, little by little, throughout the evening, pill after pill, and then I got in the shower, but by then I was starting to puke and got the runs really badly ... I think I lost consciousness at some point, and somewhere in there I had the presence of mind to call Dylan [boyfriend], who called the paramedics, and they took me to the hospital. I ended up there with a catheter and the oxygen mask and the whole thing. I looked awful and felt awful. Everybody was telling me how fortunate I was to be alive, but that made me feel worse. I sure didn't feel fortunate."

—A 28-year-old woman with bipolar I disorder, recounting her first suicide attempt

If you are cycling into a period of depression, it is unfortunately very common to have thoughts of ending your life. You may have been having these thoughts all along, but they can become more severe if your depression is getting worse. You may also find that your suicidal thoughts go along with an increase in your anxiety and worry. Some people feel suicidal chronically, not just when they are depressed. One patient said, "I know I'll kill myself someday. It's gonna happen. The only question is when."

Suicide can be accomplished in a sudden impulsive act or a carefully planned event. It usually occurs during a depressive or a mixed episode, but some people with bipolar disorder kill themselves accidentally or on impulse when they are psychotic and in the manic phase.

By some estimates, people with bipolar disorder are at 15 times the risk for committing suicide of people in the general population. Up to 15% of people with bipolar disorder die by suicide, and as many as one in three attempt suicide at least once in their lives (Novick et al., 2010). Tragically, suicidal thoughts and feelings are a part of bipolar illness, connected with its biological and genetic mechanisms. We know that levels of serotonin are lower in the brains of people who attempt or complete suicide (Mann et al., 1999). In other words, suicidal impulses are related to the neurophysiology of your disorder; they are not caused by a moral failing or weakness on your part.

Therefore, you should not feel alone with or ashamed of suicidal thoughts. Virtually every person with bipolar disorder has entertained the idea of suicide at one point or another. In fact, many people without the disorder have thought about it, even if just in passing. But among people with bipolar disorder, the thoughts often become frequent and intense and are more likely to be articulated into a plan of action (for example, to kill yourself with pills at a specific time). One patient of mine put it like this: "My suicidal thoughts are usually like a radio station that is always on but is never quite tuned in well enough to hear what's being said. When I get really depressed, though, the station comes in loud and clear, almost like someone has turned the dial."

The Desire to Escape

People with bipolar and other depressive disorders often feel hopeless, as if nothing will ever change for the better. They feel a strong need for relief from "psychic pain colored by the fear and anticipation of increasing, uncontrollable, interminable pain" (Fawcett et al., 2000, p. 147). Some people honestly want to die. But in my experience, most people with bipolar disorder want relief from the intolerable life circumstances and the emotional, mental, and physical pain that goes along with depression and anxiety. When your depression is spiraling downward and you feel a sense of dread and apprehension, you may desperately want to live, but suicide can feel like the only escape from your intolerable feelings.

Even when severe, however, suicidal thoughts can be managed and controlled medically. There is evidence that long-term treatment with lithium decreases suicide attempts and completions by people with bipolar disorder (Goodwin et al., 2003; Tondo & Baldessarini, 2000). The antidepressant, anticonvulsant, and antipsychotic drugs appear to decrease the agitation and aggressiveness that can bring about suicidal actions.

The challenge in dealing with suicidal despair is to find other ways of escaping from your intolerable feelings. As I discussed in this chapter, your options can include drug treatment, psychotherapy, the help of supportive friends or family members, and self-management techniques. Your hopelessness, pain, and emptiness are temporary, not permanent states, even though they may not seem that way at the time.

Risk Factors for Suicide

You should know about the factors that increase your probability of actually hurting or killing yourself, so that you and your doctor can determine how imminent the danger to you has become. If you plan on switching doctors, tell your new doctor about your risk factors so that he or she can determine the seriousness of your intent and hopefully be of greater help to you in a crisis.

You are at particularly high risk for committing suicide if you ...

- are male
- have bipolar disorder and are also drinking alcohol or using drugs regularly (in addition to making your illness worse, using these substances makes it unlikely that you will take your mood stabilizers regularly or seek help from others when feeling suicidal)
- have been ill for a short time and have had only a few bipolar episodes
- have panic attacks, agitation, restlessness, or other indicators of severe anxiety
- are prone to impulsive acts, such as driving recklessly or having violent outbursts
- have recently been hospitalized
- have previously tried to kill yourself
- have one or more relatives in your family tree who committed suicide or committed a violent act
- have experienced a recent stressful life event involving loss (for example, a divorce or the death of a family member)
- are isolated from friends and family members
- do not have ready access to a psychiatrist or psychotherapist, have feelings of hopelessness about your future, and/or do not feel you have strong reasons to keep living (for example, a commitment to raising children)
- have thought about a specific plan (for example, to take pills, shoot yourself, jump from a high place) and have the means to do it (access to pills or a gun) (Fawcett et al., 2000; Jamison, 2000b).

If you feel suicidal, you should always inform your psychiatrist, therapist, family members, and other significant people in your core circle. This is especially true if you have one or more of the preceding risk factors. Don't stop yourself from disclosing your suicidal thoughts because you are afraid of worrying people or hurting their feelings. Many people feel this way and then don't get the help they need. Err on the side of informing your doctors and significant others, even if you're not sure how serious you are about suicide. Later in this chapter I discuss what your doctor, therapist, friends, and/or family members can do to help you at these times.

How Can You Protect Yourself from Carrying Out Suicidal Actions?

"Anyone who suggests that coming back from suicidal despair is a straight-forward journey has never taken it."

—Jamison (2000b, p. 49)

If you have been spiraling into a depressive or mixed episode from your baseline state, or if your ongoing depression has been getting worse, you may have noticed an increase in your suicidal thoughts. These can be vague at first (for example, "I wonder what it would be like to be dead"), then more serious ("I know that I want to kill myself; I just don't know how"), then even more serious ("I've thought of various suicide plans and have settled on one, as well as a time and a place").

The feelings, thoughts, and behaviors that make up suicidal despair are quite complex and not well understood by behavioral scientists. Nonetheless, we know that there are some things you can do to protect yourself from acting on these impulses. In this chapter, you'll learn how to put together a suicide prevention plan.

Suicide prevention involves decreasing your access to the means to commit suicide and increasing your access to support systems (doctors, therapists, family members, and friends). You might wonder, at what point do these plans work, and at what point is it already too late? Keep a general caveat in mind when you develop your plan: You have more leverage in suicide prevention if you have a plan in place when you're feeling well and begin implementing it at the first emergence of suicidal thoughts or other prodromal signs of depression. Don't wait until you are really feeling desperate—don't let yourself get to that point. When suicidal thoughts and plans accompany the lowest point of a depressive or mixed episode, suicide attempts can occur by impulse.

Strategy No. 1: Get Rid of the Means to Hurt Yourself

One practical step you can take right away is to put those items you might use to kill yourself out of your reach. These include guns, sleeping pills, poisons, ropes, and sharp knives or other weapons. Give them to a trusted friend who lives apart from you, or even your psychiatrist or therapist. To avoid overdosing on your psychiatric medications, keep only a couple of days' dosages in your house and have your friend or relative (or perhaps your doctor) hold on to the rest of the pills, dispensing them as you need them. Though this practical maneuver may seem like it only scratches the surface (you are, after all, only getting rid of the means, not your intentions), it will greatly decrease the chances that you will actually kill or hurt yourself. In the same manner, limiting your access to such items as a gun decreases the chances that you will use it on yourself or someone else.

Strategy No. 2: See Your Psychiatrist and Therapist Immediately

If your next appointments with your psychiatrist and therapist are not scheduled for several weeks, call them and let them know you are at risk, or ask a member of your core circle to make the contact. If at all possible, see your doctor and therapist together (assuming they are not the same person) so that they can help you develop an integrated plan for managing your suicidal impulses, depression, anxiety, stress, and medications.

What will your doctors do to help you when you first start feeling suicidal? In all likelihood, they will start by asking you questions about your suicidal intentions, such as any plans you've been thinking about and your history of suicide attempts (if they don't already know about those). Expect to spend some time on these issues before they get to the reasons you want to kill yourself, which may be foremost in your mind. Be honest about your suicidal intentions, even if these feelings are new to you, foreign, or, in your view, shameful. Tell them how serious you are, that you may not feel safe at home, and that you have access to weapons or other means of hurting yourself.

Some people don't feel comfortable disclosing information to their doctors about their suicidal impulses. In my experience they fear that their doctor will (1) immediately hospitalize them, (2) be deeply disappointed in them and feel that the treatment plan has failed, or (3) be uncomfortable with the topic of suicide. None of these predictions is entirely a distortion on your part. In fact, your doctor may indeed hospitalize you if he or she feels the risk to your life is imminent. Keep in mind that this may be the best thing for you. Hospitalization gives you a chance to get emergency treatment, "regroup," talk to others who feel the same as you, and get your medications reevaluated and adjusted (see also Chapter 9). It will also get you away from the stimuli that may be provoking your suicidal thoughts (for example, certain family members, noises, pictures in your home, your bedroom, the computer, the telephone ringing). If you do go into the hospital, at least some of your inpatient treatment should involve suicide prevention planning for the interval following your discharge.

Some doctors are indeed more comfortable and effective in dealing with suicide risk than others. If you fear that your doctors (that is, your psychiatrist and/or psychotherapist) will be uncomfortable with your disclosure of suicidal thoughts, tell them so. You may be surprised at how forthcoming they are in expressing their concern for you. Your therapist or medical doctor has probably had experience with many other suicidal people and works best when he or she knows the truth, even if it does mean reviewing and revising his or her treatment plan. Your doctors may feel like they haven't done their job right, but it isn't your responsibility to take care of *their* feelings. Rather, it's essential that you can be open with them about your feelings of despair.

Your psychiatrist is likely to reevaluate your medication regimen. Among the options he or she will probably consider is adding an antidepressant to your regimen, switching to a different antidepressant if you are already on one, increasing the dosage of your mood stabilizer, or adding a second mood stabilizer. In extreme cases he or she may recommend electroconvulsive therapy. If you have prominent anxiety symptoms, agitation, or psychosis, your doctor may introduce an atypical antipsychotic medication or a benzodiazepine (see Chapter 6). When anxiety or agitation are controlled with drug treatment, suicidal thoughts sometimes diminish.

Try to be realistic about the speed with which your medical treatments are likely to take effect. It can be quite frustrating to have to go through a trial and error period of adjusting medications and substituting others when you're already feeling hopeless and pessimistic. You may have the impulse to give up when the first modification to your medication regimen does not immediately achieve the intended result. Your state of suicidal despair will almost certainly improve with the proper medication adjustments, but it may take several weeks before the worst symptoms go away. Nonetheless, I have been continually amazed at the degree to which even minor medication adjustments can positively affect even the most suicidal person. One client with bipolar (mixed) disorder, Gerard (age 48), tried to asphyxiate himself by locking himself in the garage and turning on his car. After a brief hospitalization, his doctor added paroxetine (Paxil, an antidepressant) to his mood stabilizer regimen. His suicidal thoughts and intentions rapidly diminished, and his depression lifted, though somewhat less rapidly.

What will your psychotherapist do? The answer depends on his or her theoretical orientation and how long he or she has been working with you. Most will try to provide emotional support and teach you ways to handle your suicidal impulses (for example, using distraction, relaxation techniques, or cognitive restructuring) and help alleviate your immediate pain. Your therapist and you may examine the antecedents, behaviors, and consequences of your suicidal thoughts and actions (perhaps using different terms). Many therapists, particularly those with a cognitive-behavioral or interpersonal orientation, view suicidal thoughts or actions as occurring in a context—as one response in a series of possible responses.

Certain events, situations, images, or memories may stimulate your suicidal thoughts or actions. In turn, these thoughts or actions are sometimes inadvertently rewarded by other people. For Maria, age 39, suicidal thoughts often came up in response to food. When depressed, she would eat voraciously and then look in the mirror, thinking she had grown fat and ugly. It was usually then that she felt suicidal. She sought reassurances about her appearance from others at these times, but these reassurances did little to alleviate her suicidal thoughts. Instead, she would become more suicidal and then call more people for reassurance. Maria's therapist assisted her in disrupting this chain of events by working directly with her on binge eating as a means of self-medicating her depression, developing alternative thinking patterns when she felt unattractive, and avoiding the pull to seek reassurance regarding her appearance. Successfully obtaining reassurance from others, he believed, was inadvertently reinforcing her suicidal thoughts rather than alleviating her distress.

Your therapist may also be able to help you frame your suicidal feelings in terms of broader life issues, such as regrets about events in the past or feelings of discouragement about your future. He or she may help you understand your suicidal impulses in terms of how they relate to the cycling of the bipolar syndrome. Finally, your therapist can help you develop a "safety plan," which can include calling him or her and/or going to the hospital when you experience your next suicidal impulse. Possibly, he or she will invite your family members, spouse/partner, or close friends to come to a session with you to make sure they're aware of your suicidal thoughts and so that they can help you design and put into place a more detailed suicide prevention plan (discussed later in this chapter, pages 252–255).

> **Effective prevention:** Many interventions and self-care techniques will be most powerful before you become actively and dangerously suicidal. Be sure to use your first suicidal thoughts as a signal that you need to see your physician and therapist on an emergency basis.

Strategy No. 3: Use Your Core Circle

"When I start thinking about the future, I go into a panic, and that's when I think about killing myself. But somehow when I get with other people, I can fantasize about how things could be, and that injects some energy into me … it gives me the feeling of purpose, like I have some effectiveness or competence, like I can channel my energy in a good way. It's not just about getting rid of loneliness, or being needy. It's a feeling of being able to make other people laugh, or affecting other people in some way, that makes me feel alive again."
—A 43-year-old man with bipolar I disorder

As you know, one theme of this book is the value of your core circle of family members, partners, and friends in helping keep you well. In Chapter 9 I talked about how members of your core circle can help keep you from escalating into a full-blown manic episode. They can also be helpful when you are feeling suicidal.

For the man quoted above, contact with other people was like an antidepressant, giving him temporary feelings of relief from painful emotions. When you are becoming suicidal, contact and support from others is absolutely critical to keep you from sinking further.

Be aware that you're more likely to reject help when you're most depressed and suicidal (Fawcett et al., 2000). You will feel vulnerable at those times and expect others to reject you. The thought that "I can't be helped, I'll be disappointed, I might even get worse" will go through your mind, contributing to your sense of hopelessness. You may start to believe that "I'm all alone with this—no one can really help me." It's important to challenge these cognitions by making yourself seek support from others, even if doing so feels useless at first. Evaluate the evidence that being with others makes you feel worse. *In all likelihood, your attempts to seek assistance will generate compassion from others, which in turn will help ease your pain.*

Start by reviewing the exercise for "Identifying Your Core Circle" in Chapter 8 (page 184). Who on your list can help you when you first start feeling suicidal? If you have been depressed or anxious for some time, whom have you relied on when you needed to "vent"? Has this person (or these people) been able to help you clarify important issues and potential solutions without bringing you down further? Have you been able to feel closer to this person as a result of confiding in him or her? Is the relationship bidirectional—does he or she also seek you out for help? One of the few positive things about depression is that it can result in your making connections with others in ways you would not typically initiate.

In evaluating your list, try to think of who is likely to be supportive in ways that you would find genuinely helpful. Is there someone on the list who can listen to you talk about wanting to die without "freaking out"? Some people with bipolar disorder find they can't discuss these matters with their parents but can do so with a sibling, a friend, a partner or spouse, or a rabbi or priest. The exact relationship you have to the person (be it family member or friend) is probably less important than whether you trust that person to listen to you calmly and attentively and acknowledge your despair, without judgment. It is also helpful to choose someone whose style is optimistic and hopeful but also realistic (that is, someone aware of the limitations imposed by your disorder and your environment). Don't choose a "Pollyanna." Finally, if you are close to a person who has some understanding of bipolar disorder (see the box in Chapter 13, "A Quick Fact Sheet on Bipolar Disorder for Family Members," on pages 285–286), or someone who has gone through periods of depression him- or herself, that person may be able to offer a unique perspective on ways to cope with your despair.

If no one on your list really fits these descriptors, try to choose the person (or persons) who comes closest. It's best to include on your list as many people as possible and not rely too heavily on any one person. Record their names on the Suicide Prevention Plan on pages 254–255.

Now think about how you can get members of your core circle to assist you.

Recall the three coping styles I mentioned at the beginning of Chapter 10 (emotion focused, cognitive, and distraction coping). First, encourage your significant others to *listen to you talk about your thoughts and feelings.* Tell them you don't need them to solve all of your problems or come up with the "bromide" that will make all the pain go away, but you do need help to focus on what's causing you pain and why. Therapists are probably best at doing this, but if you have a friend or family member who's a good listener, give him or her a chance.

Second, ask your friend or family member to *help you find a way to prevent the immediate danger to yourself.* The objective is to keep you safe. If you haven't been able to get yourself to call your doctor or therapist, ask your friend to do so. Ask him or her to take the weapons or pills off your hands. If you need to go to the hospital, ask him or her to accompany you. If you won't or can't go to the hospital, is he or she willing to stay with you, even overnight if necessary, until you feel you're out of danger? If you feel unable to take care of your kids, can that person do it temporarily or help you make other arrangements with someone who can?

Third, use *distraction.* Many people with bipolar disorder are concerned that talking about their painful emotions will be a burden to others. If you are concerned about this, consider increasing the amount of low-stress, low-demand social time you spend with your significant others or friends. These activities don't have to involve talking about your struggles. Invite them to see a movie with you, go for a walk, take a drive, have dinner, or read together. Physical or social activities that have a degree of structure and involve other people, such as those on your pleasurable activities list (Chapter 10), are especially important to do right now to take your mind away from your suicidal thoughts.

Be Aware of Others' Limitations

You may feel skeptical about the ability of members of your core circle to help you. You are probably correct that if the people you're confiding in do not have bipolar disorder themselves, they will not be able to fully understand the depth of your depression or why your suicidal thoughts are increasing in frequency. You may become distressed by friends or relatives who seem irritated with you and insist that you pull yourself out of it. Be patient with them. Their irritation probably derives from anxieties about your fate or their frustration at not being able to help more. Likewise, try not to be frustrated when they give you platitudes (for example, "We've got only one life to live, and we have to live it fully"), which people often issue when they can't think of what else to say.

Karen, age 35, complained that no one

> **Effective prevention:** People in your core circle are invaluable to your suicide prevention plan, but it's important to know what each is capable of and willing to do in this capacity. This will help you avoid asking for something that any one person can't provide.

wanted to hear about her depressive or suicidal feelings, which made her feel even greater despair. Her typical pattern was to spend hours with others talking about her sadness and then to tell them, "Now I feel a whole lot worse." It is not surprising that her friends became burned out and didn't want to help her anymore. It's important to reward or reinforce members of your core circle for their efforts from time to time. Remember, they are trying to help, even if what they do is not always helpful. They need to hear *from you* that talking to them or simply spending time with them is helping you. It probably is, even if only minimally, and it's important to tell them so.

Strategy No. 4: Reviewing Your Reasons for Living

There will be times when, alone with your suicidal thoughts and feelings, you will start to become overwhelmed by them. This is because suicide is, in part, a cognitive process. When people feel most desperate, they begin to evaluate the pros and cons of suicide as a means of solving their problems. Suicide begins to feel like a more viable alternative when you believe that nothing you do will yield a positive outcome, or that your depression or other life problems will always haunt you.

The flip side is that you will be most protected against suicide if you believe that you will be able to cope effectively with life's problems, view life as having intrinsic value, or feel that others are dependent on your existence (Linehan, 1985; Strosahl et al., 1992). In short, people are protected from suicide when they can access good reasons to live.

Marsha Linehan and her associates have developed an inventory of "Reasons for Living" (see page 250). The inventory was generated by nonsuicidal people who were asked to write down the reasons they did not kill themselves at a point when they had previously considered it, the reasons they would not do so now, and the reasons they believed other people did not. When people believe they can overcome life's problems, and when they feel a strong sense of responsibility to family and children, they are less likely to make a serious suicide attempt.

While this logic may seem obvious, it has an implication for the things you can do on your own when you start to have suicidal thoughts. When people are suicidal, they usually have a great deal of trouble accessing any positive reasons for being alive. So, when you're feeling well, generate a list of your reasons for living or reasons why you would not commit suicide if you were starting to think about it. You can then review these reasons when suicide begins to feel like a viable option.

Start by checking the items in the inventory (below) that you believe to be true. Then, in the blank spaces, add your own reasons if they are not covered in the other items. Try to do this while you're feeling reasonably stable and not seriously depressed. When you're depressed, your reasons for living may be harder to endorse, even though you might ordinarily believe in them.

You'll see that the items cover a broad spectrum of reasons, including the belief

The Reasons for Living Inventory

Check the statements below that indicate why you would *not* commit suicide if the thought were to occur to you or if someone were to suggest it to you.

_____ I have a responsibility and commitment to my family.

_____ I believe I can learn to adjust to, or cope with, my problems.

_✓_ I believe I have control over my life and destiny.

_____ I believe only God has the right to end a life.

_____ I am afraid of death.

_____ I want to watch my children as they grow.

_____ Life is all we have and is better than nothing.

_____ I have future plans I am looking forward to carrying out.

_✓_ No matter how bad I feel, I know that it will not last.

_____ I love and enjoy my family too much and could not leave them.

_____ I am afraid that my method of killing myself would fail.

_____ I want to experience all that life has to offer, and there are many experiences I have not had yet that I want to have.

_____ It would not be fair to leave the children for others to take care of.

_____ I have a love of life.

_✓_ I am too stable to kill myself.

_____ My religious beliefs forbid it.

_____ The effect on my children could be harmful.

_____ It would hurt my family too much and I would not want them to suffer.

_____ I am concerned about what others would think of me.

_✓_ I consider it morally wrong.

_____ I still have many things left to do.

_____ I have the courage to face life.

_✓_ I am afraid of the actual act of killing myself (the pain, blood, violence).

_____ I believe killing myself would not really accomplish or solve anything.

_✓_ Other people would think I am weak and selfish.

_✓_ I would not want people to think I did not have control over my life.

_✓_ I would not want my family to feel guilty afterward.

List other reasons for living: _____

_____

_____

Adapted by permission from Linehan et al. (1983). Copyright by the American Psychological Association.

that you can cope with, and overcome, your troubles, the value you put on life itself, the degree to which you feel optimistic, concerns related to your family and children, fears of disapproval by society, moral beliefs, and fears of the suicidal act itself (Linehan et al., 1983). Some of these reasons may be more relevant to you than others. Reviewing the reasons you do *not* want to kill yourself when the thought crosses your mind may help protect you from acting on a self-destructive impulse later.

Strategy No. 5: "Improving the Moment" Tools

Some people feel that their suicidal despair is always in the background even when they distract themselves from it. Suicide prevention can include learning to tolerate feelings of despair when you can't make them go away. What follows are some "improving the moment" strategies for tolerating your distress (Linehan & Dexter-Mazza, 2007).

Many people turn to religion when they are alone and feel depressed and suicidal. For some, religion is best practiced in group settings like a church, synagogue, or temple, but others prefer solitary prayer. For some, praying for strength gives them a sense of purpose and belonging. Likewise, some people find spiritual readings helpful because they put suffering into a larger perspective. For example, readings by the Dalai Lama seem quite inspirational to people in pain (*Ethics for the New Millennium,* 1999, or *The Art of Happiness,* 1998, coauthored by Howard Cutler).

If your depressed and suicidal feelings are accompanied by significant anxiety, you may benefit from self-relaxation or mindfulness exercises. Usually, relaxation involves sitting in a comfortable chair; tensing and relaxing each of your muscle groups, starting with your feet and moving up to your face; and imagining relaxing, pleasant scenes (for example, lying on a beach). Relaxation exercises often decrease the anxiety and agitation that accompany suicidal thoughts. Consult books that give you step-by-step instructions on how to relax and breathe more easily as well as how to create your own relaxation tapes (for example, Davis et al., 2000).

Take another look at the 3-minute mindful breathing exercise on page 228 in Chapter 10, which gives you a step-by-step method for "decentering" yourself (observing your emotions and physical sensations from a nonjudgmental observer's standpoint, such that you are less motivated to avoid them). Indeed, some people relate better to mindfulness exercises—exercises that make you more aware of your current sensations and experiences— than to relaxation exercises.

For others, exercise is helpful. Many people report that their mood improves significantly and suicidal thoughts diminish after they have exercised. Of course, it's hard to go and work out when you feel low in energy, apathetic, or hopeless. Try some light exercise if you feel especially lethargic, such as walking, stretching, or riding a stationary bicycle for a few minutes. When exercising, focus your attention on your body and the physical sensations that accompany the movement.

If your experience of any of these "improving the moment" tasks is positive, consider adding them to your behavioral activation list (Chapter 10). It's important to try these more than once and make them a part of your regular routine to maximize their impact.

Developing a Suicide Prevention Plan

Now try to put all of this information together into a suicide prevention plan. The form on pages 254–255 can be used as a template. At the beginning of the exercise, list your prodromal signs of depression (see the exercises in Chapter 10). Be sure to list any suicidal thoughts or impulses, including those that seem fleeting or insignificant (for example, "I start thinking about dying, but I would never do anything about it"). Then examine the list of self-management strategies that have been described in this and the prior chapter. Circle those items that seem like reasonable things for you and others to do when you experience suicidal thoughts or other signs of depression.

Next, share this exercise with your doctor/therapist and the members of your core circle, and see if they'd be willing to perform these tasks, should you go into a crisis. If a friend or family member is not willing to accept responsibility for a given item (for example, taking care of your kids, calling your therapist) consider assigning that task to another person. List each member of your core circle at the end of the exercise and indicate which items on the list can be assigned to him or her.

Keep your suicide prevention plan in a place that is readily accessible to members of your core circle. It may make sense to attach it to your mania prevention contract (Chapter 9).

Suicide is "a permanent solution to a temporary problem" (Fawcett et al., 2000, p. 147). But the intolerable feelings that go along with suicidal preoccupations can be so painful that they feel permanent. It's important to combat these states with a variety of self-management tools to help activate yourself, view your circumstances from alternate perspectives, and reengage with important sources of emotional and practical support. Try to be up front with your doctor and therapist about your suicidal impulses and take into consideration their recommendations for emergency medical treatment. Most of all, remain hopeful that your most severe depressive symptoms will eventually disappear and that you will return to a more tolerable emotional state. It's hardest to see your way out when you have hit bottom, so try to implement as many of these strategies as possible when you experience the first signs of depression or suicidal despair.

Bipolar disorder is tough to handle for both men and women even in the best of circumstances, but there are complex emotional and health problems related to the illness and its treatment that affect women more than men. In the next chapter, I discuss a number of strategies for women that will make you feel more empowered in dealing with the illness. Some of the topics covered include how to make treatment and health decisions when you are pregnant, are planning pregnancy, have just given birth, or are approaching menopause, as well as how to make the best use of mood-stabilizing medications that pose risks to your physical health. You'll see how some of the core strategies discussed throughout this book—educating yourself and others about the illness, communicating with your physician, and learning to manage the effects of stress on your mood and health—apply to the unique challenges faced by women with the disorder.

Suicide Prevention Plan

List your typical early warning signs of a depressive episode.

_____

_____

_____

_____

Circle the things *you* can do if one or more of these early warning symptoms appear, or if you have suicidal thoughts or impulses.

1. Get rid of all dangerous weapons.

2. Call your psychiatrist and psychotherapist to ask for an emergency appointment.

3. Implement your behavioral activation plan by scheduling rewarding or distracting activities.

4. Challenge negative thoughts through cognitive restructuring.

5. Ask your core circle of friends and family members for support; agree not to hurt yourself if they haven't had a chance to get back to you.

6. Practice meditation or relaxation techniques.

7. Exercise.

8. Rely on input from religious and spiritual sources.

9. Review your Reasons for Living Inventory.

Circle the things *your doctor and therapist* can do.

1. See you on an emergency basis.

2. Modify your medication regimen.

3. Arrange a hospitalization (if necessary).

4. Help you understand where your suicidal thoughts are coming from and what effects they are having on you or others.

5. Work with you on behavioral strategies for handling your painful thoughts and emotions.

Circle those things that members of *your core circle* can do.

1. Listen to you, validate your feelings, and offer suggestions.

2. Avoid being critical or judgmental.

(cont.)

3. Distract you through mutually enjoyable activities.

4. Help you take care of responsibilities that have become burdensome or difficult to perform (for example, child care).

5. Stay with you until you feel safe.

6. Call your doctor to help you arrange an appointment.

7. Take you to the hospital (if necessary).

8. Agree to store your weapons or pills away from you.

List members of your core circle and put numbers after each indicating which of items 1–8 they are willing to perform (list more than one item, if appropriate).

_____   _____

_____   _____

_____   _____

_____   _____

_____   _____

List your doctors' names and phone numbers.

_____   _____

_____   _____

_____   _____

12

For Women Only
What You Need to Know
about Bipolar Disorder and Your Health

"I had always struggled with my periods, which birth control pills to take, and how I felt about my body when I was taking mood stabilizers that made me look fat and feel stupid. But when I think back on my illness, my biggest struggle was when I had to decide whether to stay on my medications during my pregnancy. I thought I had it all figured out, but then my psychiatrist told me that if I got pregnant, he wouldn't know how to manage my medications, so I'd have to see someone else. And at the same time my OB-GYN told me that if I was planning to take medications while I was pregnant, he wouldn't treat me any longer! My husband insisted that I stop them. I didn't even know what *I* thought. So I stopped my medications and got pregnant, and then I had another episode and landed in the hospital. Fortunately my baby was born healthy. But I certainly could have used a helping hand or two."

—A 43-year-old woman with bipolar I disorder

"My boyfriend thinks I just have PMS. That doesn't even come close to capturing it. What I have is something much, much worse. It's like bipolar and PMS get multiplied several times over, and the result is an intense, panicky, really angry state, combined with a deep sadness that's weird even for me."

—A 27-year-old woman with bipolar II disorder

"My medications, which were supposed to help my depression when I went through menopause, caused me to gain a ton of weight and messed with my hormones. So I've renamed them: depa-bloat, olanza-pig, and despair-idone."

—A 52-year-old woman with bipolar II disorder

If you're a woman, bipolar disorder presents unique challenges in addition to those you read about in earlier chapters. In particular, various stages and events in a woman's reproductive life can affect and are affected by the disorder. You may face the same problems and decisions that the women quoted above encountered. Mood-stablilizing medications can affect the health of your developing baby during pregnancy (called *teratogenic risk*), but so can an untreated bipolar illness, so the risks must be carefully weighed. At significant events in your reproductive life— puberty (around age 12), pregnancy, and again at the onset of menopause (usually after 50)—the disorder may change course, requiring you to be alert for the need to modify your treatment. And the unique nature of the disorder in women sometimes calls for medications that interact with other aspects of reproductive functioning as well. All of these challenges will be addressed in this chapter.

The Course of Bipolar Disorder in Women

Knowing these facts about bipolar disorder in women will help you get the best treatment and have the best chance of managing your illness:

• *Women have longer, more frequent, and more treatment-resistant depressions than men.* As a result, you are more likely to be misdiagnosed with recurrent major depressive disorder than a man would be. You may also have to wait several years longer before being treated for bipolar disorder. As an example, women are started on lithium an average of 5½ years later than men.

• *Mixed episodes, rapid cycling, and bipolar II disorder are more common in women.* These conditions are often treated with complex combinations of medications (for example, mood stabilizers with accompanying atypical antipsychotics) that can pose particular health risks for you (for example, weight gain).

• *Women have more manic or hypomanic episodes brought on by antidepressants.* Because you're more prone to depression, your doctor is more likely to prescribe an antidepressant without an accompanying mood stabilizer, which can trigger manic, mixed, or hypomanic episodes.

• *Women are more likely to have physical disorders and pain conditions than men.* Migraine headaches, thyroid disorders, and other problems can complicate both your medication regimen and your daily life.

• *For women, mood medications are more likely to cause weight gain, insulin resistance, and elevations in blood lipids,* complicating your quality of life and affecting your well-being.

• *The disorder itself—not just the treatments for it—can affect women's functioning during pregnancy and the postpartum period, as well as the regularity of the menstrual cycle.* Bipolar disorder is also associated with weight- and insulin-related disorders like diabetes, polycystic ovarian syndrome, and menstrually related mood changes. Women with bipolar disorder are at a very high risk for postpartum depression.

• *Women are more likely to ruminate when depressed, whereas men are more likely to become aggressive or irritable. Women are more likely than men to have anxiety, panic attacks, body image problems, and eating disorders.* These comorbid conditions often require separate medications or help through psychoeducation, mutual support groups, or psychotherapy.

The good news is that you can reap the benefits of a wealth of new research findings on the biological and psychological ramifications of being a woman with bipolar disorder. (For good reviews of the science in this area, see articles by Burt & Rasgon, 2004; Cohen, 2007; Kenna et al., 2009; Marangell, 2008; Rasgon et al., 2005; and Joffe, 2007.) We now have a pretty good idea of which medications are safest during pregnancy, as well as the risks associated with stopping them altogether. This knowledge comes to us not just from studies of bipolar disorder but also from studies of conditions like epilepsy, for which anticonvulsants like divalproex (Depakote), carbamazepine (Tegretol), and lamotrigine (Lamictal) have been standard treatments for many years. Likewise, we know more than ever about the effects of mood-stabilizing medications on other reproductive functions, such as the menstrual cycle. Outside of medications, we've learned how crucial family and marital relationships are to a woman's mood stability after an episode of bipolar disorder. We know, too, that various forms of couple- and family-oriented therapy can help prevent recurrences and reduce symptoms of depression (Miklowitz, 2008a).

So, you have a lot of accumulated knowledge on your side. As you tackle the challenges that come with having bipolar disorder and being female, keep in mind the theme of this book: *successfully treating your bipolar disorder involves an ongoing collaboration between you, your doctor, and, in many cases, your family members.* Many of the treatment decisions you make will not have right or wrong answers associated with them, which can be frustrating. Also, you may have to make different decisions at different phases of your life. But knowing what the research literature does and does not say about treatment of bipolar disorder in women will help you make well-informed choices. You'll feel like you have more control over your health and that of your baby should you become pregnant, for example. Pregnancy is, in fact, the issue of greatest concern to the women with bipolar disorder I counsel, so we'll start there.

Pregnancy

"[My doctor] asked me whether or not I planned to have children ... I told him that I very much wanted to have children, which immediately led to his asking me what I planned to do about taking lithium during pregnancy. I started to tell him that it seemed obvious to me that the dangers of my illness far outweighed any potential problems that lithium might cause a developing fetus, and that

I therefore would choose to stay on my lithium. Before I finished, however, he broke in to ask me if I knew that manic–depressive illness was a genetic disease … I wasn't entirely stupid, I said, 'Yes, of course.' At that point, in an icy and imperious voice that I can hear to this day, he stated—as though he felt it were God's truth, which he no doubt felt it was—'You shouldn't have children.'

"I felt sick, unbelievably and utterly sick, and deeply humiliated. I asked him if his concerns about my having children stemmed from the fact that, because of my illness, I would be an inadequate mother or simply that he thought it was best to avoid bringing another manic–depressive into the world. Ignoring or missing my sarcasm, he replied, 'Both.'"

—Jamison (1995, p. 191)

Many women with bipolar disorder have asked me whether they should have children. I hope I have responded with more empathy and compassion than the doctor that Kay Jamison was unfortunate enough to consult. As I said in Chapter 5, there is every reason to have children if you want them and are in a position, emotionally and practically, to raise them. The chance that a child will develop bipolar disorder if one parent has it averages about 9%. In my opinion, that's not a high enough risk to influence the decision to have a child. Bipolar disorder does not carry the genetic load of conditions like Huntington's disease. When one parent has this neurodegenerative disorder, the chance that his or her child will develop it is 50%. That risk and the fact that Huntington's leads to early death makes many parents with the genetic predisposition to Huntington's decide not to have children.

Bipolar disorder presents a very different picture. It's hardly a death sentence. Even a child who inherits your biological vulnerability to bipolar illness may develop only a mild form of the disorder or possibly no disorder at all. There may also be much better treatments available once your child is an adult.

Of course, if you have doubts about whether you want to get pregnant right now, it's important to take the proper precautions to prevent it since people with bipolar disorder are vulnerable to engaging in impulsive sexual activity (see the section on contraception in this chapter). If and when you do want to plan a pregnancy, it's important to keep in mind several facts about the disorder and how to manage your illness and your treatments after you conceive.

Pregnancy Caveats

"I have experienced depression on and off since I was in high school. The only thing that has ever really worked for me is the medication I take. When I found out that I was pregnant, I told my doctor that I didn't want to keep taking medication. We stopped it, but then I started feeling down again. My feelings about the pregnancy even changed. I started resenting the baby, the ways in which my life was changing, not to mention my body and all the weight I was

gaining. During one appointment with my OB, I started crying and saying I didn't want to be pregnant anymore. I was beyond the first trimester, so he convinced me to start back on my lithium. It definitely helped, and I'm feeling better in general and more positive about the pregnancy, although I worry a lot about how I might be harming my baby with these drugs. I'm between a rock and a hard place."

—A pregnant 33-year-old woman with a history of bipolar I mixed episodes

New research: A study by Adele Viguera and colleagues (2007) at the Harvard Medical School found that 71% of pregnant women with bipolar disorder had an illness recurrence during their pregnancy. Most of the recurrences were depressive or mixed, and about half occurred during the first trimester. The rate was *twice as high* among those who discontinued, rather than continued, their medications during the pregnancy. The women who stopped their medications also spent *five times* as many weeks in states of depression or mania as those who continued their treatment.

1. *Don't believe the myth that being pregnant will protect you against recurrences of mania or depression.* In fact, as indicated in the sidebar, pregnancy can be a high-risk time for relapse, a risk that is reduced substantially by staying on your mood stabilizers.

2. *Most psychiatric medications pose at least some risks to the developing baby, but so does not taking medications.* Untreated bipolar disorder carries significant risks, such as when a pregnant woman becomes manic and abuses her health by drinking and smoking heavily, driving erratically, forgetting prenatal obstetric appointments, and not eating regularly or getting enough sleep.

3. *Beware of "alternative" treatments.* Some doctors—and often friends or family members—will encourage you to replace your prescription medications with herbal supplements, vitamins, or other over-the-counter compounds during pregnancy. Some of these compounds may indeed be beneficial to pregnancy (an example is folic acid to reduce the risk of neural tube defects). But as I said in Chapter 6, there is no evidence that "natural" compounds like omega-3 fatty acids (fish oil), flaxseed oil, St. John's wort, or valerian root can be substituted for lithium, the anticonvulsants, or the antipsychotics. Also, be wary of the common assumption that medications bought over the counter in health food stores are always safer than prescription medications.

"What Can I Expect from My Doctor If I Want to Get Pregnant?"

Once you've decided you want to conceive (regardless of whether you've been pregnant before), see your psychiatrist and your obstetrician to discuss your conception plans. Make sure the following topics are covered:

Principles for Maintaining Health and Mood Stability before and during Pregnancy

■ Keep in mind the *risk factors for poor fetal health* that all pregnant women should avoid: tobacco, alcohol, drugs, obesity, poor diet, excessive caffeine intake, and dehydration.

■ *There are no hard-and-fast rules regarding which medications to take or not take during pregnancy.* The choice—for example, whether to take lithium or divalproex—is often based on which medications have kept you stable previously.

■ If your mood is cycling up and down during your pregnancy, *continuing your prepregnancy treatment* may be the safest course of action.

■ If you decide to go off your medications, *gradual reduction* is always better than abrupt withdrawal; stopping suddenly can bring on a relapse.

■ If you are severely depressed or having a mixed episode, *electroconvulsive therapy* presents less risk to the fetus than most drugs.

■ Discuss with your physician the risks and benefits of *breast-feeding* while you are taking medications.

■ Always consider *psychotherapy* or couple counseling as an addition to your medication treatment, both during pregnancy and during the postpartum, when you are most vulnerable to recurrence.

■ *Structured daily activities* will help minimize your sleep deprivation and mood instability.

■ Keep track of your mood, medications, and, if you are not pregnant, your menstrual cycles using your *mood chart.*

Sources: Cohen (2007); Kenna et al. (2009); Viguera et al. (2007); Ward and Wisner (2007); Yonkers et al. (2004).

■ your current method of contraception

■ the reproductive risks of medications

■ your prior history of mood cycling when you've been off medications (especially during prior pregnancies)

■ how well you are responding to your current medications

■ your physical health

■ the current regularity of your menstrual cycles and your reproductive and menstrual history

■ the risks of conceiving on your current medication regimen

If you have severe bipolar disorder (for example, you have recently had a full manic or mixed episode, and you have a history of severe relapses when going off your medications), you may require treatment throughout your pregnancy. Lithium alone or in combination with an antipsychotic medication is generally safer than divalproex or carbamazepine (Cohen, 2007).

Effective treatment when planning to conceive: If your mood is stable, you may want to try a prepregnancy trial period in which you go off your medications, with instructions from your doctor on how to taper them. If all goes well during this trial, you may be able to go the first trimester without medications. If the first trimester goes well, you may then be able to have a drug-free pregnancy. Whatever you decide, base your choices on an open discussion of your concerns with your doctors (Yonkers et al., 2004).

If you have mild to moderate bipolar disorder and are currently stable (for example, you have gone a full year without an episode of major depression; you have hypomanias but not full manias), you may be able to slowly discontinue your medications before you conceive.

Most obstetricians will recommend a regular schedule of prenatal visits, a healthy diet, and childbirth classes (especially if this is your first pregnancy). They may also recommend prenatal vitamins or supplements. If you are not already in psychotherapy, consider starting therapy before you get pregnant, particularly if you are confused about what your prodromal signs of relapse look like, are having significant stress in your life (e.g., marital or couple problems), or are ambivalent about having a child (see Chapter 6 for a discussion of effective therapies for bipolar disorder). These kinds of issues are very common among women planning pregnancy, whether bipolar or not.

"What If I Am Already Pregnant?"

As many as 50% of all pregnancies are unplanned. The risk of unplanned pregnancy is even higher among women with bipolar disorder, because mania and hypomania can lead to impulsive sexual choices and because your mood-stabilizing medications can influence the effectiveness of contraceptive pills (see page 270). Take a look at Chapter 9, especially the section "Avoiding Risky Sexual Situations," when your mood is escalating. As you know, working with an OB-GYN who is familiar with mood disorders and the effects of different contraceptives on mood can be quite helpful.

The biggest problem with an unplanned pregnancy is that you may not know you're pregnant until you're well into your first trimester, when many of the medications for bipolar illness have already had their effects on the developing baby:

■ The risk of neural tube defects (for example, spina bifida, an incomplete closure of the vertebrae over the spinal cord) increases if you're taking divalproex or carbamazepine between 17 and 30 days after conception.

■ The risk of heart defects is influenced most by medications taken between 21 and 56 days after conception. Lithium may pose the greatest risk for heart abnormalities, but the chances are still very low (about 0.1–0.2%; Yonkers et al., 2004).

■ Fetal lip and palate abnormalities are influenced by medications (particularly anticonvulsants, including lamotrigine) taken between 8 and 11 weeks (8 to 20 weeks for craniofacial abnormalities).

■ In rare cases, lithium use throughout pregnancy can be associated with "floppy baby" syndrome: lethargy, blue coloration of the skin, and abnormal muscle tension.

Weighing the Medication Risks

The risks listed above are enough to convince some women to discontinue medications when they discover they're pregnant. Before you make a decision, weigh the risks of discontinuing your medications against the risks of experiencing mania or depression. Depression during pregnancy has been correlated with low birth weight and premature delivery, possibly because depressed women often have a decrease in appetite and are less likely to get adequate prenatal care. Depression late in pregnancy is associated with more C-sections and a greater need for neonatal intensive care (Chung et al., 2001). Indeed, women who are depressed often have less emotional energy to prepare for a vaginal delivery.

When manic and pregnant, some women impulsively stop their medications and endanger themselves or their baby through risky behavior like abusing substances, driving recklessly, or having multiple sexual partners. If untreated, pregnant women with bipolar illness are also at high risk for suicide.

As you see, deciding whether to stop or take medications when pregnant is a difficult choice, and often a very emo-

> **Effective prevention:** Before you decide to stop your medications, make an appointment with your psychiatrist and obstetrician to discuss your options. If you do go off them, you will need to do it gradually, through timed dose reductions. Going off your medications suddenly can greatly increase your risk of relapse and possibly put your baby at risk.

tional one. On balance, most doctors will tell you it's safer to continue your medications if your mood has been unstable prior to conceiving. But some medications are safer than others.

"Which Medications Are Safe to Take?"

No mood stabilizer or atypical antipsychotic is approved by the FDA for use during pregnancy (Cohen, 2007). Not surprisingly, exposure to only one medication is safer for the fetus than exposure to several different ones. Here are some comparisons:

• If you are choosing between lithium and divalproex, lithium is generally considered the safer of the two alternatives. Because divalproex has the highest teratogenic risk in the first trimester, it is usually best to switch to something else. You should discuss with your doctor medications other than these as well. Carbamazepine and lamotrigine appear to be somewhat better than divalproex in terms of fetal risks, but have their own complications (see below).

• As discussed in prior chapters, it's generally better to stay away from antidepressants if you have bipolar disorder because of the risks of rapid cycling or mixed episodes. But some women with bipolar disorder do well with antidepressants when given in conjunction with mood stabilizers, and it may be better to stick with them if you were taking them before the pregnancy and you've had recent, difficult periods of depression.

• Consider the option of switching from an anticonvulsant (like divalproex) to an atypical or typical antipsychotic medication, such as quetiapine (Seroquel) or even the older drug haloperidol (Haldol). These may have lower teratogenic risk than the anticonvulsants, although there are few comparison studies. The problem with some of the atypical antipsychotics (for example, risperidone [Risperdal]) is that they can elevate your prolactin levels (discussed below) or cause weight gain.

"Can Any Testing Be Done during the First Trimester?"

Some fetal abnormalities can be detected prenatally. One option includes high-resolution ultrasonography (ultrasound), which can be done at 10–13 weeks to look at the nuchal fold and nasal bone (markers of Down syndrome) and at 16–18 weeks to assess heart formation, vertebral development, facial/palate abnormalities and the status of other anatomical structures. In addition, evidence of neural tube defects in your baby is usually suggested by high levels of alpha-fetoprotein in your blood, usually tested first at 10–13 weeks and again at 15–21 weeks. Your doctor may also recommend amniocentesis (testing of the amniotic fluid for chromosomal abnormalities or fetal infections) between 16 and 21 weeks. Discuss the recommended testing regimen with your OB, ideally as soon as you start prenatal care.

"How Will I Know If I'm Depressed While I'm Pregnant?"

It can be difficult to tell whether you are depressed or just experiencing the fatigue, weight gain, sluggishness, appetite changes, and sleep disturbance that often go along with pregnancy or the postdelivery period. In fact, doctors often miss the diagnosis of depression in their pregnant patients. Nonetheless, there are important differences between the fatigue states of pregnancy and clinical depression.

Lori Altshuler and colleagues (2008) have identified seven symptoms that indicate major depression during pregnancy. These symptoms can occur during any of the three trimesters and can extend into the postpartum. Take a look at the list and check off any that you have had *most of the time* in the *past week.*

- Depressed mood ____
- Feelings of guilt ____
- Reduced time and interest in work/activities ____
- Slowness of speech and movement ____
- Feeling much worse in the morning or the evening ____
- Feeling more tired than usual ____
- Withdrawing from others ____

If you have several of these symptoms, consider seeing your psychiatrist or OB to determine whether you should restart the medications you stopped before your pregnancy or need higher dosages. If you have a therapist, you may also want to step up the frequency of sessions.

During the postpartum period, try filling out the Edinburgh Post-Natal Depression Scale, which can be found at *www.fresno.ucsf.edu/pediatrics/downloads/edinburghscale.pdf.*

"What Do I Need to Consider Later in Pregnancy and during Delivery?"

Again, weigh the medication risks against the risks of relapse if you are doing well. Consider the following issues and discuss them with your doctor when you're entering your second trimester:

- The teratogenic risks of medications continue into the second and third trimesters and can include minor physical malformations, low birth weight, premature delivery, or later behavioral problems. Many doctors, however, will recommend you stay on your medications if you were taking them during the first trimester and your mood has been stable.
- Because your body will metabolize

Effective prevention: If you are pregnant and taking lithium, divalproex, carbamazepine, or other anticonvulsants, you should have a high-resolution ultrasound at 16–18 weeks and serum alpha-fetoprotein tests to detect neural tube defects. If you take lithium, a fetal echocardiogram is recommended at 20–24 weeks.

medications differently when you are pregnant and when you deliver, you have to be alert to the signs of drug toxicity in you and your newborn. Drug toxicity can occur when you have abnormally high blood levels of a medication. Signs that you may have developed lithium toxicity include disorientation, vomiting, or dizziness; your infant's signs could include restlessness, muscle twitching, vomiting, and fever. Your doctor should take a lithium (or divalproex or carbamazepine) level as soon as possible after you deliver and may need to adjust your dosage.

- Discuss fluid intake with your doctor. Lithium can cause dehydration.
- Are you are planning to breast-feed? (See pages 267–269.)
- Are family members available to spell you and enable you to get enough sleep during the exhausting first few weeks following delivery? If not, what are your options to ensure regular sleep (as much as is realistic with a newborn)?

Treatment after Delivery

"When we first started to talk about having another child, my tendency toward postpartum depression was a big factor. Being depressed had been hard not only on me; it had been really hard on my husband too, seeing me go through it, worrying about me, having to do a lot of the child care, and dealing with the ways in which I treat him when I'm depressed. I knew I was at risk for getting depressed again if I had another baby—I wasn't sure if I should even try to get pregnant. I wanted to be a mother again, but I was afraid of what it would do to the people around me. I cried a lot. I'm glad we went ahead, but it was a hard decision."

—A 39-year-old mother with bipolar I disorder

For many women with bipolar disorder, the highest-risk time for an episode of depression or mania is during the postpartum period, usually defined as the 6 months following delivery. About 15% of women in the general population have episodes of depression at this time, but the risk is much higher among women with bipolar disorder. Between 40 and 67% of women with bipolar disorder have postpartum manic or depressive episodes. Rarely, they can develop postpartum psychosis (delusions or hallucinations; Cohen, 2007).

Not surprisingly, women who were depressed during their pregnancy are highly likely to develop postpartum depression as well. This is another reason that receiving effective treatment for depression during pregnancy is so important.

"What Is Postpartum Depression?"

Postpartum depressive episodes are not the same as the "baby blues," a 3- to 5-day period of hormonal readjustment following delivery. During those days you may cry frequently, feel intensely sad, feel inadequate as a mother and like you made a big mistake, and find it difficult to concentrate or sleep. Typically, this period lifts within 10 days after delivery. A postpartum depressive episode, in contrast, lasts for at least 2 weeks (usually much longer if untreated) and is characterized by the full syndrome of depression, with difficulty in functioning. Babies born to mothers with postpartum depression often develop emotional, cognitive, and behavioral problems, some of which can be detected even in the first few months (Forman et al., 2007; Segre et al., 2007).

The good news is that starting or restarting lithium just before or around the time of delivery, or within a day or two after delivery, reduces the rate of postpartum episodes of mania or depression from as much as 50% to 10% (Cohen, 2007). In turn, babies born to women with postpartum depression often "catch up" in terms of developmental delays once the mother's depression lifts. We know less about whether medications such as divalproex or the atypical antipsychotics have equal postpartum preventative effects.

> **Effective prevention:**
> Starting or restarting lithium just before or a day or two after delivery can help prevent postpartum depression or mania.

Some mothers experience reductions in their levels of thyroid hormone during the postpartum period. The signs of hypothyroidism include hair loss, extreme fatigue, sadness, and a low milk supply. Check with your doctor to see if a thyroid supplement would help you during the postpartum (see below).

"What If I Want to Breast-Feed?"

The health benefits of breast-feeding for the mother and infant are well known, but you may be understandably concerned about the effects of your medications on your baby. A recent review in the journal *Pediatrics* (Fortinguerra et al., 2009) concluded that most psychiatric medications are secreted in breast milk, but they differ considerably in their adverse effects on the infant.

> **Effective prevention:** All psychiatric medications are secreted in breast milk. So, if you are breast-feeding, take your medications after your infant has been fed and before he or she takes a long nap.

Lithium and the anticonvulsants can both be detected in the blood of newborns, but there is disagreement about whether they should be taken when breast-feeding. The American Academy of Pediatrics has said that lithium should not be taken at all when breast-feeding, but this recommendation is based on very limited data. In fact, one of Viguera's studies (Viguera et al., 2007) found that blood concentrations of lithium in breast-fed infants were only about 25% of those in the mother who was taking lithium, much lower than expected. Moreover, no serious growth or developmental delays or other serious adverse effects were found, and minor changes in the infant's laboratory tests did not seem to be clinically significant.

Although the actual risks of lithium or divalproex to breast-fed infants (for lithium: sedation, poor feeding, dehydration, muscle twitching; for divalproex: lethargy, sedation) appear to be low, you will feel more confident if you take a few precautions:

- Make sure you and your baby are adequately hydrated; rapid dehydration is a side effect of lithium and can appear in you or your infant as a sudden fever.

- Take your medications *after* you have finished breast-feeding or when your infant starts a long nap, so that there will be less in your breast milk the next time you feed.

- Make sure your obstetrician is monitoring your and your baby's blood levels of lithium or divalproex at least monthly to avoid any risks of toxicity, especially if your infant is under 10 weeks old.

- Talk to your doctor about simplifying your medication regimen so that you take fewer medications at the lowest possible dosages that will still help you manage your mood.

Of course, you may not be taking lithium or divalproex. Here are some additional suggestions:

- If you are taking carbamazepine, be on the lookout for decreased feeding, sedation, or spasms in your newborn. A small number of infants develop a temporary liver dysfunction.

- If you are taking lamotrigine, and especially if you started it recently, make sure to check yourself and your baby for skin rashes (see Chapter 6). The postpartum is a high-risk time for developing rashes on lamotrigine, and you will almost certainly need to stop taking it if severe itching begins.

- Antipsychotics appear to be among the safest compounds to take when breast-feeding, especially at low dosages. However, as you know from prior chapters, some of these medications (notably olanzapine [Zyprexa]) can cause you to gain a significant amount of weight, which puts you at risk for diabetes. Some breast-fed infants develop sedation and lethargy when their mothers take antipsychotics.

Breast-Feeding and Sleep Regularity

Women who breast-feed have more chaotic sleep–wake cycles than women who bottle-feed, which can place you at risk for manic relapse. The postpartum is a particularly important time for you to get regular sleep, but also one of the hardest times to make it happen.

Of course, the decision to breast-feed is a very personal and often a very emotional one, and the effects on your sleep cycles will probably not be at the forefront of your mind after you deliver. But try to weigh the benefits of breast-feeding against the risks. If you decide to breast-feed, try to enlist your family members (husband/ partner, in-laws, siblings) and others in your support system to help you with other nighttime child care tasks that can interfere with your sleep cycle (Joffe, 2007).

"What Other Treatments Are Available during the Postpartum Period?"

The postpartum is a very stressful and chaotic time for anyone. Although you are most likely enjoying the excitement and joy of having a new baby, you may also be dealing with your baby's illnesses (or those of your other children), long and sometimes conflictual visits from in-laws, and unpredictable routines. You may feel closer to your husband or partner than ever before, but, understandably, you may also be arguing more. If you had a job, you may not feel like going back, but your employer may be pressuring you to return. These stressors, along with your biological vulnerabilities, can contribute to postpartum depressive episodes.

Some women with bipolar disorder elect to take antidepressants (in addition to their mood stabilizers) during the postpartum to help deal with their anxiety and depression. If you have done well on them before, and they have not brought on mixed episodes or rapid cycling, adjunctive antidepressants are one treatment option to consider for postpartum depression. The antidepressants vary in their milk transfer rate, so discuss with your doctor which one is best for you. Some doctors recommend sertraline (Zoloft), paroxetine (Paxil), or fluvoxamine (Luvox) over fluoxetine (Prozac), citalopram (Celexa), or escitalopram (Lexapro) (Fortinguerra et al., 2009; Hale, 2002), but few studies on bipolar disorder have been done. The risks of SSRI antidepressants to your infant include sedation, nausea, and reduced feeding.

Many women resist psychotherapy during the postpartum, believing that their emotional ups and downs can be explained by hormones, sleep disturbance, or simple exhaustion. Certainly these factors will contribute to your mood states. But you may also be cycling into a depressive episode, your prior depression symptoms from the prepartum may be getting worse, or you may be developing a mixed state (depression with agitation, hypomania, or even full mania). If you have had a therapist before, now is a good time to reconnect and, possibly, resume sessions.

If you don't have the time or financial resources for individual psychotherapy, consider other alternatives for dealing with depression, such as a support group for new mothers, yoga, or meditation classes. Review Chapter 10 of this book, particularly the sections on behavioral activation (pleasant life events scheduling). Consult *The Mindful Way through Depression* (Williams et al., 2008), which includes a CD with mindfulness meditation exercises, or *Feeling Good* by David Burns (1999).

Contraceptive Choices

Planning pregnancy obviously gives you more control over the management of your disorder and the healthy development of your baby. That's one reason that effective contraception is important. But even if you never intend to become pregnant, you should know about the interactions between the psychiatric medications you're taking and oral contraceptives (birth control pills). Some of the anticonvulsant medications, including carbamazepine, oxcarbazepine (Trileptal), and topiramate (Topamax), increase the metabolism of sex hormones like estrogen and accelerate the metabolism of birth control pills. In other words, they may make your contraceptive less effective (Ward & Wisner, 2007). As a result, you may need to use a different form of contraception (for example, a diaphragm, condoms, or a birth control pill with a higher estrogen dose) if you're taking these medications and don't want to get pregnant (Joffe, 2007).

Birth control pills can also make certain medications—lamotrigine in particular—less effective by reducing the blood concentrations of the medication. So, if you are taking birth control pills, you may need to increase your dosage of lamotrigine or use another form of birth control to get the full mood-stabilizing benefit. Likewise, if you suddenly stop your birth control pills, your estrogen will drop and you may have a sudden increase in lamotrigine levels, which puts you at greater risk of rashes or Stevens–Johnson syndrome (see Chapter 6). So, make sure your doctor is aware of when you are starting or stopping oral contraceptives.

Bipolar Disorder and the Menstrual Cycle

You may find that your menstrual cycle is affected by bipolar disorder—both the biology of the illness and the medications you take to manage it. Typical menstrual abnormalities include absence of a period (amenorrhea), cycles longer than 35 days (oligomenorrhea), and cycles that are irregular from month to month. Irregular menstrual cycles, usually defined as cycles shorter than 25 days or longer than 35 days, occur in 15–20% of all women.

New research: Hadine Joffe and colleagues (2006) at Massachusetts General Hospital found that menstrual irregularities were somewhat more common among women with bipolar disorder (about 34%) than among women with depression (25%) or women without mood disorders (22%). The women with bipolar disorder were also more likely to have had an earlier onset of their menstrual irregularities.

Normal or Abnormal Irregularities?

Your doctor should be taking a detailed menstrual cycle history from you, especially if you're gaining weight on medications (see pages 274–275) or develop menstrual irregularities. There are both normal and abnormal reasons for irregular cycles. Typical reasons include just having reached puberty (younger females), breast-feeding an infant, or being close to menopause. More troubling reasons can include polycystic ovarian syndrome (see pages 272–273), elevated prolactin levels (often due to certain antipsychotic medications), hypothyroidism (see page 275), benign growths on the anterior pituitary gland, excessive exercise or weight loss, and severe psychological stress.

What Does Medication Have to Do with It?

If you've had recent irregularities in your menstrual cycle, it's important to know whether these irregularities *predated* taking medications like lithium, divalproex, and atypical antipsychotics. In studies by Natalie Rasgon and colleagues (Rasgon et al., 2000, 2005) about 50% of women with bipolar disorder who had menstrual abnormalities reported that these abnormalities started before their first medication use. But even if your menstrual problems did occur early on, your medications can worsen them because of the effects of mood stabilizers on the hypothalamic–pituitary–gonadal (HPG) axis and their peripheral effects on testosterone metabolites. Divalproex seems to have a greater effect on menstrual cycles than lithium (Joffe et al., 2006). Discuss these issues with your doctor: disrupted menstrual cycles can reduce fertility and contribute to longer-term illnesses such as osteoporosis, non-insulin-dependent diabetes, and cardiovascular disease (Kenna et al., 2009).

Mood Changes

Most women report that their mood symptoms—notably their depression and anxiety—get worse prior to and during their periods. But women with bipolar disorder have more extreme menstrually related mood variations (Rasgon et al., 2003).

> **Effective treatment:** Your mood chart can help you figure out whether any menstrual irregularities or mood changes are related to the biology of your disorder, your medications, or neither.

It can be very difficult to tell cause from effect: Do your mood changes worsen your periods or your periods worsen your moods? Do your medications make your cycles worse or better? Do birth control pills reduce your menstrually related mood changes? Again, whenever you're not sure, keep track of your cycles on your mood chart. Some women discover that their menstrual irregularities, which they thought were just an inherent feature of their physiology, are actually being worsened by medications. Other women discover that menstrual irregularities they have been attributing to their medications actually have a life of their own.

The mood chart in Chapter 8 (page 158) allows you to keep track of the beginning and end of your cycles. Take your completed charts to your next psychiatry or obstetric appointment and discuss your options. Your doctor may decide to take you off certain medications or alter the dosages to see whether your menstrual cycles (and any associated hormonal imbalances) go back to normal.

Other Physical Conditions Related to Bipolar Disorder and Its Treatments

Several endocrine (hormonal) conditions can be brought on or worsened by the medications you take for bipolar disorder. Other endocrine conditions may be part of the biology of the disorder. In some cases, both the medications and the biology of the illness combine to cause the problem. What you do to address the conditions may vary depending on what the main cause is likely to be.

Polycystic Ovarian Syndrome (PCOS)

PCOS is an endocrine disorder that increases your risk for type 2 diabetes, endometrial hyperplasia (which can presage endometrial cancer), lowered fertility, and heart disease (Kenna et al., 2009). About half of women who develop PCOS have significant weight problems (some of which are caused by the mood-stabilizing drugs they take). As the name implies, the signs of PCOS include abnormal cysts on the ovaries, but also facial acne, male pattern balding, growth of excessive facial hair, weight gain, and high levels of testosterone (Thase, 2006). The condition is diagnosed by infrequent ovulation, hyperandrogenism (an elevated level of or an increased sensitivity to the androgen steroid hormones,

> **Effective prevention of PCOS and other reproductive disorders:** Watch for the development of menstrual irregularities or significant weight gain after you start any new mood-stabilizing medication.

such as testosterone), insulin resistance, and infertility. The abnormal cysts are detected through ultrasound, and the hyperandrogenism is usually detected through blood tests of sex steroids (e.g., testosterone) and reproductive hormones (e.g., estrogen or progesterone).

PCOS affects about 1 in 20 women in the general population, but you are at a higher risk if you take divalproex. PCOS and bipolar disorder probably have some common genetic underpinnings (Jiang et al., 2009), but divalproex increases your risk substantially. The STEP-BD study (see Chapter 6) found that 10.5% of women developed irregular menstrual cycles and hyperandrogenism in their first year of taking divalproex, compared to 1.4% taking lithium or other anticonvulsants like lamotrigine (Joffe et al., 2006). Among women who then stopped taking divalproex, there was an improvement in menstrual cycles and lower levels of testosterone.

If you're taking divalproex and you experience menstrual irregularities, however, don't assume you have PCOS. Irregularities can also signal unexpected pregnancy, elevated prolactin levels (see below), stress, or the onset of menopause (all covered elsewhere in this chapter).

Other anticonvulsant medications—notably carbamazepine and oxcarbazepine (Trileptal)—may also predispose women to PCOS. Lithium and lamotrigine seem to be less frequently associated with PCOS.

At minimum, if you are on divalproex, carbamazepine, or oxcarbazepine and have developed menstrual irregularities, gained a significant amount of weight, developed facial hair, or had any of the other reproductive signs listed above, you should get your testosterone levels checked and, possibly, have an ultrasound to see if your ovaries show any polycystic changes (Isojärvi & Taubøll, 2005). If they do, in all likelihood you'll need to stop taking these anticonvulsants and switch to a different mood stabilizer (for example, lamotrigine). Your menstrual cycles may not normalize for a full year after you stop taking divalproex (Joffe, 2007).

Prolactin Elevation

Elevated levels of the hormone prolactin (hyperprolactinemia) are dangerous because they can increase your risk of breast cancer and, when you also have infrequent menstrual cycles, lead to reductions in the production of estrogen. Low levels of estrogen can in turn lead to infertility and reduce bone density, which puts you at risk for osteoporosis (Joffe, 2007). When elevated, prolactin can cause infrequent menstrual cycles, galactorrhea (breast leaking), breast enlargement, amenorrhea, migraine headaches, or decreased sexual drive (Ali & Khemka, 2008).

You are at greater risk of hyperprolactinemia if your treatment includes certain antipsychotic drugs. Between 48 and 88% of people taking risperidone develop hyperprolactinemia. The "typical" antipsychotics, such as chlorpromazine (Thorazine) and haloperidol, can also cause an elevation in prolactin levels in your blood. So, if you have a family history of breast cancer, it's particularly important to have your prolactin levels checked while taking these medications.

If you have prolactin elevation but no evidence of menstrual irregularities, you may not have to be treated for it. But if you're having active symptoms of hyperprolactinemia, you may need to stop taking your antipsychotic medication and switch to an agent less likely to cause prolactin elevation (for example, quetiapine, aripiprazole [Abilify], or ziprasidone [Geodon]). If your doctor detects low estrogen levels as well as high prolactin, a hormonal contraceptive that increases estrogen may also be recommended.

Weight Gain and the Metabolic Syndrome

Both men and women with bipolar disorder are at increased risk for developing obesity, but the risk is higher among women. *Obesity* is usually defined as a body mass index of 30 kg/m² or more; being overweight is usually defined as at least 25 kg/m² (to calculate your body mass index using pounds and inches, use the online calculator at *www.findmybmi.com*). You may have struggled with weight problems before you started taking psychiatric medications; these symptoms are suspected to be part of the illness. Nonetheless, medications can worsen preexisting weight problems.

A particularly worrisome effect of weight gain and obesity is the *metabolic syndrome,* which consists of insulin resistance or glucose intolerance (in which the body does not properly use insulin or blood sugar), hyperglycemia (excessive blood glucose), excessive fat tissue around the stomach, dyslipidemia (usually indicated by high triglycerides and low HDL and high LDL cholesterol), high blood pressure, and other symptoms. The metabolic syndrome affects between 16.7 and 49% of people with bipolar disorder and, like weight gain generally, affects more women than men (Kenna et al., 2009). Obesity and the metabolic syndrome are risk factors for serious health problems, including diabetes, hypertension, and cardiovascular problems.

The first thing you can do to protect yourself against developing the metabolic syndrome is to be aware of any weight gain on a certain medication. Whether it be an atypical antipsychotic, divalproex, or lithium, ask your doctor to check you for evidence of the metabolic syndrome (for example, testing your cholesterol and triglycerides, conducting a fasting insulin or glucose tolerance test, doing a blood lipids profile). If there is evidence that your body is reacting poorly to these medications, discuss your other treatment options with your physician (see the sidebar on this page). Some medications for bipolar disorder are better than others: for example, people with bipolar disorder generally gain more weight on the atypical antipsychotic olanzapine than on divalproex (Novick et al., 2009). Among the atypicals, ziprasidone and aripiprazole appear to be more "weight neutral" than olanzapine. Quetiapine and risperidone are both associated with weight gain, but not as much as olanzapine. Most of the atypical antipsychotics and divalproex are associated with risk of insulin resistance or hyperlipidemia (Kenna et al., 2009).

Effective treatment: If you start gaining weight, talk to your doctor about changing your medication dosage; taking your medication at a different time of day; switching to medications that have less risk of weight gain (e.g., aripiprazole, lamotrigine); or adding metformin to promote weight loss.

Among the anticonvulsants, lamotrigine appears to be better than lithium or divalproex in terms of weight gain. Although topiramate has weight-loss properties, there is less evidence for its efficacy as a mood stabilizer. If you are gaining weight, your doctor may recommend you add a drug called metformin (Glucophage), an antidiabetic agent that appears to cause weight loss with relatively few side effects.

Of course, if you have gained weight, most doctors will recommend you get regular exercise and maintain a healthy diet. We all know the importance of these lifestyle adaptations, but they can be extraordinarily difficult to implement when you are depressed, which can make you feel even more down on yourself. Try not to be critical of yourself if you can't stick to a diet or exercise plan: you may be able to return to these lifestyle habits when your mood improves.

Thyroid Disorders

Thyroid disturbances appear more often with depression than with other types of psychiatric disorders. Be alert for such conditions, particularly low production of thyroid hormones, or *hypothyroidism,* which is more common in women than men. Some women first develop thyroid problems around the time of menarche, others after giving birth, and still others as a normal part of aging. A variety of factors—autoimmune disease, iodine deficiency, genetic predisposition, and certain medications—can cause thyroid disorders.

There is some evidence that rapid cycling and hypothyroidism (both of which are more common among women) are linked, but not all studies find this. Lithium suppresses thyroid hormone and causes hypothyroidism in some people. Therefore your doctor should be checking your thyroid levels as part of your regular blood work, especially when you start a new medication.

If you have hypothyroidism, you might need a thyroid supplement, such as levothyroxine (Synthroid). Because it has been found to reduce the frequency of depressive episodes, you don't necessarily have to have an underactive thyroid to benefit from thyroid supplementation. But if you do start thyroid supplementation, be aware of the symptoms of becoming *hyperthyroid,* which can put you at risk for atrial fibrillation or osteoporosis. The symptoms of an overactive thyroid are fairly recognizable: changes in your menstrual cycle, feeling hot and sweaty, heart palpitations, having "salty skin," changes in weight or appetite, anxiety, and frequent diarrhea or bowel movements. Your doctor can measure whether you are hyperthyroid using standard blood tests. If you are, you will probably have to stop taking the supplement or change to a different form of supplementation. So, taking a thyroid supplement can be a balancing act, but when you are experiencing depression that is not responding to treatments, it can be simpler and more effective to take the supplement than to add another mood stabilizer or atypical antipsychotic into the mix.

Migraine Headaches

There is a clear link between migraine headaches and mood or anxiety (especially panic) disorders. One recent study found that the rate of bipolar disorder among women with migraines was four times higher than among women without migraines, and rates of depression were twice as high (Jette et al., 2008). Although men also develop migraines, the rate is at least twice as high among women. Girls often develop migraines around the time of their first menstrual period and then go on to have them repeatedly in the premenstrual or menstrual phases of their cycles.

Migraines are far worse than ordinary headaches: they usually begin in the morning and last for at least 4 hours, occur on only one side of the head, create a throbbing sensation, are worsened by physical activity, and often require bed rest. To treat them, you can use medications intended specifically for migraines, such as zolmitriptan (Zomig). But migraines can also be treated successfully with divalproex or other anticonvulsants. If you have migraines, avoid drugs like risperidone that elevate prolactin levels.

Lithium may improve migraines but is not considered a primary treatment for them. One of the older antidepressants, amitriptyline (Elavil), has been experimentally shown to reduce the frequency of migraines, but the difficulties of taking tricyclic antidepressants when you have bipolar disorder make this a risky option. More generally, make sure the doctor who is treating your migraines is talking to your psychiatrist about the effects of these medications on your mood and potential drug interactions with your mood stabilizers.

Menopause

"Going through menopause was absolute hell. I finally got stabilized on estrogen supplements, and then after all those years my doctor wanted to take my estrogen away. Why didn't he understand that without it I'd be a complete mess?"
—A 52-year-old woman with bipolar II disorder

Not much is known about bipolar disorder and menopause, except that menopause is a time of risk for mood swings and recurrences. One study reported that 20% of postmenopausal women with bipolar disorder reported a worsening of their mood symptoms, more typically depression than mania. About one in three women with bipolar disorder develop rapid cycling after menopause (Blehar et al., 1998).

Of course, just because your moods worsen near, during, or after menopause doesn't mean that hormones explain everything. Many women have other life changes in their late 40s and 50s, including kids mov-

Effective solution: If your mood becomes worse around the time of menopause, you may need a higher dosage of your atypical antipsychotic medication. You may also need to lower your dose of lamotrigine because of its effects on estrogen levels.

ing away from home, divorces, remarriages, illnesses, deaths of parents, and other transitions. So, if you are of perimenopausal age and start experiencing a destabilization or worsening of your mood, ask your OB-GYN for an endocrinological workup (e.g., levels of follicle-stimulating hormone, estradiol, luteinizing hormone, thyroid hormone) and talk to your psychiatrist about whether you need to adjust your medications. But also use psychotherapy or group therapy sessions to explore the effects of recent life transitions on your emotional and physical health.

Some women with bipolar disorder decide to start hormone replacement therapy, or HRT (usually estrogen and progesterone, although some women take only estrogen). There is some evidence that HRT can help stabilize moods around the time of the perimenopausal transition (Freeman et al., 2002), and it also reduces symptoms such as hot flashes. HRT also has other health benefits, such as increasing bone density, but there are case reports of women on HRT getting manic or beginning to cycle rapidly (Arnold, 2003), and it puts you at higher risk for breast cancer and heart disease. Discuss the HRT option with both your OB-GYN and

---

New Research: The Harvard Study of Moods and Cycles

This study, which involved 976 depressed and nondepressed women between ages 36 and 45 years, investigated whether depression has an effect on the *perimenopausal transition,* which is the time immediately before menopause, during which a number of biological and hormonal changes occur (Harlow et al., 2003). Perimenopause starts at an average age of 47.5 years and can last from 4 to 8 years. It is marked by a decline in ovarian function and is a time of increased risk for recurrences of depression.

Compared with women who did not have a history of depression, women with depression reported having their first menstrual period at a younger age. In a 3-year follow-up, women with a history of depression reached perimenopause sooner than women who had no depression history, particularly if their depression was severe and they were taking antidepressants for it. Women with depression also had higher follicle-stimulating hormone and luteinizing hormone levels and lower estrogen levels than their nondepressed peers.

Although no women with bipolar disorder participated, the results may have implications for you if you are approaching the age of menopause: you may develop perimenopausal symptoms earlier than your age-mates, especially if you are taking antidepressants as well as mood stabilizers. If your periods start to become irregular, shorter, involve mid-cycle spotting, or stop altogether, see your OB to have your hormone levels checked and determine whether you might be starting menopause. Some women opt for HRT at this time (see *www.nlm.nih.gov/medlineplus/hormonereplacementtherapy.html*).

your psychiatrist, and consult *www.womensmentalhealth.org* for updates in this rapidly changing area.

▪

Some of what you've learned in this chapter may discourage you and make you feel like you're "damned if you do, damned if you don't." Indeed, coping with bipolar disorder if you're a women can be a much more difficult balancing act than if you're a man, and the choices you will be asked to make will often seem quite unfair. Fortunately, you can adjust your treatment to minimize the teratogenic effects of medications during pregnancy, the effects on your menstrual cycle, and the likelihood of developing PCOS, metabolic conditions, thyroid conditions, or hyperprolactinemia. Before starting any new medication, discuss with your doctor the ways that adverse effects can be reduced. Remember that all medications, even aspirin, have long-term side effects.

The final chapter offers a different window on the question of self-management: how to cope effectively in your family and work environments after a bipolar illness episode. People with bipolar disorder often experience trouble in both settings— trouble not entirely due to their own behavior. Many of their problems derive from others' having an inadequate understanding of the disorder (see the example of Martha in Chapter 1). I will discuss several strategies that will help you feel empowered in negotiating your family, social, and work relationships. As you've seen throughout this book, managing your disorder involves acquainting others with the facts about it and being clear yourself on what will, and will not, be helpful to your recovery.

13

Succeeding at Home and at Work
Communication, Problem-Solving Skills, and Dealing Effectively with Stigma

Bipolar disorder poses significant challenges for daily life, in both your family life and your work life. When your family members first learned about your disorder, they may have been supportive, intrusive, anxious, or angry. Some may have been eager to help, while others subjected you to overt rejection. But even after everyone has seemed to adjust to life with bipolar disorder in the family, difficulties often reappear with the next bipolar episode.

Likewise, you may experience frustration in the work setting. Perhaps you want to work and be productive, but you don't know how to deal with the stigma of the disorder, the lack of understanding by employers or coworkers, or workplace demands that are incompatible with your attempts to manage your illness. We know that the symptoms of bipolar disorder affect a person's ability to function in the family or work setting (e.g., Fagiolini et al., 2005; Simoneau et al., 1998). The good news is that you can learn to negotiate the conflicts and demands of your family and work life through a variety of communication skills and self-care strategies.

Remember Martha (Chapter 1)? After her manic episode and hospitalization, her children became suspicious, withdrawn, and fearful. Her husband acted rejecting at some points and overprotective at others, before he came to a better understanding of the disorder through their couple counseling. Back at her computer programming job, Martha had problems concentrating. She found the computer screen newly confusing and forgot how to use the programs she had been so expert at using before. Her boss quickly became impatient with her low performance. Her coworkers avoided her and even seemed nervous in her presence after learning of her difficulties.

If you've recently recovered from a manic, mixed, or depressive episode, you may feel ready to reintegrate yourself into the family and the workplace, only to find that those you live and work with don't treat you the way they used to. Your loved ones may become angry and critical or overprotective. Your partner may seem hesitant to reestablish intimacy with you. At work you may feel like "It's the same old me" but get the impression that your colleagues don't see it that way. And if you really do need to adjust your work setting and work routines to help you maintain mood stability, how much can you tell them about your disorder and still get them to treat you as the confident, competent person you were before?

These issues pose undeniable challenges, but I have been continually impressed with how effectively people with bipolar disorder can learn to deal with them. Establishing close family or couple relationships is possible even after the most severe of mood disorder episodes. So is reclaiming successful work lives and reaching career aspirations. As you'll soon see, maintaining successful family and work relationships has a lot to do with how you communicate and solve problems with others and educate them as they go through their inevitable ups and downs in reacting to your disorder.

"What Family Problems Might I Encounter after an Illness Episode?"

During your period of recovery, your close relatives are going to have confusing feelings about your illness and confusing thoughts about how to help you. In the following sections I explore the most common problems that may arise.

Negative Emotional Reactions from Your Relatives

Randy, a 45-year-old plumber, had two episodes of depression and several hypomanic episodes. His most recent episode, a depression, led to the loss of his job. His wife, Cindy, had a rudimentary understanding of bipolar disorder but was fairly intolerant of his apparent inability to function. She frequently spoke to him in derogatory psychiatric lingo: "That's your mania talking"; "Last night when we got into that argument, you were totally rapid cycling"; "You're doing your ADD [attention deficit disorder] thing again." In marital sessions, however, Cindy revealed that she really didn't believe his mood problems had a biological origin. She blamed them on his "crazy, dysfunctional family," his "temperamental nature," and "unconscious, unresolved stuff with me." She also wasn't convinced by the genetic evidence that Randy's father had had bipolar disorder.

Their debates about the causes of his behavior tended to degenerate into escalating interchanges in which Cindy would berate Randy and he would try to defend himself. He typically ended up agreeing with her, just to stop the argument, but then would feel resentful and withdraw to punish her. Annoyed at his withdrawal, she would continue her attack later with the accusation that "You've never been able to deal with things directly." He began to consider going off his medications just to prove "that I can deal with all of this without anyone or anything's help."

Why is Cindy so angry? Most of the family members I have worked with are well-intentioned, caring people who honestly want to do what's best for their relative with bipolar disorder. But they don't always know what to do when he or she reacts negatively to their attempts to help. They end up feeling frustrated and burdened by the effort required of them to adapt to the disorder and then often say and do things that are critical or unhelpful.

Your relatives' reactions to your disorder, particularly during the period when you are recovering, often reflect the same styles of coping or *causal attribution* that you used at various stages of adjusting to your illness (see Chapter 4): *underidentifying* with the disorder (attributing your behavior changes to your personality or habits) or *overidentifying* with it (attributing all or most of your behaviors, even normal ones, to your illness). Highly critical relatives are often underidentifying you with the disorder, as Cindy was doing. They may believe that your biologically based, illness-related changes in behavior—including any residual mood swings from your last episode that haven't cleared up yet—are really caused by your character or morals, your unconscious motivations, or your lack of effort. If a family member believes that these factors play a causal role, he or she will also believe that you have more control over your mood swings than you really do. Your relative may then become angry and critical.

Overprotectiveness

Alternatively, you may find that your relatives want to watch you very carefully and manage your disorder to the point where you feel you're being treated like a child (overprotectiveness or overinvolvement). Relatives who are overprotective often tend to overidentify you with the disorder or label your everyday reactions as signs of your illness. For example, they say that your illness is reflected in your getting angry about things you might very well have gotten angry about before you became ill. Sometimes you and they are both right—your anger may be stimulated by real things, but your disorder makes you react with a level of emotional intensity that is out of proportion to the circumstances. Nonetheless, you may begin to register that their labeling of your behavior is making you feel worse. Relatives may remind you repeatedly to take your medications, tell you to communicate with your doctor or therapist about minor problems you have at home or at work, or even go behind your back to talk with your physician.

You may even find, as some of my clients have found, that when you confront your relatives about their overprotectiveness they use your bipolar diagnosis as a weapon against you. For example, you might express annoyance at a relative for asking too many questions about your medications, only to have him or her tell you that your reaction is a sign of your illness. You can get into a vicious cycle in which you complain about their intrusiveness, your relatives react as if you are cycling into an episode, you get more annoyed with their labeling of you as mentally ill, their beliefs about your cycling become more confirmed, and then they become increasingly critical or overprotective.

Problems with Intimacy

Now let's consider a different kind of emotional reaction that often arises between spouses or romantic partners during the recovery period: a discomfort with physical intimacy in your partner's relationship with you. Your spouse's discomfort may not be associated with criticism or overprotectiveness; instead, you may experience him or her as emotionally withdrawn. Physical intimacy may have stopped altogether during, or shortly after, your last episode (as Martha experienced with her husband after her hospitalization), or it may have gradually diminished over time after multiple episodes.

It is quite common for relationships to be at a vulnerable point during the recovery period, even if the episode was only a minor one. Many spouses feel angry about events that occurred during the episode and don't feel comfortable being close.

If you are currently hypomanic, you may have an increased sex drive, but your spouse may have pulled away because of mistrust related to your disorder (for example, an increase in your irritability). The opposite can also occur: You may be depressed, and your spouse may want to reestablish physical contact, but you may feel under pressure, uncomfortable with your body, or bad about yourself as a sexual partner.

Effective solution: The first step in dealing effectively with family members after an episode is to educate them about your disorder. This is generally a good idea even if your family is functioning well, but it is especially important during your recovery period following an episode, when negative emotions are often at their peak.

If you've been well for some time, you may have an easier time negotiating intimacy with your partner. But even clients of mine who have remained well complain that basic issues of trust between them and their partners were violated by their earlier illness states and that emotional and physical intimacy has been hard to reestablish. If you are experiencing one or more of these problems, you are certainly not alone. Fortunately, these couple problems can be addressed using a number of relationship-rebuilding skills, outlined in the next few sections.

Tools for Improving Family Relationships after an Episode

Educating Your Family

Your relatives may harbor many misconceptions about the illness, its treatments, or what the future holds for all of you. This can happen even if they have interacted with your doctors, read any of the popular books on the subject, and listened to your explanations.

Flawed or incomplete information about bipolar disorder can cause your loved ones to be critical or overprotective of you. Make copies of the box on pages 285–286, which summarizes the basic facts about bipolar disorder, so that you have it available for all family members (whether or not they have been with you during episodes), including your adult or teenage children, parents, siblings, and other extended relatives.

It is important to have a common language when communicating with close relatives about your symptoms or changes in functioning. Hidden within the different terms your family members use in discussing your behavior are often subtle differences in beliefs about what causes you to behave in these ways. Acquainting your relatives with the facts about the disorder may make them think twice about what causes your mood swings. For example, your family members will be more supportive of you if they understand that increases in your irritability are a sign of the disorder's cycling rather than evidence that "you've gotten mean" or "you're more hostile than you used to be" or "you've got a temper problem." Likewise, they should come to understand that you are suffering from "depressed mood" or "fatigue" or "concentration problems" rather than "mental laziness" or "a pessimistic outlook on life."

Family members who know the basic facts about bipolar disorder will also be more supportive of your efforts to maintain consistency in your treatment. Well-meaning relatives who do not understand the disorder may view drug treatment or psychotherapy as crutches, or believe that you're being too watchful over your health and moods. They may give you direct or indirect messages about how they liked you better before you began your medicine or therapy. These messages may make you feel even more ambivalent than you already feel about your treatments. Your family needs to know why you are taking medications, attending psychotherapy, and engaging in self-management tasks like sleep–wake regulation.

Spend some time answering their questions after they have read the fact sheet. Depending on their age or education level, they may have trouble understanding how you have experienced certain symptoms, where in the family tree the illness may have originated, or why you are taking a certain combination of medications (for example, a mood stabilizer *and* an antidepressant). If you are sharing information about your disorder with your school-age children, try to see if you can simplify it to fit their developmental level. One man explained to his 6-year-old son, "You know how happy you get during your birthday parties? I get that way sometimes for a whole week, and then it gets hard for me to do my work." One woman explained to her 7-year-old, "You know how when you get excited, you can usually calm yourself down? When Daddy gets excited, he gets going really fast and he can't calm down right away." Another woman explained to her daughters that when she became sad she couldn't turn it off like they could. "You know how when you're upset and someone tells you a joke, you feel better? Mommy gets upset, but things like jokes won't get her over it right away—she needs more time." She also made it clear to them that they should not blame themselves when she became depressed or withdrawn.

Use age-appropriate terms when describing your disorder. Kids relate better to terms such as "happy," "excited," "amped," "wired," "sad," or "bummed" than to "manic" or "depressed." You may have to explain the disorder to them in several different ways and at different times, however. Following a lengthy discussion of the disorder, one parent reported hearing her 9-year-old son say to one of his friends, "My mother has a bipolar in her head!"

Helping Your Relatives Understand the Medical Bases of Your Disorder

It's important that your close relatives understand that at least a portion of your behavior is biologically and chemically determined. When they finally come to accept this, they will probably become less angry or hostile, as Rebecca did:

> "I had bought concert tickets and was looking forward to the event for weeks. The night we were supposed to go, my husband said he wasn't going to go, that he was too tired and depressed. I was enraged—it just seemed like something he should've known before. It felt like he was doing it to hurt me and disappoint me. I had really wanted us to do this together. I called to cancel the babysitter and the next day went to the ticket office for a refund, feeling like I was arguing from a position of weakness. To my surprise, I told them, 'My husband has a medical illness.' Somehow, that cut through my anger. It helped me do away with the feeling that he was doing something to hurt me. That was how I decided to explain it to myself and to the outside world."

Rebecca's realization that her husband skipped the concert not necessarily because he didn't want to go but because he could not go made her feel less resentful of the limitations his illness placed on their lives. Understand, however, that the frustration and dissatisfaction that such limitations cause will not evaporate over-

A Quick Fact Sheet on Bipolar Disorder for Family Members

What Is Bipolar Disorder?

Having bipolar disorder means that I may have severe mood swings, in which I go from very high and energized (manic) to very low, unmotivated, and lethargic (depressed). My high periods may last from a few days to a month or more. My low periods may last much longer, from several weeks to several months. About 1 in every 50 people in the United States has bipolar disorder. It most often affects a person for the first time in adolescence or young adulthood.

What Are the Symptoms?

My main symptoms during a high period may include feeling *overly happy* and excited or overly *irritable* and *angry.* I may also feel like I can do things that no one else can do (grandiosity). I may sleep less than usual or not at all, do many things at once, have more energy, talk faster and express many ideas (some realistic and some unrealistic), and be easily distracted. I may do things that are impulsive when manic, like spend a great deal of money unwisely or drive recklessly.

I may experience the symptoms of depression at other times, which can include feeling very sad, down, irritable, or anxious, losing interest in people or things, sleeping too much or being unable to sleep, having little or no appetite, having trouble concentrating or making decisions, feeling fatigued or low in energy, moving or talking slowly, feeling very bad or guilty about myself, or contemplating suicide or actually carrying out suicide attempts.

How Does Bipolar Disorder Affect the Family?

My bipolar disorder may affect my ability to relate to others in our family or in the work setting, especially when I become ill. Our family or relationship problems may be most apparent during or just after my episode of mania or depression, but then will probably improve as I get better. We can resolve our family conflicts through good communication and problem solving, emotional support for each other, and encouragement. We may want to get the additional help of a family or couple counselor or a family support group.

What Causes Bipolar Disorder?

Having bipolar disorder means that I have dysregulations in the emotional regulation "circuitry" of the brain, especially the amygdala and the prefrontal cortex. Nobody chooses

(cont.)

A Quick Fact Sheet on Bipolar Disorder for Family Members (*cont.*)

to become bipolar. It's possible that I inherited these imbalances from my blood relatives, although not necessarily from my parents. My mood swings may also be affected by life stress or sudden changes in my sleep–wake habits.

How Is Bipolar Disorder Treated?

My treatment will probably include mood-stabilizing medications such as lithium, divalproex (Depakote), or lamotrigine (Lamictal), or atypical antipsychotic medications like risperidone (Risperdal), quetiapine (Seroquel), aripiprazole (Abilify), ziprasidone (Geodon), or olanzapine (Zyprexa). I may also take antidepressant medications or drugs to control my anxiety or problems with thinking. These medications require that I see a psychiatrist regularly to make sure my side effects don't get out of hand and, for some medications, to get my blood levels tested. I may also benefit from individual therapy, family counseling sessions, or support groups. Therapy may help me to learn more about my disorder, learn to prevent relapses, monitor moods and sleep–wake cycles, and function better in the family and workplace. If I am one of the many people with bipolar disorder who have problems with drugs or alcohol, mutual support programs like Alcoholics Anonymous may also help me and our family.

What Does the Future Hold?

It is likely that I will have high and low mood episodes in the future. But there is every reason to be hopeful. With the help of a regular program of medication, therapy, and support from others, my mood disorder episodes can become less frequent, less extreme, and less disruptive. With help and support, I can accomplish many of my goals for my family and work life.

---

night. Family members need time and practice to come to grips with the changes in their lives. Consider the way that Evan's relationship with his father evolved:

> "For years, he didn't understand, and we could barely talk to each other. I'd shout and scream and spread my self-loathing all over him, and of course he'd get pissed off. Then I'd get depressed and even less able to deal with him. But after my second wife and I split and then I lost my job, I finally told him I had bipolar disorder, and we were really open about it. I just told him, 'Dad, this is one of the main reasons we've had so many problems between us.' I explained how it's a chemical thing and that it wasn't about how he raised me, and he

didn't believe me at first. But in another way it made sense to him—he's got a scientific mind and it put so many different things into place ... my temper, my job stuff, my problems when I was a teenager. When he came to accept it and we could talk about it, he was able to pull back and think about his own responses to me. And I've gotten a lot calmer and less reactive to him ... we get along much better now."

It's unlikely that your relatives will immediately adopt a medical view of your disorder—it took Evan's father quite some time. But with repeated exposure to educational information, your relatives may begin to reevaluate their belief that you are behaving out of ill will or negative intentions. This was the case for Gray, who, with his wife, Arlene, was getting marital therapy to help adapt to Arlene's bipolar disorder.

Arlene: When I get depressed, it's like a veil just comes over me. It's not at all like when you get tired after work. It's like being numb, like a ton of cement sitting on my heart.

Gray: I know, honey, but I just don't think the answer is to mope. You've gotta get out there and deal with things.

Therapist: Arlene, can you say more about what that depression is like, and what you think causes it?

Arlene: It's probably something chemical. It feels physical; it doesn't feel like lack of effort. I know how frustrated you get, Gray, but you have to realize it's not something I want either. If I could pull myself out, I would—in a minute.

Communication Skills for Reducing Criticism and Conflict

In the interchange between Arlene and Gray, Arlene made an effort to validate her husband's point of view. *Effective communication is a very important component of managing your family or marital relationships and can even help facilitate your recovery from your illness episode.* In one of our studies of family-focused therapy, one of the most consistent changes, over time, among patients whose bipolar disorder improved was an enhanced ability to communicate with their spouse or parents (Simoneau et al., 1999). The following is a selection of communication skills you can try out when dealing with criticism, tension, or conflict in your close relationships.

Although the skills look easy on the surface, they can be difficult to apply and require regular practice. Certainly, couples and families not affected by bipolar disorder have to practice regularly to make these communication skills work for them. Yet the stress of family life after an episode requires you to be even more skillful in your communication than you would ordinarily have to be. And when your mood is swinging up and down and you feel that your relatives are unfairly jumping on you, using new communication skills can be doubly hard. These skills require that you step back when you feel the heat rising and put yourself in another person's place. As with many self-management strategies, familiarizing yourself with these skills when you are well makes them easier to use when you are ill.

Skill No. 1: Active Listening

After dealing with an episode of bipolar disorder or any other kind of significant stressor, you will have trouble listening to the feelings, objections, or troubles of other family members. This difficulty is quite understandable. But if your family members don't feel that you or others in the family care enough to listen, they will probably be unwilling to perform some of the other tasks that are essential to your recovery (for example, keeping the home environment low key). So, if your parents, spouse, or kids are responding to you negatively or with criticism, consider helping them modulate their anger by listening and expressing an understanding of their position, even if you do not agree with it. This is a technique called active listening, and attempts to use it will almost certainly change the outcome of what would otherwise be unproductive interchanges. The box on this page lists the steps.

In active listening, you become less active in the speaking part of communication than you might be used to, and you become more active on the listening end. You don't just sit there and hear. You maintain eye contact with the person speaking to you, offer nonverbal acknowledgments like a nod of the head, paraphrase or otherwise check out what you've heard (otherwise known as *reflective listening*), and ask questions designed to get the speaker to clarify his or her point of view. This is a good skill to use whenever you talk with your family members, but it will be especially helpful when arguments start to escalate. There is nothing like validating someone else's point of view in the middle of an argument to reduce his or her anger—it's hard to be mad at someone who is making a genuine attempt to understand you.

Active listening requires that you avoid any implication of blaming the other person. That is, stay away from any reflective statements or questions that imply the other person is at fault for his or her reactions or that involve name-calling. For example, the statement "So you feel that if you're mean to me, I'll change for the better" is not really a reflective statement but more of an accusation. The question "Why would you want to be a nag if you are trying to get me to do something on my own?" may feel like a reasonable question, but it will not help resolve the disagreement. It's hard to avoid saying things like that when you're angry or irritable. But if you stay at the level of asking simple, straightforward questions and paraphrasing exactly what you have heard from your relative (even word for word, if necessary), you will be less likely to say something to cause him or her to take offense.

Steps of Active Listening

■ Look at the speaker.

■ Attend to what is said.

■ Nod your head or say "uh-huh."

■ Ask clarifying questions.

■ Check out what you heard (paraphrase).

Adapted by permission from Miklowitz (2008b). Copyright by The Guilford Press.

Consider the following interchange between Randy and Cindy. Randy is practicing the skill of active listening.

Randy: You were pretty mad at me this morning. What was up? [clarifying question]

Cindy: I tried to get you to talk about that tax-related thing, and you just blew me off. Why do I keep trying?

Randy: (*pausing*) So you were frustrated with me. You wanted me to get it done. [paraphrasing]

Cindy: (*still irritated*) Yes, of course I did! And I had asked you a million times.

Randy: (*Nods.*) Yes, I understand how that would be frustrating. But partly it's because I'm having a tough time. Were you concerned that I wouldn't get it done? [clarifying question]

Cindy: (*Softens.*) Maybe I came down too hard on you, but the question is, when are we gonna do it? The 15th is coming up pretty quick.

Randy's reflective listening and validation of Cindy's point of view helped reduce her irritation and the antagonism that had built up between them. Ideally, this discussion would then merge into problem solving, another skill that will help you negotiate a more productive relationship with your spouse or parent (explained later in this section). But active listening doesn't always have its intended effect, as is discussed in the troubleshooting tips also later in this section.

Skill No. 2: Positive Requests for Change

Another way to reduce tension and avoid the verbal attacks that can turn into full-scale war is to phrase your comments to family members as *positive requests for change* (Falloon et al., 1984). This involves stating, *specifically and diplomatically,* what you'd like to see happen differently in your interactions with your relative. Criticisms tell people what they have done wrong—"I resent that you always bring up my illness when my friends are around"—and naturally generate defensiveness. Stating the same thought in a positive way—"It's very important to me that when we're with our friends we talk about things of importance to us other than my illness"—is almost certain to reduce any defensiveness, even though it's not guaranteed to prevent it altogether. If you're not entirely sure of the difference between the two, note that positive requests usually ask someone to do something new and positive, whereas criticisms usually involve telling someone to stop doing something.

After being hospitalized for a mixed episode of her bipolar disorder, Carol returned to her apartment, only to discover that her father, Roy, was constantly coming over unannounced, and then criticizing her for how messy she kept her living room. This surveillance was a particularly sensitive issue for Carol, who felt strongly that her autonomy and independence were important to her recovery. Roy, however, had become hypervigilant and worried that she would descend into another illness episode. He felt that his concerns were justified by the fact that she'd had several recent mood episodes.

Carol began saying things like "Just don't come over here anymore" or "Why don't you leave me alone?" to which her father responded, "I do it because I don't think you can take care of yourself." During family-focused treatment sessions, her therapist encouraged her to try transforming her criticisms into positive requests for change. At first she had trouble with this communication tool, saying things like "Dad, could you leave me alone more? That'd make my life much better." With coaching, she was able to word her request more diplomatically, and her father responded more positively as a result:

Carol: Dad, will you please call me before you're going to come over? That'd give me the chance to clean up first.

Therapist: Good, Carol. And how would that make you feel?

Carol: I'd like it, and I'd probably feel grateful that you cared about me and what I need. It'd also be nice to see you.

Therapist: That was excellent. Roy, what did you think about what Carol just said?

Roy: Much better, easier to hear. And I might even do it? (*Laughs.*) [From Miklowitz (2008b)]

Your family members are often doing their best to try to help you. They may benefit from knowing, in a constructive way, what they can do differently. Making positive requests in this way may feel artificial at first, but it will help you make your needs known without alienating your relatives.

Making a Positive Request

■ Look at your family member.

■ Say exactly what you would like him or her to do.

■ Tell him or her how it would make you feel.

■ Use phrases such as:

"I would like you to ____."

"I would really appreciate it if you would ____."

"It's very important to me that you help me with the ____."

Adapted by permission from Miklowitz (2008b). Copyright by The Guilford Press.

Skill No. 3: Problem Solving to Defuse Family Conflicts

Some of the arguments you have with your family members can be reduced to a specific problem that can be solved. As you know, bipolar disorder sometimes generates practical problems that need to be addressed as a family or couple, particularly in the aftermath of an illness episode. These can include financial problems, difficulties related to resuming your work or family roles (for example, child rearing), problems related to your treatments or medications, or relationship and living situation conflicts. Often, these unresolved but relatively specific problems fuel your relatives' expressions of criticism or resentment. The more you can help direct conversations with your family members toward identifying and solving specific problems, the less tension there will be during your recovery period.

The steps in the Problem-Solving Worksheet on pages 292–293 provide a structure for resolving your disagreements. Let's imagine, for example, that you got into an argument with your spouse about the lack of intimacy in your relationship since your last episode of bipolar disorder. You might find yourself getting increasingly irritated, especially if you were unclear about what your spouse wanted. First, discuss the definition of this problem (Step 1) with your spouse: Can the broad issue of intimacy be redefined as a more specific problem (for example, lack of time spent together away from the kids)? Try to get him or her to slow down and help you define what the disagreement is about. Use your listening skills to help your spouse define what is really bothering him or her.

Next, encourage your spouse or other family members to suggest as many solutions as possible to the problem you've defined (Step 2). Let's imagine you've defined it as lack of time spent together. Potential solutions could include cordoning off an

Problem–Solving Worksheet

Step 1: Define "What is the problem?" Talk and listen, ask questions, and get everybody's opinion.

_____

_____

_____

Step 2: List all possible solutions, even ones that don't seem feasible. Do not evaluate the pros or cons of any solution yet.

1. _____

2. _____

3. _____

4. _____

5. _____.

Step 3: Discuss and list the advantages and disadvantages of each possible solution.

Advantages   _Disadvantages_

1. _____   _____

2. _____   _____

3. _____   _____

4. _____   _____

5. _____   _____

Step 4: Choose the best possible solution or solutions, and list. Include combinations of possible solutions.

_____

_____

Step 5: Plan how to carry out the chosen solutions, and set a date to implement them.

Date _____

List who will do what.

_____

_____

(cont.)

List what resources you'll need (for example, money, a babysitter, access to a car, reservations).

_____

_____

Step 6: Implement the chosen solution and praise each other's efforts.

Step 7: After you've implemented the solution, go back to Step 1 and decide whether the problem was solved. If not, try to redefine the problem and come up with solutions that will work better.

hour or more of your time during the evening when the kids are not allowed to disturb you, arranging a weekly night out together, exercising together once or twice a week, or having one meal at home each week without the kids present. When generating solutions, be careful not to evaluate whether they are good or bad ideas just yet. It's important to get all of the ideas out on the table first.

In Step 3, weigh the advantages and disadvantages of each proposed solution. For example, a weekly night out together has the advantage of being fun and pleasurable; its disadvantages might include its costs, or feeling too tired at the end of the day to enjoy it. Then try to choose one solution or a combination of solutions based on your mutual discussion of the pros and cons of each possibility (Step 4). For example, you may agree that going out once a week is too costly but that a meal at home together, while the kids are at a babysitter's house, achieves the same objective (bringing the two of you closer) without the cost.

In Step 5, think about the tasks involved in making the solution work. In this example, you'll need to choose a night to have dinner together, buy food to cook, and arrange a babysitter. You will find it easier to implement the solution—and the result will probably be more satisfying—if you divide up the tasks such that you do some of them and your spouse does some of them.

In Step 6, try implementing your solutions and see if the original problem has been addressed. Problem solving does not guarantee that you'll come up with a solution that will work. Nonetheless, give some encouragement or praise to your spouse for his or her willingness to work with you, even if you don't feel the problem is solved yet. For example, say, "I'm really glad you're working with me to solve this. It makes me feel good that you care." Your relatives need to know when they are doing things right, and it's important to tell them so as often as possible.

You may go through a problem-solving exercise only to discover that the original problem was not defined adequately in the first place. For example, the problem might be the lack of personal, intimate conversations between you and your spouse rather than simply not having enough time away from the kids. If so, try redefining the problem and going through the solution steps again (Step 7). You may be more successful the second time around.

Some families or couples find it useful to select a weekly time to sit down and solve problems that have cropped up during the week. Often, they deal with problems such as household chores, managing finances, or planning social events. The structure that a regular meeting provides helps assure that certain nagging disagreements, even if trivial, get resolved.

Communicating and Problem Solving with Relatives Who Are Overprotective

"Bipolar illness is so taxing emotionally to the family, and most families don't have the skills for knowing how to deal with it. We feel overwhelmed and our skills are exceeded, and we can't get answers from the mental health system. All the while we see our loved one in pain. Who wouldn't get overprotective under those circumstances?"

—A 34-year-old son who takes care of his bipolar mother during her manic and depressive episodes

Communication and problem solving can also help you negotiate the difficulties that arise when your relatives start to overmonitor your behavior. Your first task is to try to understand the source of their responses. If you've been ill recently, your relative is probably very concerned that you'll become ill again. He or she may fear that you will kill yourself, hurt someone, impulsively leave the family, spend a lot of money, or otherwise damage yourself or others. This anxiety can result in a desire to control things, which often leads to overprotective behavior.

Use active listening as you gently encourage your relatives to recognize and verbalize their fears about your future, if they haven't made these clear to you already. Reassure them that you'll work hard to manage your disorder on your own. For example, you might say, "I know you're afraid I'm going to become ill again and that things will be hard for our family [validating their feelings]. I am taking care of myself, though, and the best way you can help me is to let me do as much as I can on my own." They may be relieved to hear you say this. You may also be able to use your positive request skills to set appropriate boundaries with them, as Carol did with her father.

In addition, consider the role of problem solving when dealing with relatives who overmonitor your behavior. Can you develop agreements with them in which you do something to allay their anxiety, and they, in turn, agree not to watch you so closely? Bart, 18, was being constantly reminded by his mother, Greta, to take his medication and get his blood level checked. He got his revenge in a rather unproductive way: leaving lithium tablets around the house for her to find (for example, on the kitchen floor, behind the toilet, under her pillow). Greta then became more annoyed and anxious and increased her monitoring of his behavior. Bart said that he was willing to take his medication and even have his blood level checked, but not if it meant that his mother "follows me around with pills in her hand." Understandably, he wanted to feel like taking medication was his own decision. Greta expressed doubt that he would take medication without her vigilance. She complained, "How can I know if he's taking it if I don't ask?"

Through problem solving, Bart and his mother generated a list of possible scenarios: Bart taking full responsibility for his medication; Greta taking all the responsibility; Greta reminding him only once per day; Greta having more phone contact with his physician. Eventually they agreed that Greta would place Bart's four daily lithium tablets on a plate for him in the morning. He was to agree to take them during the day, and she was to agree not to mention his medication unless she found pills on the plate or lying around the house by the day's end. They also agreed that she could see his lithium level report at the end of each month. This agreement worked well for both of them.

What if it is your spouse who is behaving in an overprotective way? Some of my clients say that their spouses feel less anxious if they are allowed to attend the drug monitoring visits with the psychiatrist. There are some advantages to doing this: Your spouse will feel more secure if he or she has input into your care and has a connection with your physician (which can be helpful in emergencies). Your spouse may also remember certain of the physician's recommendations that have slipped your mind (and likewise, you may recall things that your spouse has forgotten). If you decide to go this route, you may want to establish some agreements ahead of time about what role you want your spouse to play in these medication visits. For example, you might say, "I want to invite you to my next medication session, but I need to do most of the talking about my state and what the medication is doing. You can chime in, but it's really me who has to describe my own experiences." Your spouse may feel less of a need to closely monitor your behavior if his or her opinions are regularly incorporated into your treatment plan.

Troubleshooting Your Use of Communication and Problem-Solving Skills

Putting communication and problem-solving skills into practice during your postepisode recovery period presents some challenges. As I mentioned previously, even the healthiest of families can have trouble communicating clearly and efficiently. But when you are also dealing with dysregulations in your mood and thought processes, it can be even harder to step back and phrase your statements to your relatives in the ways that I've outlined, or to take a step-by-step approach to problem solving. You will probably feel easily provoked and impatient. As a result you may quickly abandon the skills when in conflict with relatives, which will then keep the negative cycles going.

There are several things you can do to address problems in implementing these skills. First, try to flag those instances when you are getting too upset to listen effectively or solve problems, and then diplomatically exit the situation. Consider the scenario in which your relative is being critical and accusatory and the thought "this is so unfair" keeps going through your mind. *If you feel the heat rising and can tell that the conversation is going in a negative direction, ask for a "time-out."* For example, you might say, "I don't think I can discuss this right now. Let's talk later when we're both calmed down." A time-out gives you breathing room so that you can think about what you do and don't want to say to your parent, spouse, or sibling. It also enables you to examine what is happening that is making you so upset. You may want to resolve the disagreement with your relative later or perhaps just drop it, if it doesn't seem worth the cost of another argument. There may be a period after the time-out when things are awkward and icy in your household, but this probably would have occurred anyway if you had let the argument continue along its destructive path.

Here's another difficulty you might experience: You know the steps of a skill (for example, making a positive request) but then forget them as soon as an argument starts. It is hard to remember to draw on communication skills when you are angry and in the midst of a conflict with someone who is angry at you. When you recall the conversation later on, you may think of a number of things you could have said to help defuse the argument.

Effective parenting solutions: If you have children, you will probably find that their behavior often provokes you and leads you to outbursts of rage, which get worse if your mood is already unstable. Some children think that getting their parent upset is like winning a game! If your child is getting under your skin, and there is no second parent or grandparent who can step in, consider the following:

- Use *problem-solving strategies* early in the argument; get your child thinking about options other than immediately getting what he or she wants.
- Use the "three-volley" rule: when you have expressed your point of view and been rebuffed three times, your part of the conversation has ended.
- *Exit the situation* when you feel yourself getting angry (for example, your face getting hotter, your breathing shallower, your heart racing); agree with yourself that you don't need to "win" the confrontation to prove your authority.
- Spend some time apart until he or she and you calm down; use *self-relaxation* or *mindfulness breathing exercises* during the interval.
- *Revisit the issue with your child later,* when you feel more in control of your emotions.

If this difficulty sounds familiar, practice using the skills first with people outside the family who don't provoke you and with whom you're generally comfortable. For example, make a positive request of a coworker ("I'd really appreciate it if you could cover for me next weekend so that I can take some time off"), or try paraphrasing the statements of a friend who has described to you a problem he or she is having (for example, "Sounds like you're going through a rough time").

> **Effective solution:** You may find that by practicing a skill in nonthreatening circumstances, it becomes easier to remember to apply it when the stakes are higher.

Now consider the scenario in which you are doing your best with the communication tools but there seems to be little impact on your relationship. You may feel annoyed that you are the only one who is trying to communicate or solve problems effectively, whereas others seem to keep doing whatever they've been doing. For example, you may be quite diplomatic in asking your close relatives to change their behavior, yet the way they ask you to do the same continues to sound challenging and demeaning. Of course, if you were to ask your family members for their view of this problem, they might say that they try to be diplomatic but that you get very defensive in return.

If you find yourself in this stalemate, consider the long-term benefits of "unilateral change." In other words, try to change your own behavior in relation to your relatives first, with the expectation that, with time, they will change their behavior toward you. In other words, keep trying! Your repeated attempts at problem solving or diplomacy (for example, continuing to validate other people's emotions even when they refuse to do so for you) will eventually have an impact on their responses, especially if you are able to stick with the formats outlined for active listening and making positive requests for change. Of course, this requires a high tolerance for frustration, but there is potentially a high payoff as well.

To increase the chances that your relatives will improve their way of communicating with you, be sure to praise them for even minor attempts on their part (for example, "Thanks for asking me if I was upset after our conversation. I'm glad you noticed that it bothered me"). The chances are high that, over repeated discussions with your relatives, they will do or say something helpful or that shows an awareness of your viewpoint. Be ready to acknowledge their attempts to make things better, even if these attempts seem overshadowed by everything else they did that made you feel worse.

You may feel that the communication or problem-solving strategies outlined here are artificial or superficial. If you are still hypomanic or energized, it may feel stifling to talk in this very measured, careful way. What hap-

> **Effective solution:** The cardinal rule of behavior modification is that people increase the frequency of those behaviors that get rewarded by others.

pened to the exciting, spontaneous interchanges you used to have with your partner or your siblings? Remember that you are trying to improve life during a specific interval—your recovery period. This period requires that you be extra efficient in your communication and problem-solving styles, above and beyond what is required of others who do not have to cope with bipolar disorder. Think of incorporating these skills as trying on a new pair of shoes. At first they won't fit or feel comfortable. If they're still uncomfortable after you've worn them for a while, you may decide you don't like them and take them off. But they have the potential to work well for you if you break them in. Practicing the skills repeatedly will eventually make them feel like second nature and will probably lead to changes in the way that your family members respond to you. As you recover and your family relationships improve, you may be able to return to more spontaneous ways of communicating or making your needs known.

Reestablishing Physical Intimacy with Your Partner after an Episode

In the previous section, you saw an example of problem solving as related to emotional intimacy in a couple's relationship. As for physical intimacy, you and your partner will probably need some time to get reacquainted with each other after an episode. If you both would like to reinitiate a physical relationship, consider getting the help of a couple counselor who specializes in sex therapy. Traditional sex therapists encourage couples to take part in *sensate focus* exercises that they do together at home.

After Mara's bipolar mixed episode, she and her husband, Kevin, abandoned their sex life, deciding that "our primary goal as a couple is Mara's recovery." In their marital sessions, they both recognized that sex had become frightening to them and that the illness had become an excuse for not dealing directly with each other. Once they agreed that they wanted to reestablish a romantic life, their counselor encouraged them to take small steps, in between sessions, toward greater intimacy. They started by going out together on an evening date one week, giving each other back rubs the following week, hugging and kissing the next, taking a bath together the next, and gradually working back up to a sexual relationship. This relaxed, step-by-step approach was very important for Mara and Kevin in regaining the trust and intimacy they had shared prior to her episode.

You may feel that the guidance of a couple therapist is not necessary. But many couples do have significant anxiety concerning sex. If so, a therapist can teach you relaxation and desensitization techniques (like those above) to practice with your spouse between sessions.

The most important point to remember is that anxiety or discomfort about being close is a natural part of coping as a couple with bipolar disorder, particularly during the recovery period. Many couples can overcome this discomfort by moving slowly, not expecting too much from each other at first, and being willing to try again if their first attempts at sexual intimacy are not as satisfying as they had hoped.

Bipolar Disorder and the Work Setting

Louise, a 35-year-old woman with bipolar I disorder, had a manic episode that led to a short (5-day) hospitalization. Prior to the development of her episode, she had worked as a paralegal in a law firm. The trigger for her hospitalization appeared to have been a legal case. The firm had insisted that she work late at night for several weeks to help prepare the attorneys' arguments for the case.

Her illness episode kept her out of work for almost a month. When she had mostly recovered, she returned to her job. She decided not to tell her employers that she had been in the hospital and instead explained that she had had an unnamed physical illness, and did not elaborate further. But she became physically uncomfortable, easily fatigued, and irritable after her second week on the job when her employers started to increase her work load again. They expected her to work late shifts one night and early morning shifts the next. She found that she couldn't function mentally at work the morning after a night shift. Even worse, they assigned her a new task upon arriving at work in the morning: calling clients who were delinquent on their bills or who hadn't responded to letters. She summarized her experience this way:

> "It was a bad idea for me to do something like that first thing in the morning. It made it hard for me to even get up to go to this job. My body was slow, my mind was slow. It took me a long time to come out of my haze. If I got to work at 9, I had to be up by 6 just to get my mind rolling. I felt rushed, irritable, then depressed. My boss got controlling and started criticizing my work. ... I got stressed out and anxious, and then I would try to calm down and couldn't. I tried to make myself busy, but then I felt even more lethargic and couldn't get the job done."

Louise was on the verge of quitting her job when she decided to have an open conversation about her bipolar disorder with one of the partners in the law firm, a woman who, she felt, had been on her side. Louise apologized for her irritability and explained that she needed more consistent work hours, adding that the unpleasant tasks she had been assigned in the morning were better off assigned to the afternoon. The law partner was unwilling to compromise on the amount of work assigned to Louise or the quality she expected. But given that Louise was a valued employee, the partner did compromise on some other issues: limiting the number of late nights she would have to work, allowing her to do some of her work at home, and deferring the unpleasant tasks until later in the day. These adjustments made a big difference to Louise. She eventually decided to cut to a half-time work week, which was much better for her from the standpoint of mood stability and health.

If you have bipolar disorder, you can still be successful in your chosen career. A survey done by the Center for Psychiatric Rehabilitation at Boston University discovered that out of 500 professionals and managers (including nurses, newspaper reporters, corporate executives, lawyers, and professors), previously diagnosed with a serious psychiatric illness, 73% were able to maintain full-time employment in their chosen occupations (Ellison et al., 2008). Of the respondents to the survey, 62% had worked in their position for more than 2 years, and 69% had increased their levels of responsibility in their jobs. Most (84%) were taking some kind of psychiatric medication, and two-thirds had been hospitalized three or more times.

Above all, many respondents said that getting back to their jobs was important to their recovery. Nonetheless, as the story of Louise illustrates, people with bipolar disorder face significant challenges in the workplace. Some of these challenges arise from the stigma of bipolar disorder and the reactions of others. But for most of my clients, the bigger challenge is finding a job that is satisfying but also helps keep them from mood cycling. It is difficult to balance severely fluctuating moods with a stable work life, as Louise found. Jobs that permit this balance are hard to find, but they do exist or can be created.

Maintaining a stable mood is essential to functioning well at your job. This is, of course, another reason to stay consistent with your medication regimen. But it is equally true that working within a supportive environment is important to maintaining your mood stability. The key is finding the right balance of stability in work hours, levels of stress, levels of stimulation, and satisfaction with the directions in which your job is taking you. I am optimistic that you can find this balance. In this section, I discuss some self-care strategies to help you get back into the working world after an episode.

"How Will Bipolar Disorder Affect My Job Performance?"

"I was hypomanic all last weekend, really pushing the envelope. Me and the guys were up partying and drinking until 3 in the morning both Friday and Saturday nights, and then I slept until 11 the next day, even though I knew it was a bad idea because I had to get up at 6 for work on Monday. I forgot to take my medications on Sunday morning, and I didn't sleep that well Sunday night. By Monday I was tired, grouchy, withdrawn, snappy with my boss, and just really wasn't all that efficient. My boss reacted, mentioned that I seemed like I was in a bad mood, hinted that maybe in those circumstances I should just take the day off. He didn't know about my bipolar disorder. I could just feel the old 'authority figure' stuff coming up again, but I also recognized I was having a depression hangover of sorts. I took it easy after work Monday afternoon, did some low-stress stuff like talking on the phone and going for a run, had dinner and went to bed at the usual time. I slept fine and was back in the swing of things by Tuesday. I apologized to my boss and everything was OK

after that, but I realized that, at some point, I might have to tell him about my problems."

—A 27-year-old man with bipolar II disorder

As is true for most people, your mood state will influence your day-to-day job performance. This man's cycle of sleep deprivation, alcohol use, and overstimulation followed by irritability, lethargy, and depression could have described almost anyone. The difference is that this cycle is magnified in bipolar disorder, and the intensity of your resulting mood can affect your work performance more than would be the case for the average person.

How are bipolar symptoms expressed in the work setting? Manic or hypomanic reactions can take the form of flying off the handle at things that normally wouldn't annoy you or being preoccupied by so many ideas that concentrating on your job becomes difficult. You may start more projects than you can possibly complete, darting from task to task without accomplishing what you originally set out to do (multitasking). During hypomanic intervals, you may be particularly prone to arguments with irritating coworkers or confrontations with your boss (a client said, "I usually just *think* my coworkers are idiots. When I'm manic, I also *tell* them so").

When you're in a depressed phase, your physical state resembles a severe case of the flu. At these times you will not be able to expect as much from yourself, nor will others. Your thinking and physical responsiveness (for example, your typing speed) may be slower. You may also suffer from considerable anxiety, which can interfere with your concentration. As always, you can use your mood chart to anticipate when you are entering one of these phases of mood disorder.

On the other side, some people report that their bipolar disorder enhances their job performance. Many persons with bipolar disorder work in high-level business or government positions and are known for their high work output (see the sidebar on this page). They report that when they have a major writing project to do, an oral presentation, or an important sales meeting, they use the "adrenaline rush" of hypomania to their advantage. You'll recall from Chapter 7 the link between mania and creativity or productivity.

New research: A group of economists at Oregon State University found that people with bipolar disorder were more likely than people without bipolar disorder to be employed in creative occupations, such as artist, musician, or writer (Tremblay et al., 2010).

In my experience, people with bipolar disorder benefit from hypomania in the work setting only if they can harness it. Harnessing hypomania includes learning to recognize when you are moving or speaking too fast, setting limits on yourself when work starts to make you overly goal driven, trying to accomplish only one task at a time, accepting feedback from others about how you are coming across, and backing off when people seem to be reacting to your intensity. It may indeed be possible to translate your increased energy into work productivity, but also be aware of when you need to slow down and take a break.

Self-Disclosure in the Workplace: "Should I Tell People about My Illness?"

Can bipolar disorder be kept a secret? In my experience and that of many of my colleagues, people with bipolar disorder usually adopt one of four solutions regarding disclosure:

1. They tell everybody about it, including their boss and coworkers.
2. They tell one or more trusted coworkers who do not carry positions of authority over them.
3. They do not tell anybody, but do admit to bipolar disorder on their work-sponsored health insurance claims (leaving open the possibility that their employer could find out).
4. They do not tell anyone at work, and they do not use their work-sponsored insurance to cover their psychiatric costs.

There is no single solution that is right for everybody. Let me go through the pros and cons of telling employers or coworkers about your disorder, to help you decide which option seems best for you in your current or future work environment.

What Are the Disadvantages of Disclosing?: The Risk of Job Discrimination

If you are currently employed, the most obvious disadvantage of disclosing your disorder is that you may get fired or demoted or denied a promotion or a raise. Likewise, telling a prospective employer about your disorder introduces the possibility that he or she will decide against hiring you, without telling you why.

Some people with bipolar disorder, including some of my clients, have reported job discrimination. It is unclear how often this occurs. In a study by Nicholas Glozier (1998) of the Institute of Psychiatry in London, 80 British personnel directors were asked to evaluate two hypothetical job candidates who, based on a written profile, were described in an identical manner (for example, as having a good prior work record). One was described as having had a diagnosis of depression and the other as having diabetes. Personnel directors were less likely to hire the applicant with depression and more likely to believe that his or her performance in an executive job would be impaired relative to a person with diabetes. In other words, we have a long way to go in educating employers about depression and bipolar disorders, their similarity to other medical disorders, and how they will, and will not, affect job performance. It is not clear whether an unwillingness to hire a hypothetical candidate translates into discrimination once a real person with depression or bipolar disorder is hired.

If you are fired or are not hired because of your bipolar disorder, the law is on your side. *In the United States, under the Americans with Disabilities Act (Department of Justice, 2009;* www.ada.gov/pubs/ada.htm*), it is unlawful to discriminate against a "qualified individual with a disability," meaning a person who, "with or without reasonable accommodation, can perform the essential functions of the employment position that such individual holds or desires" (p. 9).* Bipolar disorder does qualify as a disability, which is defined as "a physical or mental impairment that substantially limits one or more of the major life activities of such individual" (p. 7). Discrimination refers to prejudicial behavior on the employer's part in job application procedures, hiring practices, promotion or discharge, pay, or training. You cannot legally be denied an equal job for equal pay, be segregated from others, or classified such that your opportunities for advancement are limited (for example, demoted to working in the mail room) because of your disorder.

If you are qualified for a job, "reasonable accommodations" can be required of the employer. For a person with bipolar disorder these may include modified work schedules (for example, consistent work shifts), job reassignments to positions more suitable to your stress tolerance level, or restructuring your work environment to avoid overstimulation (see examples in the following case and in the box on pages 308–309). Of course, the employer has to know about your disorder to make reasonable accommodations. Your employer cannot legally fire you or refuse to hire you because you need a reasonable accommodation, unless he or she can prove that such an accommodation would prove an undue hardship for the business (for example, place the firm deeply in debt, require moving to another facility).

Consider the experience of Janine, a 37-year-old woman who worked at an advertising firm.

> Janine was a valued employee of her firm because of her high productivity. She said that she had always been somewhat hypomanic by nature and that this hypomania had served her well in her high-demand workplace. Her first major bipolar episode was a depression with symptoms of paranoia that developed gradually and significantly interfered with her work productivity. She took a leave of absence but didn't know at the time that she had bipolar disorder. Following successful medical treatment with mood stabilizers and an antipsychotic agent, she wrote a letter to her firm explaining what had happened. Upon learning of her disorder, her employer dismissed her. She consulted an attorney and challenged this move on legal grounds. After several back-and-forth legal communications, she was invited back to work at the firm, but was told she could do so only if she found a job in a different department. She did find a job within the same firm but was unhappy there and eventually decided to leave. She is now working in another firm that is more sympathetic to her needs.

Proving that job discrimination occurred can be difficult. If you think you are being discriminated against because of the disclosure of your disorder (whether it was you or someone else who made the disclosure), I would advise you to consult an attorney and the Equal Employment Opportunities Commission. They can help you determine if a legal action should be taken against your current or former employer.

Janine could have continued to pursue her legal case but decided that she did not want to work in a firm that held these attitudes toward her. Deciding whether or not to pursue a legal case is very much a personal and often a family decision. Consider its potential impact on your mood stability as well as the likely outcome of the case (for example, being reinstated in your old position, which you may no longer want or feel comfortable in). Be prepared for a long period of frustrations and high economic costs before your case is resolved. Nonetheless, after weighing all of the relevant factors you may well decide that pursuing your case is worth it.

"Can My Employer Ask Whether I Have Bipolar Disorder?"

The Americans with Disabilities Act makes it clear that employers are not to ask direct questions about your disability or require their own psychiatric examination for a job application or during the course of your employment, "unless such examination or inquiry is shown to be job-related and consistent with business necessity" (p. 7). They can require a medical examination after a job offer has been made, if one is required of all new employees, or as part of an employee health program. An example would be a physical exam required for all new personnel at a nursing home.

Your employer would have to prove that inquiring about your mental health status is essential to knowing whether you can perform your job duties or whether you would endanger others. In most cases, having bipolar disorder does not mean that others are at risk, unless you have a documented history of violence or also have an alcohol or drug abuse problem. These associated problems could jeopardize the safety of others (for example, if you work at a child care facility, operate heavy machinery, or drive a vehicle).

If the business to which you're applying does require a medical exam, it has to collect this information in a form that can be treated as a confidential medical record, meaning that you would have to give a signed release of information before your records were sent to anyone. However, the doctor or nurse who examines you can inform a supervisor or manager of work accommodations required by your disorder, as revealed in the medical exam. Likewise, if your firm has safety or first-aid personnel, they may be informed that your bipolar disorder could require emergency treatment. These disclosures may or may not occur in your work setting and, in any case, cannot legally be used to discriminate against you.

What should you do if your current or potential employer asks about your psychiatric history, either directly or on a job application? You can say that you don't wish to answer the question (or leave the question blank) or point out that the question is inappropriate (Court & Nelson, 1996). If your employer presses you, you don't have to lie about having the disorder. Just say you'd rather not discuss this matter or that you want to get a consultation before you discuss it.

A potential employer can refuse to hire you upon learning of your disorder, but only if he or she can prove that the disorder will interfere with your job functions and that no reasonable accommodations can be made. In most cases, he or she will have a tough time proving these points just because you have bipolar disorder. Of course, you would need to initiate legal action against your prospective employer to make your case.

Disadvantages of Disclosure: Dealing with Stigma at Work

If your coworkers learn that you have a mood disorder, you may experience a feeling of stigma—the sense that your behavior is being viewed negatively in light of your illness. Usually this stigma will be most salient to you right after a major bout of mania or depression, in part because you will still be depressed or hypomanic and possibly more attuned to the reactions of others. But even people whose bipolar disorder has been stable can feel stigmatized at work. For example, imagine that your illness is "leaked" by a fellow coworker who tells others in the office. Julie, age 55, became quite angry with a coworker one day, and the coworker left the office crying. Julie had earlier disclosed her illness to a woman in the office whom she considered to be a close friend. After the incident this friend told others in the office about Julie's illness, as a way of explaining why Julie had responded so seemingly irrationally. After that, Julie felt that others viewed her with apprehension.

The stigma you experience at work may feel similar to the stigma you experience in your family. For example, coworkers may interpret problems in your work as stemming from your illness, even when you can point to other employees who have the same problems (for example, being late with assignments, reacting irritably to a disorganized or harsh boss). You may also find that your coworkers become distant or overly cautious in their interactions with you. Coworkers may even react by doting on you or becoming overly solicitous (for example, frequently asking if you want to talk about your problems, repeatedly reminding you that "I'm there for you"). All of these responses can feel unhelpful. To be fair, coworkers, like family members, are often struggling to figure out how best to respond to your disorder.

On a more hopeful note, mood disorders carry less of a stigma than they used to. Because of the bravery of many public figures who have talked openly about their experiences of bipolar disorder or unipolar depression (for example, Kay Jamison, Carrie Fisher, Patty Duke, Jane Pauley, Margot Kidder, Mike Wallace, William Styron), and because of events such as the National Depression Screening Day, the public has an increased awareness and a greater acceptance of mood disorders. As a result, you may get more understanding from others than you expected.

What Are the Advantages of Disclosing?

There are arguments in favor of being open about your disorder as well. First, disclosing can be destigmatizing and increase your own acceptance of the illness. You may feel that bipolar disorder is not so shameful if you tell a coworker and he or she does not have a strong negative reaction. Upon learning of your disorder, a coworker may admit to having experienced depression or having a family member or friend who has bipolar disorder. Some of my clients have chosen one trusted person at work to tell about the disorder. Sharing this kind of personal information helps to increase mutual trust and can create an atmosphere of support within the work setting. But deciding to whom you disclose requires careful thought. In *An Unquiet Mind*, Kay Jamison describes the reactions of others upon learning of her disorder, which varied from empathic acceptance to outright rejection and insensitivity.

When considering whether or not to disclose your disorder to a coworker or employer, first ask yourself several questions (Court & Nelson, 1996):

"Why do I want him or her to know?"

"How will it make my life at work easier—will it lead to a specific work accommodation?"

"Will it be helpful for someone to know about my disorder if there is an emergency at work?"

"Will I feel closer to this coworker—is he or she a potential friend?"

"Will explaining about my disorder help me explain absences or lapses in my work productivity to my boss?"

"If there is no reason to expect that the illness will impair my work, why does he or she need to know?"

There are ways to tell people of your disorder without actually using the label *bipolar*. For example, your disorder can be described as "a chemical imbalance that affects my mood" or "a medical problem related to my energy level that can affect my work and concentration." Simple explanations like these may be all that employers or coworkers require to understand why your work performance has shifted, or why you have been irritable, withdrawn, or absent lately.

Disclosing to your boss early on may set the stage for later changes in the structure or demands of your job (see the box on pages 308–309). You may have more legal protection if you disclose your bipolar disorder when you are well. If your employer knows ahead of time, you can problem-solve with him or her about what accommodations seem reasonable during your period of illness and once you have begun to recover (as Louise did).

There may be instances when you feel you must disclose the disorder to your boss, such as when you've had multiple absences or a clear deterioration in your work productivity. Some people decide to wait to see if their performance actually does slip and then disclose the disorder to the boss when asking for time off or other work adjustments. This can be a sensible plan, but timing is important: Your boss may feel annoyed by this disclosure if it occurs in the midst of trying to meet an important deadline. Also, when you are in an active period of illness, you may not be able to tell if your work performance has changed or if you need accommodations.

> **Effective solution:** If you decide to disclose your disorder to someone at work and it seems appropriate, use the Quick Fact Sheet (on pages 285–286) intended for family members to help you explain the illness to this coworker.

Self-Care Strategies for Coping Effectively in the Work Setting

Adjusting the Work Setting to Your Disorder

There is virtually no research literature on what kinds of jobs are best for people with bipolar disorder. We suspect that people with the disorder should avoid jobs that involve sudden bursts of social stimulation with little down time in between (for example, being a waitress at a bar with a "happy hour"), frequent travel across time zones, or consistently stressful interactions with others (for example, working in a hospital emergency room or at the complaint desk at the phone company). We also suspect that people with the disorder do better with consistent work hours and predictable workdays than in jobs requiring shifting schedules (for example, working on weekdays one week and then weekends the next, or working evening shifts followed immediately by morning ones). Jobs in restaurants, manufacturing, nursing, and retail sales often require variable shifts, whereas jobs in accounting, computer programming, banking, and schools are usually more consistent. But if the jobs in the former category appeal to you, you may not have to rule them out. Pursue them but try to determine whether you can obtain some of the accommodations listed in the box on pages 308–309.

What constitutes *reasonable accommodations*? These are innovations or modifications in your job requirements or work schedule that give you a better shot at successful employment. Reasonable accommodations are usually requested by you as the employee, and are generally not offered up front by the employer. Remember that your employer cannot be expected to provide accommodations without knowing about your disorder and why these accommodations are required.

The box lists examples of accommodations that might be reasonable to request of an employer. These items are not meant to reflect the adjustments that all people with bipolar disorder should expect. Rather, they are meant as examples of things you can ask for. Try to determine which of these are negotiable for you and which are not. It is highly unlikely that any employer would grant all or even a majority of

Reasonable Workplace Accommodations for Persons with Bipolar Disorder

Work Hours

■ Working regular daily or nightly hours rather than variable night/day work shifts

■ Being assigned work shifts that fit best with your circadian rhythms (for example, 10 A.M.–7 P.M. instead of 8 A.M.–5 P.M.; working 3-hour shifts for 5 days rather than 5-hour shifts for 3 days)

■ Avoiding work early in the morning if you suffer from "medication hangovers"

■ Reducing work hours or changing from full-time to part-time

■ Being excused from, or getting reductions in, overtime work

■ Completing some of your tasks at home versus at work

Stress Management

■ Being allowed to share responsibilities for projects with others

■ Being placed in an office or cubicle that has a degree of distance from noise and stimulation

■ Working in well-lit, uncrowded rooms

■ Being excused from certain work assignments that historically have been triggers for your mood swings

■ Obtaining support or counseling from an employee assistance program

■ Leaving work for breaks or lunch to decompress, exercise, walk, or use self-relaxation techniques

■ Taking a greater number of short breaks rather than two long breaks during an 8-hour work shift

Absences from Work

■ Being granted brief absences for medical appointments, with chances to make up the hours

■ Being granted extended leaves of absence with a doctor's note

■ Being allowed to leave work early when having difficult mood swings or anxiety/stress reactions

---

Reasonable Workplace Accommodations for Persons with Bipolar Disorder (*cont.*)

Communication with Your Employer about Performance Evaluations

▪ Having regular and open communication with your employer about your job performance

▪ Hearing what you're doing right as well as what you're doing wrong

▪ Being judged by overall productivity and task completion as well as number of hours worked

▪ Revisiting these accommodations from time to time to determine if they are enabling you to be productive and remain stable

---

them (and some may be against the nature or policies of the firm). Nonetheless, your employer might approve enough of these adjustments to help you function better at work. Note that some accommodations would also benefit employees who do not have bipolar disorder but who are seeking ways to manage stress.

It is not always possible to know in advance which accommodations will work for you, but your employer will probably be most open to these requests once you have been offered the job and are in the negotiation phase. Some of the items (for example, changing from full-time to part-time work, negotiating leaves of absence, the style of employer/employee performance evaluations, asking that your office be moved) may need to be negotiated later, once you have worked at the job for a period of time and have identified problems with the existing structure.

Ralph, 52, worked as the primary short-order cook in a restaurant, where he supervised two other cooks. He determined that he was prone to hyperactivity, irritability, and inefficiency on nights when the restaurant activity reached a certain volume. With the support of his employer, he learned to delegate the task of supervising food preparation to one of the other cooks at those times. He would then continue his shift as the secondary cook and would take over again as primary cook the next day.

Tina, age 59, worked for a research firm that assigned employees to closely interconnected cubicles. One of her coworkers insisted on listening to his radio while working, which was not against company policy but was very disturbing to Tina. She became unable to concentrate. She tried to reason with the coworker, who expressed mock sympathy and then went back to playing his radio. She became more and more irritated and noticed that her thoughts began to race.

She eventually consulted her boss about the problem without explaining that she had bipolar II disorder. Her boss felt that Tina was a good employee and decided to let her move to a smaller room where she would have less contact with others. This adjustment helped Tina restore her previous level of productivity.

Beth, a 44-year-old woman with bipolar I disorder, discovered that her mood swings were at their worst at the onset of her menstrual period. She worked at a news office with variable shifts; she had been unable, for a variety of financial and personal reasons, to obtain regular hours. Despite the loss of pay, she decided to ask to be excused from 8-hour work shifts in the 2 days prior to the onset of her menstrual period. She resumed work at her normal pace once the worst mood swings associated with her menstrual cycle were over.

Balancing Work Time against Down Time

One work-related difficulty I've heard expressed by a number of people with bipolar disorder is the feeling of being wired and driven at work and then feeling spent, exhausted, or depressed once home for the night. Their problems are compounded on the weekend if there is little to do and they feel like their body and brain have shut down. As a result, some people feel hypomanic when they're working and depressed when they're not.

This form of cycling is most likely to happen when you start a new job. Like most other new employees, you probably want to perform at your peak and begin pushing yourself hard. But a cycle can occur in which you try to produce at your maximum and are quickly rewarded with praise, compensation, or advancement by an appreciative boss. This reward may make you drive yourself even harder, leading to more reward but also more hypomania or even mania. As I mentioned in Chapter 5, goal attainment events (events that involve reward or advancement and that increase your drive toward other goals) are particularly potent in precipitating manic episodes (Johnson et al., 2000). Unfortunately, these manic states often lead into a depressive or mixed episode, along with negative thoughts and feelings about your capabilities ("I used to be able to accomplish so much"). In turn, your boss, who may not know about your disorder, may compare your performance when depressed to the way you performed when you first started the job (rather than to the performance of other workers in his or her firm). He or she may wonder what happened to you.

When you first start a job, try to take a more cautious, measured approach. Turn in a consistent work performance and get your footing in the new job, but don't try to be a superstar at the outset. Know when you are overstressing yourself. It's better to be a consistent employee than a "start-stop" employee, on whom others are unsure they can depend.

When you get home from work, allow yourself to relax but also introduce some structure (see Chapter 8) and a degree of low-key stimulation. Avoid scheduling lots of demanding social activities for weekday evenings. During weekends, avoid "sleep bingeing" (for example, sleeping 12 or more hours and getting up late) to counteract your fatigue from getting up at 6 A.M. every morning during the week. Instead, keep your bedtimes and wake times during the weekend to within 1 hour of your times during the week. Plan a social activity or exercise for the mornings during the weekend to assure that you'll be out of bed by a certain time. That way, your internal clock will stay regulated as you transition from the work week to the weekend.

> **Effective prevention:** When you start a new job, keep a regular daily and nightly routine and set limits on the workload you initially accept. These adjustments can help keep the job from triggering hypomania during the workday and depression after work.

These recommendations may sound rigid, but they will help you function in the early stages of your new job. Once you have worked at a job for a while and have settled into a routine, you may be able to introduce more flexibility into your daily habits without sacrificing mood stability. This balance varies considerably from person to person, so take your time to find the solution that works best for you.

Using Vocational Rehabilitation Support

If you have been having trouble finding a job that is suitable for you, or trouble keeping jobs, you may want to consider vocational counseling. Most states have a division of vocational rehabilitation devoted to helping people with disabilities. Generally, you will not have to pay for these services. To locate these services in your area, call the local mental health center or your city or town's chamber of commerce, or look in the phone book under "State" in the government listings.

Vocational rehabilitation specialists can help you develop a plan for finding and performing successfully in a job. These plans are focused on what you want to achieve (for example, part-time versus full-time employment; people-oriented versus more solitary work settings). Rehabilitation can involve *vocational testing* (for example, questionnaires regarding your interests, environments you enjoy, or job skills); training in *job-seeking skills* (for example, writing a résumé, making initial telephone calls to an employer, and effective interviewing strategies); and *job development* (locating jobs in the community or sometimes even designing them to fit your aptitudes and skills).

Job coaching is often the most active component of vocational rehabilitation. A job coach goes with you to a new job site, helps you learn the required tasks, and encourages you to stay motivated. He or she can facilitate communication between you and your boss. A job coach may help explain your disorder to your supervisor and clarify any special considerations you may require (for example, a work envi-

ronment with as few distractions as possible).

Employers may listen and respond
more readily to a job coach than to an
employee.

> **Effective solution:** A job coach can be a valuable intermediary, handling difficult communications between you and your supervisor.

Jamal, a 25-year-old man with bipolar I disorder, became stressed by his job at an auto parts store after being switched from one sales area to another. He didn't like his new supervisor, whom he found sarcastic and unsympathetic to the limitations imposed by his disorder. Just as he was about to quit, Jamal's job coach interceded and explained the disorder to this supervisor. They agreed on rules for their working relationship and strategies by which Jamal could tempo-rarily leave the setting when he felt overwhelmed by it. He eventually left this job and found a new one, but he felt empowered by the fact that by the time he left, his supervisor had changed his style of dealing with him.

Job coaches can also be helpful if you need a leave of absence from work. If you need to be hospitalized for a manic or depressive episode, you may not be in a con-dition to ask your employer for a leave. A job coach can write a letter or call your employer to advocate on your behalf.

Applying for Disability

If you have had a series of illness episodes or unremitting symptoms and have been unable to function at work, you may want to apply for disability payments. If you have previously paid for short-term or long-term private disability insurance through your employer, you may be eligible for payments with an accompanying doctor's order. You may also apply for disability payments through the Social Secu-rity Administration. Social Security payments are not large (for example, about $500 per month), but they can help support you during a period of work disability.

Usually, you apply for disability through a liaison at your local Social Security Office. The application process can be long (about 6 months) and frustrating. The procedure usually requires that your doctor and psychotherapist provide medical records and answer questions about your ability to work. If you are in touch with a vocational rehabilitation counselor, he or she may be able to acquaint you with the application procedures or recommend someone who can. Because of the length of the process, you may be more stable by the time your payments arrive than you were when you first applied!

Receiving disability payments does not mean you have to abandon the idea of working in the future. You can be on disability for a period of time (for example, during a long-term depression that is not responding well to medications) and then reconsider the working world once you have recovered. ***Being on disability should*** *not have to be stigmatizing or shameful.* In fact, many people with bipolar disorder and other medical disorders conclude that they need this kind of support. In the Boston University survey of professionals and managers, one-third had received disability payments at some point in their past (Ellison & Russinova, 2001).

Despite the toll that bipolar disorder can take on your family and work life, I strongly believe that you can learn to cope effectively in both settings. As you've just seen, coping involves being comfortable with your own understanding of the disorder, educating others about it, knowing your limitations, setting appropriate expectations for yourself, and trying to adjust your environment to maximize the chances that you'll function at your best. Remember to rely on the help of others (friends, family, and coworkers) for support when it seems appropriate. Constance Hammen and her colleagues at UCLA (2000) found that the people who did best within the work setting were those who had strong social and relationship support outside of work.

Bipolar disorder poses many challenges that are hard for anyone, except those suffering from it, to understand. Now that you have arrived at the end of this book, I hope you have become convinced that the strategies recommended here—learning as much as you can about the disorder, getting consistent medical treatment, taking advantage of psychotherapy, relying on social supports, and using self-management tools—can help you cope with the disorder on a day-to-day basis. As articulately expressed by one client who has been stable for some time, "I have learned to manage my disorder rather than being managed by it."

Mood Chart

MOOD

Rate with 2 marks each day to indicate best and worst (if applicable)

		Psychotic Symptoms Strange Ideas, Hallucinations	
Elevated	Severe	Significant Impairment NOT ABLE TO WORK	X
	Mod.	Significant Impairment ABLE TO WORK	
	Mild	Without significant impairment	
WNL	MOOD NOT DEFINITELY ELEVATED OR DEPRESSED.	NO SYMPTOMS Circle date to indicate menses	
Depressed	Mild	Without significant impairment	
	Mod.	Significant Impairment ABLE TO WORK	
	Severe	Significant Impairment NOT ABLE TO WORK	

Hours Slept Last Night	X

0 = none
1 = mild
2 = moderate
3 = severe

Anxiety	
Irritability	X

Month/Year _____

Daily Notes

Weight: _____

TREATMENTS
(Enter number of tablets taken each day)

Verbal Therapy	
Lithium	____ mg
Benzodiazepine	____ mg
Anticonvulsant Depakote	_____ ____ mg
Antidepressant	____ mg
	____ mg
Antipsychotic	____ mg
	____ mg

Name _____

Adapted by permission of Gary Sachs, MD (Copyright 1993).

Resources for People
with Bipolar Disorder

National and International Organizations

The following are comprehensive organizations that offer not just a wealth of online services and information but also in many cases community outreach services and phone/mail contacts.

National Alliance on Mental Illness (800-950-NAMI [6264]; *www.nami.org*) is a grass-roots self-help support and advocacy organization for people with severe mental illnesses (including bipolar disorder, recurrent depression, and schizophrenia), their family members, and friends. NAMI offers parent support groups all over the United States and a structured educational program taught by parents of people with severe psychiatric disorders called "Family to Family."

Child and Adolescent Bipolar Foundation (847-492-8519; *www.bpkids.org*), a parent-led organization, provides information and support to family members, health care professionals, and the public concerning bipolar disorders in the young. CABF advocates for health services and research on the nature, causes, and treatment of early-onset bipolar disorder. Particularly useful is information on how to locate a mental health provider who sees children with bipolar disorder in your area. The Learning Center provides examples of mood charts, articles on how to prepare for initial doctor visits, and information on research studies.

Depression and Bipolar Support Alliance (800-826-3632; *www.dbsalliance.org*) is devoted to educating consumers and their family members about mood disorders, decreasing the public stigma of these illnesses, fostering self-help, advocating for research funding, and improving access to care. DBSA has chapters in many cities that offer free, peer-led support groups.

International Society for Bipolar Disorders (412-802-6940; *www.isbd.org*) aims to promote awareness of bipolar conditions in society at large, educate mental health professionals, foster research on bipolar disorder, and promote international collaborations. Its journal, *Bipolar Disorders: An International Journal of Psychiatry and Neurosciences,* is becoming a primary outlet for new research on the diagnosis, etiology, and treatment of bipolar conditions. ISBD publishes a newsletter and has several online chat rooms, including an "ask the experts" exchange.

Juvenile Bipolar Research Foundation (866-333-JBRF; *www.bpchildresearch.org*) is the first charitable organization dedicated solely to the support of research on the etiology, treatment, and prevention of juvenile-onset bipolar disorder. JBRF has organized a consortium of collaborative research groups and individual investigators from a number of medical schools and treatment centers around the country. Through its website, parents can learn about and volunteer for research studies that are sponsored by the foundation. Information is provided concerning educational forums for parents and teachers; how to subscribe to professional e-mail Listservs for family members, physicians, and therapists; and new research findings pertinent to childhood-onset bipolar disorder.

MDF the Bipolar Organization (Castle Works, 21 St. George's Road, London SE1 6ES; 08456 340 540 [United Kingdom only]; 0044 207793 2600 [international]; *www.mdf.org.uk*) is a user-led charitable organization that offers self-help groups, publications, and other practical information for those living with bipolar disorder. There is a useful link for employment services and an "eCommunity" with online message boards.

Mental Health America (800-969-6642; crisis line: 800-273-TALK; *www.nmha.org*) is the oldest and largest nonprofit organization in the United States that addresses all aspects of mental health and illness. Research information, legislative updates, and practitioner referrals are available on its website.

National Alliance for Research on Schizophrenia and Depression (516-829-0091; *www.narsad. org*) is the largest donor-supported, nongovernment organization dedicated to raising and distributing funds for research into the nature, causes, treatments, and prevention of severe mental illnesses, including bipolar disorder, schizophrenia, depression, and severe anxiety disorders. Its website includes up-to-date information about the diagnosis and treatment of severe psychiatric disorders.

National Institute of Mental Health Publications (866-615-6464; *www.nimh.nih.gov/publicat/ index.cfm*) provides up-to-date information on the symptoms, course, causes, and treatment of bipolar disorder. Separate sections are devoted to child and adolescent bipolar illness, suicide, medical treatments and their side effects, co-occurring illnesses, psychosocial treatments, sources of help for individuals and families, and clinical research studies.

National Network of Depression Centers (734-332-3914 or 734-332-3989; *nndc.org*; e-mail: nndc@nndc.org) is a collection of comprehensive care centers for depression and bipolar disorder across the United States, coordinated by the University of Michigan. It consists of a network of universities committed to implementing consistent, state-of-the-art treatment protocols and research.

Websites

The following are Internet-only resources. They offer a variety of information and often interactive features such as chat rooms and forums, but have no physical presence in the community and no phone contact (e-mail contact is available where noted).

Bipolar Child (*www.bipolarchild.com*), developed by Demitri and Janis Papolos, offers up-to-date research findings pertaining to children with a bipolar disorder, a newsletter on new treatment approaches, samples of individualized educational programs, information on upcoming conferences, and tips on how to start a support group.

Bipolar Disorder Sanctuary (*www.mhsanctuary.com/bipolar*) includes educational articles on bipolar disorder, an "ask the therapist" discussion forum, first-person accounts, chat rooms for patients and family members, a clinician's forum, links to new research studies, and an online bookstore.

Bipolar Significant Others (*www.bpso.org*) is a website and an e-mail exchange group in which members—relatives or friends of persons with bipolar disorder—share information about the illness, provide support to one another, and problem-solve about issues related to the impact of the illness on families and intimate relationships. The website contains much helpful information on treatment, book reviews, and links.

Bipolar World (*www.bipolarworld.net*) provides information on bipolar diagnosis, treatments, and suicide, an "ask the doctor" link, personal stories, information on disabilities and stigma, community and family support, relevant books, a bipolar message board, and chat rooms.

Depression Central Website (*www.psycom.net/depression.central.bipolar.html*) is an informational website that offers links to the Mayo Clinic's bipolar disorder home page; answers frequently asked questions about bipolar disorder; discusses treatment guidelines; gives up-to-date information on topics such as novel treatment approaches, use of lithium during pregnancy, sleep deprivation, differential diagnosis, adjunctive therapy, suicide, and seasonal mood disorders; and provides a self-screening tool.

Harbor of Refuge Organization, Inc. (*www.harbor-of-refuge.org*) provides peer-to-peer support for individuals diagnosed with bipolar disorder who are undergoing treatment. There is a discussion forum/chat room. Information is provided on self-care and illness management strategies.

Internet Mental Health (*www.mentalhealth.com/dis/p20-md02.html*) is another informational website. A strength of this site is the direct linkage between specific topics and relevant published research abstracts. It is a particularly good site for new research on medications. Downloadable self-rated mood questionnaires and mood charts are available.

McMan's Depression and Bipolar Web (*www.mcmanweb.com*) is a comprehensive website with substantial links to current research, essays on first-person experiences, and an opinion page. The webmaster, John McManamy, is an award-winning mental health journalist and author.

Medline Plus Health Information (*www.nlm.nih.gov/medlineplus/bipolardisorder.html*) offers links to National Institute of Mental Health publications and clinical trials. It includes overviews of current bipolar research and information regarding children, teenagers, and seniors with the disorder. A link to the Medline search engine for the most recent research articles on bipolar disorder is provided.

Pendulum Resources (*www.pendulum.org*) offers information about the DSM-IV diagnostic criteria, current medical treatments, books favored by mental health consumers and family members, articles on how to cope with depression or bipolar disorder in yourself or a loved one, writings and poetry by people with bipolar disorder, links to other relevant sites, and updates on research studies. One section compiles abstracts of research studies relevant to specific topics relating to bipolar disorder.

Books on Bipolar Disorder or Depression

Books on mood disorders can be informational, self-help guides or first-person accounts.

Informational Guides

Addis, M. E., & Martell, C. R. (2004). *Overcoming depression one step at a time: The new Behavioral Activation approach to getting your life back.* Oakland, CA: New Harbinger.

Amador, X., & Johanson, A. L. (2000). *I am not sick I don't need help!* Peconic, NY: Vida Press.

Basco, M. R. (2005). *The bipolar workbook: Tools for controlling your mood swings.* New York: Guilford Press.

Bauer, M., Ludman, E., Greenwald, D. E., & Kilbourne, A. M. (2009). *Overcoming bipolar disorder: A comprehensive workbook for managing your symptoms and achieving your life goals.* Oakland, CA: New Harbinger.

Birmaher, B. (2004). *New hope for children and teens with bipolar disorder.* New York: Three Rivers Press.

Brondolo, E., & Amador, X. (2007). *Break the bipolar cycle: A day-by-day guide to living with bipolar disorder.* New York: McGraw-Hill.

Burns, D. D. (1999). *The feeling good handbook.* New York: Plume.

Carlson, T. (2000). *The life of a bipolar child: What every parent and professional needs to know.* Duluth, MN: Benline Press.

Copeland, M. E., & McCay, M. (2002). *The depression workbook: A guide for living with depression and manic depression* (2nd ed.) Oakland, CA: New Harbinger.

Court, B. L., & Nelson, G. E. (1996). *Bipolar puzzle solution: A mental health client's perspective.* Philadelphia: Taylor & Francis.

Fast, J. A., & Preston, J. D. (2004). *Loving someone with bipolar disorder: Understanding and helping your partner.* Oakland, CA: New Harbinger.

Fawcett, J., Golden, B., & Rosenfeld, N. (2000). *New hope for people with bipolar disorder.* Roseville, CA: Prima Health.

Findling, R. L., Kowatch, R. A., & Post, R. M. (2002) *Pediatric bipolar disorder.* Boston: Boston Medical Publishers.

Frank, E. (2005). *Treating bipolar disorder: A clinician's guide to interpersonal and social rhythm therapy.* New York: Guilford Press.

Fristad, M. A., & Goldberg Arnold, J. S. (2004). *Raising a moody child: How to cope with depression and bipolar disorder.* New York: Guilford Press.

Geller, B., & DelBello, M. P. (Eds.). (2003). *Bipolar disorder in childhood and early adolescence.* New York: Guilford Press.

Goodwin, F. K., & Jamison, K. R. (2007). *Manic–depressive illness* (2nd ed.). New York: Oxford University Press.

Greenberger, D., & Padesky, C. A. (1995). *Mind over mood.* New York: Guilford Press.

Jamison, K. R. (1993). *Touched with fire: Manic–depressive illness and the artistic temperament.* New York: Macmillan.

Jamison, K. R. (2000). *Night falls fast: Understanding suicide.* New York: Vintage Books.

Jamison, K. R. (2004). *Exuberance: The passion for life.* New York: Knopf.

Lynn, G. T. (2000). *Survival strategies for parenting children with bipolar disorder.* London: Jessica Kingsley.

Miklowitz, D. J. (2008). *Bipolar disorder: A family-focused treatment approach* (2nd ed.). New York: Guilford Press.

Miklowitz, D. J., & George, E. L. (2008). *The bipolar teen: What you can do to help your teen and your family.* New York: Guilford Press.

Mondimore, F. M. (1999). *Bipolar disorder: A guide for patients and families.* Baltimore: Johns Hopkins University Press.

Papolos, D. F., & Papolos, J. (2006). *The bipolar child: The definitive and reassuring guide to childhood's most misunderstood disorder* (3rd ed.). New York: Broadway Books.

Phelps, J. (2006). *Why am I still depressed?: Recognizing and managing the ups and downs of bipolar II and soft bipolar disorder.* New York: McGraw-Hill.

Stahl, S. M., & Muntner, N. (2000). *Essential psychopharmacology of depression and bipolar disorder.* Cambridge, UK: Cambridge University Press.

Torrey, E. F., & Knable, M. B. (2002). *Surviving manic depression: A manual on bipolar disorder for patients, families, and providers.* New York: Basic Books.

Waltz, M. (2000). *Bipolar disorders: A guide to helping children and adolescents.* Sebastopol, CA: O'Reilly & Associates.

Whybrow, P. C. (1998). *A mood apart: The thinker's guide to emotion and its disorders.* New York: HarperCollins.

Wilens, T. E. (1999). *Straight talk about psychiatric medications for kids.* New York: Guilford Press.

Williams, M., Teasdale, J., Segal, Z., & Kabat-Zinn, J. (2007). *The mindful way through depression: Freeing yourself from chronic unhappiness.* New York: Guilford Press.

Woolis, R., & Hatfield, A. (1992). *When someone you love has a mental illness: A handbook for family, friends, and caregivers.* Los Angeles: Tarcher.

First-Person Accounts

Behrman, A. (2002). *Electroboy: A memoir of mania.* New York: Random House.

Greenberg, M. (2008). *Hurry down sunshine: A father's story of love and madness.* New York: Vintage Press.

Hinshaw, S. P. (2002). *The years of silence are past: My father's life with bipolar disorder.* Cambridge, UK: Cambridge University Press.

Hornbacher, M. (2009). *Madness: A bipolar life.* Mariner Books.

Jamison, K. R. (1995). *An unquiet mind.* New York: Knopf.

Pauley, J. (2005). *Skywriting: A life out of the blue.* New York: Ballantine Books.

Simon, L. (2002). *Detour: My bipolar road trip in 4-D.* New York: Washington Square Press.

Solomon, A. (2001). *The noonday demon: An atlas of depression.* New York: Touchstone.

Steele, D. (2000). *His bright light: The story of Nick Traina.* Des Plaines, IL: Dell.

Styron, W. (1992). *Darkness visible: A memoir of madness.* New York: Vintage Books.

Weiland, M. F., & Warren, L. (2009). *Fall to pieces: A memoir of drugs, rock 'n' roll, and mental illness.* New York: William Morrow.

References

Akiskal, H. S., Kilzieh, N., Maser, J. D., Clayton, P. J., Schettler, P. J., Shea, M. T., et al. (2006). The distinct temperament profiles of bipolar I, bipolar II and unipolar patients. *Journal of Affective Disorders, 92*(1), 19–33.

Akiskal, H. S., Mendlowicz, M. V., Jean-Louis, G., Rapaport, M. H., Kelsoe, J. R., Gillin, J. C., et al. (2005). TEMPS-A: Validation of a short version of a self-rated instrument designed to measure variations in temperament. *Journal of Affective Disorders, 85*(1–2), 45–52.

Ali, J., & Khemka, M. (2008). Hyperprolactinemia: Monitoring children on long-term risperidone. *Current Psychiatry, 7*(11), 64–72.

Altman, E., Rea, M., Mintz, J., Miklowitz, D. J., Goldstein, M. J., & Hwang, S. (1992). Prodromal symptoms and signs of bipolar relapse: A report based on prospectively collected data. *Psychiatry Research, 41*, 1–8.

Altshuler, L. L., Cohen, L. S., Vitonis, A. F., Faraone, S. V., Harlow, B. L., Suri, R., et al. (2008). The Pregnancy Depression Scale (PDS): A screening tool for depression in pregnancy. *Archives of Women's Mental Health, 11*(4), 277–285.

Altshuler, L., Suppes, T., Black, D., Nolen, W. A., Keck, P. E. J., Frye, M. A., et al. (2003). Impact of antidepressant discontinuation after acute bipolar depression remission on rates of depressive relapse at 1-year follow-up. *American Journal of Psychiatry, 160*, 1252–1262.

American Psychiatric Association. (2000). *Diagnostic and statistical manual of mental disorders* (4th ed., text rev.). Washington, DC: American Psychiatric Press.

Amsterdam, J. D., Wang, G., & Shults, J. (2010). Venlafaxine monotherapy in bipolar type II depressed patients unresponsive to prior lithium monotherapy. *Acta Psychiatrica Scandinavica, 121*(3), 201–208.

Andreasen, N. C. (2008). The relationship between creativity and mood disorders. *Dialogues in Clinical Neuroscience, 10*(2), 251–255.

Arnold, L. M. (2003). Gender differences in bipolar disorder. *Psychiatric Clinics of North America, 26*, 595–620.

Baker, T. B., McFall, R. M., & Shoham, V. (2008). Current status and future prospects of clinical psychology. *Psychological Science in the Public Interest, 9*(2), 67–103.

Baldessarini, R. J., Tondo, L., & Hennen, J. (2003). Lithium treatment and suicide risk in major affective disorders: Update and new findings. *Journal of Clinical Psychiatry, 64*(Suppl. 5), 44–52.

Barnett, J. H., & Smoller, J. W. (2009). The genetics of bipolar disorder. *Neuroscience, 164*(1), 331–343.

Bauer, M., Ludman, E., Greenwald, D. E., & Kilbourne, A. M. (2009). *Overcoming bipolar disorder: A comprehensive workbook for managing your symptoms and achieving your life goals.* Oakland, CA: New Harbinger.

Beck, A. T., Rush, A. J., Shaw, B. F., & Emery, G. (1987). *Cognitive therapy of depression.* New York: Guilford Press.

Benedetti, F., Serretti, A., Colombo, C., Barbini, B., Lorenzi, C., Campori, E., et al. (2003). Influence of CLOCK gene polymorphism on circadian mood fluctuation and illness recurrence in bipolar depression. *American Journal of Medical Genetics B: Neuropsychiatric Genetics, 123B*(1), 23–26.

Birmaher, B., Axelson, D., Goldstein, B., Strober, M., Gill, M. K., Hunt, J., et al. (2009). Four-year longitudinal course of children and adolescents with bipolar spectrum disorders: The Course and Outcome of Bipolar Youth (COBY) study. *American Journal of Psychiatry, 166*(7), 795–804.

Blehar, M. C., DePaulo, J. R. J., Gershon, E. S., Reich, T., Simpson, S. G., & Nurnberger, J. I. J. (1998). Women with bipolar disorder: Findings from the NIMH Genetics Initiative sample. *Psychopharmacology Bulletin, 34*(3), 239–243.

Bowden, C. L. (2009). Anticonvulsants in bipolar disorder: Current research and practice and future directions. *Bipolar Disorders, 11*(Suppl. 2), 20–33.

Brown, E. B., McElroy, S. L., Keck, P. E. J., Deldar, A., Adams, D. H., Tohen, M., et al. (2006). A 7-week, randomized, double-blind trial of olanzapine/fluoxetine combination versus lamotrigine in the treatment of bipolar I depression. *Journal of Clinical Psychiatry, 67*(7), 1025–1033.

Burns, D. D. (1999). *Feeling good: The new mood therapy* (Rev. ed.). New York: Avon Books.

Burt, V. K., & Rasgon, N. (2004). Special considerations in treating bipolar disorder in women. *Bipolar Disorders, 6,* 2–13.

Cade, J. F. J. (1949). Lithium salts in the treatment of psychotic excitement. *Medical Journal of Australia, 36,* 349–352.

Calabrese, J. R., Fatemi, S. H., Kujawa, M., & Woyshville, M. J. (1996). Predictors of response to mood stabilizers. *Journal of Clinical Psychopharmacology, 16*(Suppl. 1), 24–31.

Calabrese, J. R., Suppes, T., Bowden, C. L., Sachs, G. S., Swann, A. C., McElroy, S. L., et al. (2000). A double-blind, placebo-controlled, prophylaxis study of lamotrigine in rapid-cycling bipolar disorder. Lamictal 614 Study Group. *Journal of Clinical Psychiatry, 61,* 841–850.

Calabrese, J. R., Vieta, E., El-Mallakh, R., Findling, R. L., Youngstrom, E. A., Elhaj, O., et al. (2004). Mood state at study entry as predictor of the polarity of relapse in bipolar disorder. *Biological Psychiatry, 56,* 957–963.

Carlson, G. A., & Goodwin, F. K. (1973). The stages of mania: A longitudinal analysis of the manic episode. *Archives of General Psychiatry, 28,* 221–228.

Carreno, T., & Goodnick, P. J. (1998). Creativity and mood disorder. In P. J. Goodnick (Ed.), *Mania: Clinical and research perspectives* (pp. 11–36). Washington, DC: American Psychiatric Press.

Chang, K., Adleman, N. E., Dienes, K., Simeonova, D. J., Menon, V., & Reiss, A. (2004). Anomalous prefrontal-subcortical activation in familial pediatric bipolar disorder: A functional magnetic resonance imaging investigation. *Archives of General Psychiatry, 61*(8), 781–792.

Chengappa, K. N. R., Rathore, D., Levine, J., Atzert, R., Solai, L., Parepally, H., et al. (1999). Topiramate as add-on treatment for patients with bipolar mania. *Bipolar Disorders, 1,* 42–53.

Chung, T. K., Lau, T. K., Yip, A. S., Chiu, H. F., & Lee, D. T. (2001). Antepartum depressive symptomatology is associated with adverse obstetric and neonatal outcomes. *Psychosomatic Medicine, 63*(5), 830–834.

Cohen, L. S. (2007). Treatment of bipolar disorder during pregnancy. *Journal of Clinical Psychiatry, 68*(Suppl. 9), 4–9.

Colom, F., Vieta, E., Martinez-Aran, A., Reinares, M., Benabarre, A., & Gasto, C. (2000). Clinical factors associated with treatment noncompliance in euthymic bipolar patients. *Journal of Clinical Psychiatry, 61,* 549–555.

Colom, F., Vieta, E., Martinez-Aran, A., Reinares, M., Goikolea, J. M., Benabarre, A., et al. (2003). A randomized trial on the efficacy of group psychoeducation in the prophylaxis of recurrences in bipolar patients whose disease is in remission. *Archives of General Psychiatry, 60,* 402–407.

Colom, F., Vieta, E., Tacchi, M. J., Sanchez-Moreno, J., & Scott, J. (2005). Identifying and improving non-adherence in bipolar disorders. *Bipolar Disorders, 7*(5), 24–31.

Connolly, J. J. (2009). *America's Top Doctors* (8th ed.). New York: Castle Connolly.

Coryell, W. (2009). Maintenance treatment in bipolar disorder: A reassessment of lithium as the first choice. *Bipolar Disorders, 11*(Suppl. 2), 77–83.

Coryell, W., Scheftner, W., Keller, M., Endicott, J., Maser, J., & Klerman, G. L. (1993). The enduring psychosocial consequences of mania and depression. *American Journal of Psychiatry, 150,* 720–727.

Court, B. L., & Nelson, G. E. (1996). *Bipolar puzzle solution: A mental health client's perspective.* Philadelphia: Taylor & Francis.

Dalai Lama. (1999). *Ethics for the new millennium.* New York: Riverhead Books.

Dalai Lama & Cutler, H. C. (1998). *The art of happiness: A handbook for living.* New York: Riverhead Books.

Davis, M., McKay, M., & Eshelman, E. R. (2000). *The relaxation and stress reduction workbook.* Oakland, CA: New Harbinger.

Denicoff, K. D., Smith-Jackson, E. E., Disney, E. R., Ali, S. O., Leverich, G. S., & Post, R. M. (1997). Comparative prophylactic efficacy of lithium, carbamazepine, and the combination in bipolar disorder. *Journal of Clinical Psychiatry, 58,* 470–478.

Drevets, W. C. (2001). Neuroimaging and neuropathological studies of depression: Implications for the cognitive-emotional features of mood disorders. *Current Opinions in Neurobiology, 11*(2), 240–249.

Dubovsky, S. L., & Buzan, R. (1999). Mood disorders. In R. E. Hales, S. Yudofsky, & J. Talbott (Eds.), *American Psychiatric Press Textbook of Psychiatry* (3rd ed., pp. 479–566). Washington, DC: American Psychiatric Press.

Ehlers, C. L., Kupfer, D. J., Frank, E., & Monk, T. H. (1993). Biological rhythms and depression: The role of zeitgebers and zeitstorers. *Depression, 1,* 285–293.

Ellison, M., & Russinova, Z. (2001). *Employment outcomes of professionals and managers with serious mental illness: Findings from a national survey.* Unpublished manuscript. Center for Psychiatric Rehabiliitation, Boston University, Boston, MA.

Ellison, M. L., Russinova, Z., Lyass, A., & Rogers, E. S. (2008). Professionals and managers with severe mental illnesses: Findings from a national survey. *Journal of Nervous and Mental Disease, 196*(3), 179–189.

Epstein, L., & Mardon, S. (2006). *The Harvard Medical School guide to a good night's sleep.* New York: McGraw-Hill.

Espie, C. (2006). *Overcoming insomnia and sleep problems.* London: Constable & Robinson.

Fagiolini, A., Kupfer, D. J., Masalehdan, A., Scott, J. A., Houck, P. R., & Frank, E. (2005). Functional impairment in the remission phase of bipolar disorder. *Bipolar Disorders, 7*(3), 281–285.

Falloon, I. R. H., Boyd, J. L., & McGill, C. W. (1984). *Family care of schizophrenia: A problem-solving approach to the treatment of mental illness.* New York: Guilford Press.

Fawcett, J., Golden, B., & Rosenfeld, N. (2000). *New hope for people with bipolar disorder.* Roseville, CA: Prima Health.

Forman, D. R., O'Hara, M. W., Stuart, S., Gorman, L. L., Larsen, K. E., & Coy, K. C. (2007). Effective treatment for postpartum depression is not sufficient to improve the developing mother–child relationship. *Development and Psychopathology, 19*(2), 585–602.

Fortinguerra, F., Clavenna, A., & Bonati, M. (2009). Psychotropic drug use during breastfeeding: A review of the evidence. *Pediatrics, 124*(4), e547–556.

Frank, E. (2005). *Treating bipolar disorder: A clinician's guide to interpersonal and social rhythm therapy.* New York: Guilford Press.

Frank, E., Kupfer, D. J., Thase, M. E., Mallinger, A. G., Swartz, H. A., Fagiolini, A. M., et al. (2005). Two-year outcomes for interpersonal and social rhythm therapy in individuals with bipolar I disorder. *Archives of General Psychiatry, 62*(9), 996–1004.

Freeman, M. P., Smith, K. W., Freeman, S. A., McElroy, S. L., Kmetz, G. E., Wright, R., et al. (2002). The impact of reproductive events on the course of bipolar disorder in women. *Journal of Clinical Psychiatry, 63*(4), 284–287.

Frye, M. A., Grunze, H., Suppes, T., McElroy, S. L., Keck, P. E. J., Walden, J., et al. (2007). A placebo-controlled evaluation of adjunctive modafinil in the treatment of bipolar depression. *American Journal of Psychiatry, 164*(8), 1242–1249.

Geddes, J. R., Burgess, S., Hawton, K., Jamison, K., & Goodwin, G. M. (2004). Long-term lithium therapy for bipolar disorder: Systematic review and meta-analysis of randomized controlled trials. *American Journal of Psychiatry, 161*(2), 217–222.

Geddes, J. R., Calabrese, J. R., & Goodwin, G. M. (2009). Lamotrigine for treatment of bipolar depression: Independent meta-analysis and meta-regression of individual patient data from five randomised trials. *British Journal of Psychiatry, 94*(1), 4–9.

Geddes, J. R., Goodwin, G. M., Rendell, J., Azorin, J. M., Cipriani, A., Ostacher, M. J., et al. (2010). Lithium plus valproate combination therapy versus monotherapy for relapse prevention in bipolar I disorder (BALANCE): A randomised open-label trial. *Lancet, 375*(9712), 385–395.

Geller, B., Williams, M., Zimerman, B., Frazier, J., Beringer, I., & Warner, K. L. (1998). Prepubertal and early adolescent bipolarity differentiated from ADHD by manic symptoms, grandiose delusions, ultra-rapid or ultraradian cycling. *Journal of Affective Disorders, 51,* 81–91.

George, E. L., Miklowitz, D. J., Richards, J. A., Simoneau, T. L., & Taylor, D. O. (2003). The comorbidity of bipolar disorder and axis II personality disorders: Prevalence and clinical correlates. *Bipolar Disorders, 5,* 115–122.

Ghaemi, N., Sachs, G. S., & Goodwin, F. K. (2000). What is to be done? Controversies in the diagnosis and treatment of manic–depressive illness. *World Journal of Biological Psychiatry, 1*(2), 65–74.

Gitlin, M. J., Swendsen, J., Heller, T. L., & Hammen, C. (1995). Relapse and impairment in bipolar disorder. *American Journal of Psychiatry, 152*(11), 1635–1640.

Glovinsky, P., & Spielman, A. (2006). *The insomnia answer: A personalized program for identifying and overcoming the three types of insomnia.* New York: Perigee Trade Books.

Glozier, N. (1998). Workplace effects of the stigmatization of depression. *Journal of Occupational and Environmental Medicine, 40,* 793–800.

Goldberg, J. F. (2000). Treatment of bipolar disorders. *Psychiatric Clinics of North America, 7,* 115–149.

Goldberg, J. F., Burdick, K. E., & Endick, C. J. (2004). Preliminary randomized, double-blind, placebo-controlled trial of pramipexole added to mood stabilizers for treatment-resistant bipolar depression. *American Journal of Psychiatry, 161*(3), 564–566.

Goldberg, J. F., & Garno, J. L. (2009). Age at onset of bipolar disorder and risk for comorbid borderline personality disorder. *Bipolar Disorders, 11*(2), 205–208.

Goodwin, F. K., Fireman, B., Simon, G. E., Hunkeler, E. M., Lee, J., & Revicki, D.et al. (2003).

Suicide risk in bipolar disorder during treatment with lithium and divalproex. *Journal of the American Medical Association, 290,* 1467–1473.

Goodwin, F. K., & Jamison, K. R. (2007). *Manic–depressive illness* (2nd ed.). New York: Oxford University Press.

Gotlib, I. H., & Krasnoperova, E. (1998). Biased information processing as a vulnerability factor for depression. *Behavior Therapy, 29,* 603–617.

Greenberger, D., & Padesky, C. A. (1995). *Mind over mood.* New York: Guilford Press.

Grof, P., Alda, M., Grof, E., Fox, D., & Cameron, P. (1993). The challenge of predicting response to stabilizing lithium treatment: The importance of patient selection. *British Journal of Psychiatry, 163,* 16–19.

Hale, T. (2002). Using antidepressants in breastfeeding mothers. Retrieved July 5, 2009, from *www.kellymom.com/health/meds/antidepressants-hale10-02.html.*

Hammen, C., Gitlin, M., & Altshuler, L. (2000). Predictors of work adjustment in bipolar I patients: A naturalistic longitudinal follow-up. *Journal of Consulting and Clinical Psychology, 68,* 220–225.

Harlow, B. L., Wise, L. A., Otto, M. W., Soares, C. N., & Cohen, L. S. (2003). Depression and its influence on reproductive endocrine and menstrual cycle markers associated with perimenopause: The Harvard Study of Moods and Cycles. *Archives of General Psychiatry, 60*(1), 29–36.

Harrow, M., Grossman, L. S., Herbener, E. S., & Davies, E. W. (2000). Ten-year outcome: Patients with schizoaffective disorders, schizophrenia, affective disorders and mood-incongruent psychotic symptoms. *British Journal of Psychiatry, 177,* 421–426.

Harvey, A. G. (2008). Sleep and circadian rhythms in bipolar disorder: Seeking synchrony, harmony, and regulation. *American Journal of Psychiatry, 165*(7), 820–829.

Hillegers, M. H., Reichart, C. G., Wals, M., Verhulst, F. C., Ormel, J., & Nolen, W. A. (2005). Five-year prospective outcome of psychopathology in the adolescent offspring of bipolar parents. *Bipolar Disorders, 7*(4), 344–350.

Hirschfeld, R. M., Williams, J. B., Spitzer, R. L., Calabrese, J. R., Flynn, L., Jr., K. P. E., et al. (2000). Development and validation of a screening instrument for bipolar spectrum disorder: The Mood Disorder Questionnaire. *American Journal of Psychiatry, 157,* 1873–1875.

Isojärvi, J. I., Taubøll, E., and Herzog, A. G. (2005). Effect of antiepileptic drugs on reproductive endocrine function in individuals with epilepsy. *CNS Drugs, 19*(3), 207–223.

Jamison, K. R. (1993). *Touched with fire: Manic–depressive illness and the artistic temperament.* New York: Macmillan.

Jamison, K. R. (1995). *An unquiet mind.* New York: Knopf.

Jamison, K. R. (2000a). *Night falls fast: Understanding suicide.* New York: Vintage Books.

Jamison, K. R. (2000b). Suicide and bipolar disorder. *Journal of Clinical Psychiatry, 61*(Suppl. 9), 47–56.

Jamison, K. R. (2005). *Exuberance: The passion for life.* New York: Vintage Press.

Jette, N., Patten, S., Williams, J., Becker, W., & Wiebe, S. (2008). Comorbidity of migraine and psychiatric disorders: A national population-based study. *Headache, 48*(4), 501–516.

Jiang, B., Kenna, H. A., & Rasgon, N. L. (2009). Genetic overlap between polycystic ovary syndrome and bipolar disorder: The endophenotype hypothesis. *Medical Hypotheses, 73*(6), 996–1004.

Joffe, H. (2007). Reproductive biology and psychotropic treatments in premenopausal women with bipolar disorder. *Journal of Clinical Psychiatry, 68*(9), 10–15.

Joffe, H., Cohen, L. S., Suppes, T., McLaughlin, W. L., Lavori, P., Adams, J. M., et al. (2006). Valproate is associated with new-onset oligoamenorrhea with hyperandrogenism in women with bipolar disorder. *Biological Psychiatry, 59*(11), 1078–1086.

Joffe, H., Kim, D. R., Foris, J. M., Baldassano, C. F., Gyulai, L., Hwang, C. H., et al. (2006).

Menstrual dysfunction prior to onset of psychiatric illness is reported more commonly by women with bipolar disorder than by women with unipolar depression and healthy controls. *Journal of Clinical Psychiatry, 67*(2), 297–304.

John, H., & Sharma, V. (2009). Misdiagnosis of bipolar disorder as borderline personality disorder: Clinical and economic consequences. *World Journal of Biological Psychiatry, 10*(4, Pt. 2), 612–615.

Johnson, S. L. (2005a). Life events in bipolar disorder: Towards more specific models. *Clinical Psychology Review, 25*(8), 1008–1027.

Johnson, S. L. (2005b). Mania and dysregulation in goal pursuit. *Clinical Psychology Review, 25,* 241–262.

Johnson, S. L., Cuellar, A., Ruggero, C., Perlman, C., Goodnick, P., White, R., et al. (2008). Life events as predictors of mania and depression in bipolar I disorder. *Journal of Abnormal Psychology, 117,* 268–277.

Johnson, S. L., Sandrow, D., Meyer, B., Winters, R., Miller, I., Solomon, D., et al. (2000). Increases in manic symptoms following life events involving goal-attainment. *Journal of Abnormal Psychology, 109,* 721–727.

Johnson, S. L., Winett, C. A., Meyer, B., Greenhouse, W. J., & Miller, I. (1999). Social support and the course of bipolar disorder. *Journal of Abnormal Psychology, 108,* 558–566.

Joyce, P. R. (1985). Illness behaviour and rehospitalisation in bipolar affective disorder. *Psychological Medicine, 15,* 521–525.

Judd, L. L., Akiskal, H. S., Schettler, P. J., Coryell, W., Endicott, J., Maser, J. D., et al. (2003). A prospective investigation of the natural history of the long-term weekly symptomatic status of bipolar II disorder. *Archives of General Psychiatry, 60,* 261–269.

Judd, L. L., Akiskal, H. S., Schettler, P. J., Endicott, J., Maser, J., Solomon, D. A., et al. (2002). The long-term natural history of the weekly symptomatic status of bipolar I disorder. *Archives of General Psychiatry, 59,* 530–537.

Just, N., Abramson, L. Y., & Alloy, L. B. (2001). Remitted depression studies of tests of the cognitive vulnerability hypotheses of depression onset: A critique and conceptual analysis. *Clinical Psychology Review, 21,* 63–83.

Keck, P. E. Jr., McElroy, S. L., Strakowski, S. M., Bourne, M. L., & West, S. A. (1997). Compliance with maintenance treatment in bipolar disorder. *Psychopharmacology Bulletin, 33,* 87–91.

Kenna, H. A., Jiang, B., & Rasgon, N. L. (2009). Reproductive and metabolic abnormalities associated with bipolar disorder and its treatment. *Harvard Review of Psychiatry, 17,* 138–146.

Kessler, R. C., Chiu, W. T., Demler, O., & Walters, E. E. (2005). Prevalence, severity, and comorbidity of 12-month DSM-IV disorders in the National Comorbidity Survey Replication. *Archives of General Psychiatry, 62,* 617–627.

Ketter, T. A., Post, R. M., Denicoff, K., Pazzaglia, P. J., Marangell, L. B., George, M. S., et al. (1998). Carbamazepine. In P. J. Goodnick (Ed.), *Mania: Clinical and research perspectives* (pp. 263–300). Washington, DC: American Psychiatric Press.

Kochman, F. J., Hantouche, E. G., Ferrari, P., Lancrenon, S., Bayart, D., & Akiskal, H. S. (2005). Cyclothymic temperament as a prospective predictor of bipolarity and suicidality in children and adolescents with major depressive disorder. *Journal of Affective Disorders, 85*(1–2), 181–189.

Kocsis, J. H., Shaw, E. D., Stokes, P. E., Wilner, P., Elliot, A. S., Sikes, C., et al. (1993). Neuropsychological effects of lithium discontinuation. *Journal of Clinical Psychopharmacology, 13* (268–275).

Kraguljac, N. V., Montori, V. M., Pavuluri, M., Chai, H. S., Wilson, B. S., & Unal, S. S. (2009).

Efficacy of omega-3 Fatty acids in mood disorders: A systematic review and metaanalysis. *Psychopharmacology Bulletin, 42*(3), 39–54.

Krampe, R. T., & Ericsson, K. A. (1996). Maintaining excellence: Deliberate practice and elite performance in young and older pianists. *Journal of Experimental Psychology: General, 125*, 331–359.

Kwapil, T. R., Miller, M. B., Zinser, M. C., Chapman, L. J., Chapman, J., & Eckblad, M. (2000). A longitudinal study of high scorers on the hypomanic personality scale. *Journal of Abnormal Psychology, 109*, 222–226.

Lewinsohn, P. M., Munoz, R. F., Youngren, M. A., & Zeiss, A. M. (1992). *Control your depression*. New York: Fireside/Simon & Schuster.

Lewinsohn, P. M., Seeley, J. R., & Klein, D. N. (2003). Bipolar disorders during adolescence. *Acta Psychiatrica Scandinavica, 418*(Suppl.), 47–50.

Lewis, L. (2000). A consumer perspective concerning the diagnosis and treatment of bipolar disorder. *Biological Psychiatry, 48*, 442–444.

Lewis, M. A., & Rook, K. S. (1999). Social control in personal relationships: Impact on health behaviors and psychological distress. *Health Psychology, 18*(1), 63–71.

Linehan, M. M. (1985). The reasons for living inventory. In P. A. Keller & L. G. Ritt (Eds.), *Innovations in clinical practice: A source book* (pp. 321–330). Miami, FL: Professional Resource Exchange.

Linehan, M. M., Comtois, K. A., Murray, A. M., Brown, M. Z., Gallop, R. J., Heard, H. L., et al. (2006). Two-year randomized controlled trial and follow-up of dialectical behavior therapy vs. therapy by experts for suicidal behaviors and borderline personality disorder. *Archives of General Psychiatry, 63*(7), 757–766.

Linehan, M. M., & Dexter-Mazza, E. T. (2007). Dialectical behavior therapy for borderline personality disorder. In D. H. Barlow (Ed.), *Clinical handbook of psychological disorders* (4th ed., pp. 365–420). New York: Guilford Press.

Linehan, M. M., Goodstein, J. L., Nielsen, S. L., & Chiles, J. A. (1983). Reasons for staying alive when you are thinking of killing yourself: The Reasons for Living Inventory. *Journal of Consulting and Clinical Psychology, 51*, 276–286.

Lish, J. D., Dime-Meenan, S., Whybrow, P. C., Price, R. A., & Hirschfeld, R. M. (1994). The National Depressive and Manic-Depressive Association (NDMDA) survey of bipolar members. *Journal of Affective Disorders, 31*, 281–294.

Machado-Vieira, R., Manji, H. K., & Zarate, C. A. J. (2009). The role of lithium in the treatment of bipolar disorder: Convergent evidence for neurotrophic effects as a unifying hypothesis. *Bipolar Disorders, 11*(Suppl. 2), 92–109.

MacQueen, G., Parkin, C., Marriott, M., Bégin, H., & Hasey, G. (2007). The long-term impact of treatment with electroconvulsive therapy on discrete memory systems in patients with bipolar disorder. *Journal of Psychiatry and Neuroscience, 32*(4), 241–249.

Malhi, G. S., Adams, D., & Berk, M. (2009). Medicating mood with maintenance in mind: Bipolar depression pharmacotherapy. *Bipolar Disorders, 11*(Suppl. 2), 55–76.

Malkoff-Schwartz, S., Frank, E., Anderson, B., Sherrill, J. T., Siegel, L., Patterson, D., et al. (1998). Stressful life events and social rhythm disruption in the onset of manic and depressive bipolar episodes: A preliminary investigation. *Archives of General Psychiatry, 55*, 702–707.

Manji, H. (2009). The role of synaptic and cellular plasticity cascades in the pathophysiology and treatment of mood and psychotic disorders. *Bipolar Disorders, 11*(Suppl. 1), 2–3.

Manji, H. K., Quiroz, J. A., Payne, J. L., Singh, J., Lopes, B. P., Viegas, J. S., et al. (2003). The underlying neurobiology of bipolar disorder. *World Psychiatry, 2*(3), 136–146.

Mann, J. J., Oquendo, M., Underwood, M. D., & Arango, V. (1999). The neurobiology of suicide risk: A review for the clinician. *Journal of Clinical Psychiatry, 60*(Suppl. 2), 7–11.

Mansell, W., & Pedley, R. (2008). The ascent into mania: A review of psychological processes associated with the development of manic symptoms. *Clinical Psychology Review, 28*(3), 494–520.

Marangell, L. B. (2008). Current issues: Women and bipolar disorder. *Dialogues in Clinical Neuroscience, 10*(2), 229–238.

Marangell, L. B., Suppes, T., Zboyan, H. A., Prashad, S. J., Fischer, G., Snow, D., et al. (2008). A 1-year pilot study of vagus nerve stimulation in treatment-resistant rapid-cycling bipolar disorder. *Journal of Clinical Psychiatry, 69*(2), 183–189.

Marlatt, G. A., & Donovan, D. M. (2007). *Relapse prevention: Maintenance strategies in the treatment of addictive behaviors* (2nd ed.). New York: Guilford Press.

Martell, C. R., Dimidjian, S., & Herman-Dunn, R. (2010). *Behavioral activation for depression: A clinician's guide.* New York: Guilford Press.

Mayberg, H. S., Lozano, A. M., Voon, V., McNeely, H. E., Seminowicz, D., Hamani, C., et al. (2005). Deep brain stimulation for treatment-resistant depression. *Neuron, 45*(5), 651–660.

McCrady, B. S. (2007). Alcohol use disorders. In D. Barlow (Ed.), *Clinical handbook of psychological disorders* (4th ed., pp. 492–546). New York: Guilford Press.

McDonald, W. M. (2000). Epidemiology, etiology, and treatment of geriatric mania. *Journal of Clinical Psychiatry, 61*(Suppl. 13), 3–11.

Merikangas, K. R., Akiskal, H. S., Angst, J., Greenberg, P. E., Hirschfeld, R. M. A., Petukhova, M., et al. (2007). Lifetime and 12-month prevalence of bipolar spectrum disorder in the National Comorbidity Survey replication. *Archives of General Psychiatry, 64*(5), 543–552.

Miklowitz, D. J. (2004). The role of family systems in severe and recurrent psychiatric disorders: A developmental psychopathology view. *Development and Psychopathology, 16,* 667–688.

Miklowitz, D. J. (2008a). Adjunctive psychotherapy for bipolar disorder: State of the evidence. *American Journal of Psychiatry, 165*(11), 1408–1419.

Miklowitz, D. J. (2008b). *Bipolar disorder: A family-focused treatment approach* (2nd ed.). New York: Guilford Press.

Miklowitz, D. J., Alatiq, Y., Geddes, J. R., Goodwin, G. M., & Williams, J. M. G. (2010). Thought suppression in bipolar disorder. *Journal of Abnormal Psychology, 119*(2), 355–365.

Miklowitz, D. J., & George, E. L. (2008). *The bipolar teen: What you can do to help your teen and your family.* New York: Guilford Press.

Miklowitz, D. J., George, E. L., Richards, J. A., Simoneau, T. L., & Suddath, R. L. (2003). A randomized study of family-focused psychoeducation and pharmacotherapy in the outpatient management of bipolar disorder. *Archives of General Psychiatry, 60,* 904–912.

Miklowitz, D. J., Goldstein, M. J., Nuechterlein, K. H., Snyder, K. S., & Mintz, J. (1988). Family factors and the course of bipolar affective disorder. *Archives of General Psychiatry, 45,* 225–231.

Miklowitz, D. J., & Scott, J. (2009). Psychosocial treatments for bipolar disorder: Cost-effectiveness, mediating mechanisms, and future directions. *Bipolar Disorders, 11*(Suppl. 2), 110–122.

Miklowitz, D. J., Simoneau, T. L., George, E. L., Richards, J. A., Kalbag, A., Sachs-Ericsson, N., et al. (2000). Family-focused treatment of bipolar disorder: 1-year effects of a psychoeducational program in conjunction with pharmacotherapy. *Biological Psychiatry, 48,* 582–592.

Miller, W. R., & Rollnick, S. (2002). *Motivational interviewing: Preparing people for change* (2nd ed.). New York: Guilford Press.

Millett, K. (1990). *The loony-bin trip.* New York: Simon & Schuster.

Mondimore, F. M. (1999). *Bipolar disorder: A guide for patients and families.* Baltimore: Johns Hopkins University Press.

Monk, T. H., Flaherty, J. F., Frank, E., Hoskinson, K., & Kupfer, D. J. (1990). The social rhythm metric: An instrument to quantify daily rhythms of life. *Journal of Nervous and Mental Disease, 178,* 120–126.

Morris, C. D., Miklowitz, D. J., Wisniewski, S. R., Giese, A. A., Allen, M. H., & Thomas, M. R. (2005). Care satisfaction, hope, and life functioning among adults with bipolar disorder: Data from the first 1,000 participants in the Systematic Treatment Enhancement Program. *Comprehensive Psychiatry, 46,* 98–104.

Newberg, A. R., Catapano, L. A., Zarate, C. A., & Manji, H. K. (2008). Neurobiology of bipolar disorder. *Expert Reviews in Neurotherapeutics, 8*(1), 93–110.

Newman, C., Leahy, R. L., Beck, A. T., Reilly-Harrington, N., & Gyulai, L. (2001). *Bipolar disorder: A cognitive therapy approach.* Washington, DC: American Psychological Association.

Nierenberg, A. A., Burt, T., Matthews, J., & Weiss, A. P. (1999). Mania associated with St. John's wort. *Biological Psychiatry, 46*(12), 1707–1708.

Novick, D., Gonzalez-Pinto, A., Haro, J. M., Bertsch, J., Reed, C., Perrin, E., et al. (2009). Translation of randomised controlled trial findings into clinical practice: Comparison of olanzapine and valproate in the EMBLEM study. *Pharmacopsychiatry, 42*(4), 145–152.

Novick, D. M., Swartz, H. A., & Frank, E. (2010). Suicide attempts in bipolar I and bipolar II disorder: A review and meta-analysis of the evidence. *Bipolar Disorders, 12*(1), 1–9.

O'Reardon, J. P., Solvason, H. B., Janicak, P. G., Sampson, S., Isenberg, K. E., Nahas, Z., et al. (2007). Efficacy and safety of Transcranial Magnetic Stimulation in the acute treatment of major depression: A multisite randomized controlled trial. *Biological Psychiatry, 62,* 1208–1216.

Otto, M. W., Reilly-Harrington, N., Knauz, R. O., Henin, A., Kogan, J. N., & Sachs, G. S. (2008). *Living with bipolar disorder: A guide for individuals and families.* New York: Oxford University Press.

Pavuluri, M. N., Birmaher, B., & Naylor, M. W. (2005). Pediatric bipolar disorder: A review of the past 10 years. *Journal of the American Academy of Child & Adolescent Psychiatry, 44*(9), 846–871.

Perlis, R. H., Ostacher, M. J., Miklowitz, D. J., Hay, A., Nierenberg, A. A., Thase, M. E., et al. (2010). Clinical features associated with poor pharmacologic adherence in bipolar disorder: Results from the STEP-BD study. *Journal of Clinical Psychiatry, 71*(3), 296–303.

Perlis, R. H., Ostacher, M. J., Patel, J., Marangell, L. B., Zhang, H., Wisniewski, S. R., et al. (2006). Predictors of recurrence in bipolar disorder: Primary outcomes from the Systematic Treatment Enhancement Program for Bipolar Disorder (STEP-BD). *American Journal of Psychiatry, 163*(2), 217–224.

Phillips, M. L., Ladoucer, C. D., & Drevets, W. C. (2008). A neural model of voluntary and automatic emotion regulation: Implications for understanding the pathophysiology and neurodevelopment of bipolar disorder. *Molecular Psychiatry, 13,* 833–857.

Post, R. M., Altshuler, L. L., Leverich, G. S., Frye, M. A., Nolen, W. A., Kupka, R. W., et al. (2006). Mood switch in bipolar depression: Comparison of adjunctive venlafaxine, bupropion and sertraline. *British Journal of Psychiatry, 189,* 124–131.

Post, R. M., Frye, M. A., Denicoff, K. D., et al. (1998). Beyond lithium in the treatment of bipolar illness. *Neuropsychopharmacology, 19,* 206–219.

Post, R. M., & Leverich, G. S. (2006). The role of psychosocial stress in the onset and progression of bipolar disorder and its comorbidities: The need for earlier and alternative modes of therapeutic intervention. *Development and Psychopathology, 18*(4), 1181–1211.

Rasgon, N. L., Altshuler, L. L., Fairbanks, L., Elman, S., Bitran, J., Labarca, R., et al. (2005). Reproductive function and risk for PCOS in women treated for bipolar disorder. *Bipolar Disorders, 7*(3), 246–259.

Rasgon, N. L., Altshuler, L. L., Gudeman, D., Burt, V. K., Tanavoli, S., Hendrick, V., et al.

(2000). Medication status and polycystic ovary syndrome in women with bipolar disorder: A preliminary report. *Journal of Clinical Psychiatry, 61*(3), 173–178.

Rasgon, N., Bauer, M., Glenn, T., Elman, S., & Whybrow, P. C. (2003). Menstrual cycle related mood changes in women with bipolar disorder. *Bipolar Disorders, 5*(1), 48–52.

Rea, M. M., Tompson, M., Miklowitz, D. J., Goldstein, M. J., Hwang, S., & Mintz, J. (2003). Family focused treatment vs. individual treatment for bipolar disorder: Results of a randomized clinical trial. *Journal of Consulting and Clinical Psychology, 71*, 482–492.

Regier, D. A., Farmer, M. E., Rae, D. S., Locke, B. Z., Keith, S. J., Judd, L. L., et al. (1990). Comorbidity of mental disorders with alcohol and other drug abuse: Results from the Epidemiologic Catchment Area (ECA) Study. *Journal of the American Medical Association, 264*, 2511–2518.

Rosa, A. R., Fountoulakis, K., Siamouli, M., Gonda, X., & Vieta, E. (2009). Is anticonvulsant treatment of mania a class effect? Data from randomized clinical trials. *CNS Neuroscience Therapeutics, Dec 15 (EPub ahead of print)*.

Roybal, K., Theobold, D., Graham, A., DiNieri, J. A., Russo, S. J., Krishnan, V., et al. (2007). Mania-like behavior induced by disruption of CLOCK. *Proceedings of the National Academy of Sciences USA, 104*(15), 6406–6411.

Rush, A. J., Trivedi, M. H., Ibrahim, H. M., Carmody, T. J., Arnow, B., & Klein, D. N. (2003). The 16-item quick inventory of depressive symptomatology (QIDS), clinician rating (QIDS-C), and self-report (QIDS-SR): A psychometric evaluation in patients with chronic major depression. *Biological Psychiatry, 54*(5), 573–583.

Sachs, G. (2000, December). *Barriers to Concordance*. Paper presented at the Bipolar Disorder Thoughtleader Summit, Boston, MA.

Sachs, G., & Lafer, B. (1998). Child and adolescent mania. In P. J. Goodnick (Ed.), *Mania: Clinical and research perpectives* (pp. 37–62). Washington, DC: American Psychiatric Press.

Sachs, G. S., Nierenberg, A. A., Calabrese, J. R., Marangell, L. B., Wisniewski, S. R., Gyulai, L., et al. (2007). Effectiveness of adjunctive antidepressant treatment for bipolar depression. *New England Journal of Medicine, 356*(17), 1711–1722.

Sachs, G. S., Thase, M. E., Otto, M. W., Bauer, M., Miklowitz, D., Wisniewski, S. R., et al. (2003). Rationale, design, and methods of the systematic treatment enhancement program for bipolar disorder (STEP-BD). *Biological Psychiatry, 53*, 1028–1042.

Sapolsky, R. M. (2000). The possibility of neurotoxicity in the hippocampus in major depression: A primer on neuron death. *Biological Psychiatry, 48*, 755–765.

Scherk, H., Pajonk, F. G., & Leucht, S. (2007). Second-generation antipsychotic agents in the treatment of acute mania: A systematic review and meta-analysis of randomized controlled trials. *Archives of General Psychiatry, 64*(4), 442–455.

Schlaepfer, T. E., Cohen, M. X., Frick, C., Kosel, M., Brodesser, D., Axmacher, N., et al. (2008). Deep brain stimulation to reward circuitry alleviates anhedonia in refractory major depression. *Neuropsychopharmacology, 33*(2), 368–377.

Schloesser, R. J., Huang, J., Klein, P. S., & Manji, H. K. (2008). Cellular plasticity cascades in the pathophysiology and treatment of bipolar disorder. *Neuropsychopharmacology Reviews, 33*(1), 110–133.

Schneck, C. D., Miklowitz, D. J., Miyahara, S., Wisniewski, S., Gyulai, L., Allen, M. H., et al. (2008). The prospective course of rapid cycling bipolar disorder. *American Journal of Psychiatry, 165*(3), 370–377.

Segal, Z. V., Williams, J. M. G., & Teasdale, J. D. (2002). *Mindfulness-based cognitive therapy for depression: A new approach to preventing relapse*. New York: Guilford Press.

Segre, L. S., O'Hara, M. W., Arndt, S., & Stuart, S. (2007). The prevalence of postpartum depression: The relative significance of three social status indices. *Social Psychiatry and Psychiatric Epidemiology, 42*(4), 316–321.

Seligman, M. E. P., Reivich, K., Jaycox, L., & Gillham, J. (1996). *The optimistic child: A proven program to safeguard children from depression and build lifelong resilience.* New York: HarperCollins.

Shaw, E. D., Mann, J. J., & Stokes, P. E., & Manevitz, A. Z. (1986). Effects of lithium carbonate on associational productivity and idiosyncrasy in bipolar outpatients. *American Journal of Psychiatry, 143,* 1166–1169.

Simoneau, T. L., Miklowitz, D. J., Richards, J. A., Saleem, R., & George, E. L. (1999). Bipolar disorder and family communication: Effects of a psychoeducational treatment program. *Journal of Abnormal Psychology, 108,* 588–597.

Simoneau, T. L., Miklowitz, D. J., & Saleem, R. (1998). Expressed emotion and interactional patterns in the families of bipolar patients. *Journal of Abnormal Psychology, 107,* 497–507.

Smith, L. A., Cornelius, V., Warnock, A., Tacchi, M. J., & Taylor, D. (2007). Pharmacological interventions for acute bipolar mania: A systematic review of randomized placebo-controlled trials. *Bipolar Disorders, 9*(6), 551–560.

Smoller, J. W., & Finn, C. T. (2003). Family, twin, and adoption studies of bipolar disorder. *American Journal of Medical Genetics, Part C: Seminars in Medical Genetics, 123*(1), 48–58.

Solomon, A. (2002). *The Noonday Demon: An Atlas of Depression.* New York: Scribner.

Stoll, A. L., Severus, W. E., Freeman, M. P., Rueter, S., Zboyan, H. A., Diamond, E., et al. (1999). Omega 3 fatty acids in bipolar disorder: A preliminary double-blind, placebo-controlled trial. *Archives of General Psychiatry, 56,* 407–412.

Strakowski, S. M., DelBello, M. P., Fleck, D. E., & Arndt, S. (2000). The impact of substance abuse on the course of bipolar disorder. *Biological Psychiatry, 48,* 477–485.

Strakowski, S. M., Keck, P. E., McElroy, S. L., West, S. A., Sax, K. W., Hawkins, J. M., et al. (1998). Twelve-month outcome after a first hospitalization for affective psychosis. *Archives of General Psychiatry, 55,* 49–55.

Strosahl, K., Chiles, J. A., & Linehan, M. (1992). Prediction of suicide intent in hospitalized parasuicides: Reasons for living, hopelessness, and depression. *Comprehensive Psychiatry, 33,* 366–373.

Styron, W. (1992). *Darkness visible: A memoir of madness.* New York: Vintage Books.

Suppes, T., Dennehy, E. B., & Gibbons, E. W. (2000). The longitudinal course of bipolar disorder. *Journal of Clinical Psychiatry, 61,* 23–30.

Terman, M., & Terman, J. S. (1999). Bright light therapy: Side effects and benefits across the symptom spectrum. *Journal of Clinical Psychiatry, 60,* 799–808.

Thase, M. E. (2006). Pharmacotherapy of bipolar depression: An update. *Current Psychiatry Reports, 8*(6), 478–488.

Thase, M. E. (2010). Pharmacotherapy for adults with bipolar depression. In D. J. Miklowitz & D. Cicchetti (Eds.), *Understanding bipolar disorder: A developmental psychopathology perspective* (pp. 445–465). New York: Guilford Press.

Thompson, T. (1996). *The beast: A journey through depression.* New York: Plume.

Tohen, M., Chengappa, K. N., Suppes, T., Zarate, C. A. J., Calabrese, J. R., Bowden, C. L., et al. (2002). Efficacy of olanzapine in combination with valproate or lithium in the treatment of mania in patients partially nonresponsive to valproate or lithium monotherapy. *Archives of General Psychiatry, 59,* 62–69.

Tohen, M., Kryzhanovskaya, L., Carlson, G., DelBello, M. P., Wozniak, J., Kowatch, R., et al. (2005). Olanzapine in the treatment of acute mania in adolescents with bipolar I disorder: A 3-week randomized double-blind placebo-controlled study. *Neuropsychopharmacology, 30*(Suppl. 1), 176.

Tohen, M., & Vieta, E. (2009). Antipsychotic agents in the treatment of bipolar mania. *Bipolar Disorders, 11*(2), 45–54.

Tohen, M., Vieta, E., Calabrese, J., Ketter, T. A., Sachs, G., Bowden, C., et al. (2003). Efficacy of olanzapine and olanzapine-fluoxetine combination in the treatment of bipolar I depression. *Archives of General Psychiatry, 60,* 1079–1088.

Tondo, L., & Baldessarini, R. J. (2000). Reducing suicide risk during lithium maintenance treatment. *Journal of Clinical Psychiatry, 61*(Suppl. 9), 97–104.

Tondo, L., Baldessarini, R. J., & Floris, G. (2001). Long-term clinical effectiveness of lithium maintenance treatment in types I and II bipolar disorders. *British Journal of Psychiatry, 41*(Suppl.), s184–s190.

Tremblay, C. H., Grosskopf, S., & Yang, K. (2010). Brainstorm: Occupational choice, bipolar illness and creativity. *Economics and Human Biology, 8*(2), 233–241.

U.S. Department of Justice. (2009). Americans with Disabilities Act of 1990, as Amended. Retrieved March 10, 2010, from *www.ada.gov/pubs/ada.htm.*

Viguera, A. C., Newport, D. J., Ritchie, J., Stowe, Z., Whitfield, T., Mogielnicki, J., et al. (2007). Lithium in breast milk and nursing infants: Clinical implications. *American Journal of Psychiatry, 164*(2), 342–345.

Viguera, A. C., Whitfield, T., Baldessarini, R. J., Newport, D. J., Stowe, Z., Reminick, A., et al. (2007). Risk of recurrence in women with bipolar disorder during pregnancy: Prospective study of mood stabilizer discontinuation. *American Journal of Psychiatry, 164*(12), 1817–1824.

Ward, S., & Wisner, K. L. (2007). Collaborative management of women with bipolar disorder during pregnancy and postpartum: Pharmacologic considerations. *Journal of Midwifery and Women's Health, 52*(1), 3–13.

Weiss, R. D., Greenfield, S. F., Najavits, L. M., Soto, J. A., Wyner, D., Tohen, M., et al. (1998). Medication compliance among patients with bipolar disorder and substance use disorder. *Journal of Clinical Psychiatry, 59,* 172–174.

Weiss, R. D., Griffin, M. L., Kolodziej, M. E., Greenfield, S. F., Najavits, L. M., Daley, D. C., et al. (2007). A randomized trial of integrated group therapy versus group drug counseling for patients with bipolar disorder and substance dependence. *American Journal of Psychiatry, 164*(1), 100–107.

Willcutt, E., & Mcqueen, M. (2010). Genetic and environmental vulnerability to bipolar spectrum disorders. In D. J. Miklowitz & D. Cicchetti (Eds.), *Understanding bipolar disorder: A developmental psychopathology perspective* (pp. 225–258). New York: Guilford Press.

Williams, J. B. W. (1988). A structured interview guide for the Hamilton Depression Rating Scale. *Archives of General Psychiatry, 45,* 742–747.

Williams, J. M., Alatiq, Y., Crane, C., Barnhofer, T., Fennell, M. J., Duggan, D. S., et al. (2008). Mindfulness-based Cognitive Therapy (MBCT) in bipolar disorder: Preliminary evaluation of immediate effects on between-episode functioning. *Journal of Affective Disorders, 107*(1–3), 275–279.

Williams, M., Teasdale, J., Segal, Z., & Kabat-Zinn, J. (2007). *The mindful way through depression: Freeing yourself from chronic unhappiness.* New York: Guilford Press.

Wong, G., & Lam, D. (1999). The development and validation of the coping inventory for prodromes of mania. *Journal of Affective Disorders, 53,* 57–65.

Wurtzel, E. (1994). *Prozac nation.* New York: Riverhead Books.

Yonkers, K. A., Wisner, K. L., Stowe, Z., Leibenluft, E., Cohen, L., Miller, L., et al. (2004). Management of bipolar disorder during pregnancy and the postpartum period. *American Journal of Psychiatry, 161*(4), 608–620.

Young, R. C., Biggs, J. T., Ziegler, V. E., & Meyer, D. A. (1978). A rating scale for mania: Reliability, validity, and sensitivity. *British Journal of Psychiatry, 133,* 429–435.

Zubin, J., & Spring, B. (1977). Vulnerability: A new view of schizophrenia. *Journal of Abnormal Psychology, 86,* 103–126.

Index

impulsive, self-destructive, or addictive behaviors and, 26–28
missing while on medication, 138–139
mood charting and, 161–163
mood stabilizers and, 106
other disorders that could explain, 42–53
overview, 15–17, 185–187
periods between manic and depressive states and, 16
prevention and, 196–201, 209–213, 210f–211f
progression of episodes and, 35–37, 36f
relapse prevention and, 187–189
self-evaluation and, 38–39
severity of, 16
social support and, 189–191
thinking and perception changes, 23–24
warning signs of, 191–196, 194f
in women, 257
work settings and, 301, 310
Marijuana use, 178–179. *See also* Drug use
Medical records, diagnosis and, 40–41
Medication. *See also* Antidepressant medications; Concordance with medication; Mood stabilizer medications
accepting your diagnosis and, 69
acute versus preventative treatment, 100–101, 102f
ADHD and, 45–46
alcohol and drug use and, 106, 177
anticonvulsants, 109–114, 121
atypical antipsychotics, 114, 116–117
benefits of, 99–100
benzodiazepines, 120–122
biological factors and, 7, 88
bipolar disorder in women and, 257, 258, 271, 275
borderline personality disorder and, 48, 49
breast feeding and, 267–269
calcium channel blockers, 122
contraceptive choices and, 270
depression and, 216
diagnosis and, 31
discontinuing, 134–152
effectiveness of, 144–145
length of time you'll need, 101–103
missing high periods while on, 138–139
mood charting and, 158, 165–166
neuroenhancers, 121–122
omega-3 fatty acid plan (fish oil), 122
other options, 120–122
overview, 98–99, 286f
pregnancy and, 259–260, 261, 263–266
prolactin elevation and, 273
pros and cons of, 148, 149–151
protecting yourself from suicidal actions and, 245
rapid cycling and, 35
relapse prevention and, 187–188, 205–206
remembering to take, 147–148
research regarding, 99
schizophrenia and, 50
side effects of, 140–143
sleep disturbances and, 174
substance-induced mood disorder and, 53

suicidal thoughts and, 241–242
taking regularly, 133–134
thyroid supplements, 120–122
weight gain and the metabolic syndrome, 274–275
Memory
electroconvulsive therapy and, 123–124
during mania, 24
medication concordance and, 147–148
treatment and, 128
Menopause, 276–278
Menstrual cycle
bipolar disorder in women and, 270–272
mood charting and, 166
overview, 257
polycystic ovarian syndrome (PCOS) and, 272–273
Metabolic syndrome, 274–275
Migraine headaches, 275–276
Mindfulness breathing exercise, 228, 251
Mirtazapine (Remeron), 118. *See also* Antidepressant medications
Misdiagnosis, 42–53
Mixed episodes
diagnosis and, 31–35
mood stabilizers and, 106
overview, 16
in women, 257
Modafinil (Provigil), 122. *See also* Medication
Molecular factors, 76
Money management, 196–198
Monoamine oxidase inhibitors (MAOIs), 118, 120. *See also* Antidepressant medications
Mood charting
bipolar disorder in women and, 271
overview, 158–167, 159f, 314f
pleasurable activities and, 226
pregnancy and, 261
Mood disorders, 78
Mood spiral, 222–224
Mood stabilizer medications. *See also* Medication
antidepressants and, 117–118
Depakote (divalproex sodium), 109–111
diagnosis and, 31
Lamictal (lamotrigine), 111–112
lithium, 31, 100, 104–109
overview, 103–104, 115t
pregnancy and, 264
schizophrenia and, 50
side effects of, 140–143
Tegretol (carbamazepine), 112–114
Trileptal (oxcarbazepine), 113–114
types of, 104–114
Mood states. *See also* Normal mood; Symptoms of bipolar disorder
accepting your diagnosis and, 61
bipolar disorder in women and, 271–272
bipolar I disorder and, 32–33
cognitive restructuring method, 232–239, 235f
depression and, 222–224
doctor's assessment of, 21
genetic factors and, 79–80
missing high periods while on medication and, 138–139

About the Author

David J. Miklowitz, PhD, is Professor of Psychiatry at the University of California, Los Angeles (UCLA), School of Medicine, and Senior Clinical Researcher at Oxford University, United Kingdom. He directs the Integrative Study Center in Mood Disorders and the Child and Adolescent Mood Disorders Program at the UCLA Semel Institute. Dr. Miklowitz's numerous publications include the award-winning book for professionals *Bipolar Disorder: A Family-Focused Treatment Approach*. He lives with his wife in Los Angeles.